Fundamentals for Nursing
Review Module Edition 8.0

CONTRIBUTORS

Sheryl Sommer, PhD, RN, CNE
VP Nursing Education & Strategy

Janean Johnson, MSN, RN
Nursing Education Strategist

Karin Roberts, PhD, MSN, RN, CNE
Nursing Education Coordinator

Sharon R. Redding, EdD, RN, CNE
Nursing Education Specialist and Content Project Coordinator

Lois Churchill, MN, RN
Nursing Education Specialist

Lisa Davila, MS, RN
Nursing Education Specialist

Norma Jean Henry, MSN/Ed, RN
Nursing Education Specialist

Mary Jane Janowski, MA, BSN, RN
Nursing Resource Specialist

Audrey Knippa, MS, MPH, RN, CNE
Nursing Education Coordinator

EDITORIAL AND PUBLISHING

Derek Prater
Spring Lenox
Michelle Renner
Mandy Tallmadge
Kelly Von Lunen

CONSULTANTS

Mary-Jane Araldi, MSN, RN
Pam DeMoss, MSN, RN
Nancy Glab, MSN, RN
Justina Higgins, RN, MSN, PLNC, HCE, CHC
Dedra D. Merrill, RN BSN
Gale Sewell PhD(c), MSN, RN, CNE

Intellectual Property Notice

Important Notice to the Reader

User's Guide

Welcome to the Assessment Technologies Institute® Fundamentals Review Module Edition 8.0. The mission of ATI's Content Mastery Series® review modules is to provide user-friendly compendiums of nursing knowledge that will:

- Help you locate important information quickly.

- Assist in your learning efforts.

- Provide exercises for applying your nursing knowledge.

- Facilitate your entry into the nursing profession as a newly licensed RN.

Organization

This review module is organized into units covering the NCLEX® major client needs categories: Safe, Effective Care Environment, Health Promotion and Maintenance, Psychosocial Integrity, and Physiological Integrity. Chapters within these units conform to one of four organizing principles for presenting the content:

- Nursing concepts

- Growth and development

- Procedures

Nursing concepts chapters begin with an overview describing the central concept and its relevance to nursing. Subordinate themes are covered in outline form to demonstrate relationships and present the information in a clear, succinct manner.

Growth and development chapters cover expected growth and development, including physical and psychosocial development and age-appropriate activities, and health promotion, including immunizations, health screenings, nutrition, and injury prevention.

Procedures chapters include an overview describing the procedure(s) covered in the chapter. These chapters will provide you with nursing knowledge relevant to each procedure, including indications, interpretations of findings, nursing actions, and complications.

Application Exercises

Questions are provided at the end of each chapter so you can practice applying your knowledge. The Application Exercises include NCLEX-style questions, such as multiple-choice and multiple-select items, and questions that ask you to apply your knowledge in other formats, such as by using an ATI Active Learning Template. After the Application Exercises, an answer key is provided, along with rationales for the answers.

NCLEX® Connections

To prepare for the NCLEX-RN, it is important for you to understand how the content in this review module is connected to the NCLEX-RN test plan. You can find information on the detailed test plan at the National Council of State Boards of Nursing's Web site: https://www.ncsbn.org/. When reviewing content in this review module, regularly ask yourself, "How does this content fit into the test plan, and what types of questions related to this content should I expect?"

To help you in this process, we've included NCLEX Connections at the beginning of units and sections and with each question in the Application Exercises Answer Keys. The NCLEX Connections at the beginning of each unit will point out areas of the detailed test plan that relate to the content within the section or unit. The NCLEX Connections attached to the Application Exercises Answer Keys will demonstrate how each exercise fits within the detailed content outline.

These NCLEX Connections will help you understand how the detailed content outline is organized, starting with major client needs categories and subcategories and followed by related content areas and tasks. The major client needs categories are:

- Safe and Effective Care Environment
  - Management of Care
  - Safety and Infection Control
- Health Promotion and Maintenance
- Psychosocial Integrity
- Physiological Integrity
  - Basic Care and Comfort
  - Pharmacological and Parenteral Therapies
  - Reduction of Risk Potential
  - Physiological Adaptation

An NCLEX Connection might, for example, alert you that content within a unit is related to:

- Basic Care and Comfort
  - Assistive Devices
    - Assess client use of assistive devices.

QSEN Competencies

As you use the review modules, you will note the integration of the Quality and Safety Education for Nurses (QSEN) competencies throughout the chapters. These competencies are integral components of the curriculum of many nursing programs in the United States and prepare you to provide safe, high-quality care as a newly licensed RN. Icons appear to draw your attention to the six QSEN competencies:

- Safety: The minimization of risk factors that could cause injury or harm while promoting quality care and maintaining a secure environment for clients, self, and others.
- Patient-Centered Care: The provision of caring and compassionate, culturally sensitive care that addresses clients' physiological, psychological, sociological, spiritual, and cultural needs, preferences, and values.

- Evidence-Based Practice: The use of current knowledge from research and other credible sources, on which to base clinical judgment and client care.

- Informatics: The use of information technology as a communication and information-gathering tool that supports clinical decision-making and scientifically based nursing practice.

- Quality Improvement: Care related and organizational processes that involve the development and implementation of a plan to improve health care services and better meet clients' needs.

- Teamwork and Collaboration: The delivery of client care in partnership with multidisciplinary members of the health care team to achieve continuity of care and positive client outcomes.

Icons

Icons are used throughout the review module to draw your attention to particular areas. Keep an eye out for these icons:

 This icon is used for NCLEX connections.

 This icon is used for content related to safety and is a QSEN competency. When you see this icon, take note of safety concerns or steps that nurses can take to ensure client safety and a safe environment.

 This icon is a QSEN competency that indicates the importance of a holistic approach to providing care.

 This icon, a QSEN competency, points out the integration of research into clinical practice.

 This icon is a QSEN competency and highlights the use of information technology to support nursing practice.

 This icon is used to focus on the QSEN competency of integrating planning processes to meet clients' needs.

 This icon highlights the QSEN competency of care delivery using an interprofessional approach.

 This icon indicates that a media supplement, such as a graphic, animation, or video, is available. If you have an electronic copy of the review module, this icon will appear alongside clickable links to media supplements. If you have a hardcopy version of the review module, visit www.atitesting. com for details on how to access these features.

Feedback

ATI welcomes feedback regarding this review module. Please provide comments to: comments@atitesting.com.

TABLE OF CONTENTS

UNIT 1 ## Safe, Effective Care Environment

SECTION: MANAGEMENT OF CARE

› Health Care Delivery Systems
› The Interprofessional Team
› Ethical Responsibilities
› Legal Responsibilities
› Information Technology
› Delegation and Supervision
› Nursing Process
› Critical Thinking and Clinical Judgment
› Admissions, Transfers, and Discharge

NCLEX® CONNECTIONS

When reviewing the chapters in this unit, keep in mind the relevant sections of the NCLEX® outline, in particular:

Client Needs: Management of Care

› Relevant topics/tasks include:
  » Collaboration with Interprofessional Team
    › Identify the need for interprofessional conferences.
  » Delegation
    › Utilize the five rights of delegation.
  » Ethical Practice
    › Recognize ethical dilemmas and take appropriate action.
  » Information Technology
    › Use information technology to enhance the care provided to the client.
  » Legal Rights and Responsibilities
    › Identify legal issues affecting the client.

chapter 1

Overview

- Health care delivery systems incorporate interactions between health care providers and clients within the constraints of financing mechanisms and regulatory agencies.

- Health care systems include the individuals who participate, the settings in which health care takes place, the agencies that regulate health care, and mechanisms that provide financial support.

- Most nurses deliver care within the context of health care systems. As these systems continue to become more business-driven and less service-oriented, the challenge to nursing today is to retain its caring values while practicing within a cost-containment structure.

Components of Health Care Systems

COMPONENTS OF HEALTH CARE SYSTEMS	
Participants	
› Consumers (clients)	
› Providers	
» Licensed providers such as:	
› Registered nurses	
› Licensed practical nurses (also known as licensed vocational nurses)	
› Advanced practice nurses	
› Medical doctors	
› Pharmacists	
› Dentists	
› Dietitians	
› Physical, respiratory, and occupational therapists	
» Unlicensed providers, such as assistive personnel	
Settings	
› Hospitals	› Hospices
› Homes	› Providers' offices
› Skilled-nursing, assisted-living, and extended-care facilities	› Ambulatory care clinics
› Community/health departments	› Occupational health clinics
› Adult day care centers	› Stand-alone surgical centers
› Schools	› Urgent care centers

COMPONENTS OF HEALTH CARE SYSTEMS
Regulatory agencies

› U.S. Department of Health and Human Services

› U.S. Food and Drug Administration (FDA)

› State and local public health agencies

› State licensing boards – to ensure that health care providers and agencies comply with state regulations

› The Joint Commission (formerly JCAHO) – to set quality standards for accreditation of health care facilities

› Professional Standards Review Organizations (PSROs)

› Utilization review committees – to monitor for appropriate diagnosis and treatment of hospitalized clients

Health care financing mechanisms

› Public federally funded programs

» Medicare is for clients 65 years of age or older and for those with permanent disabilities.

» Medicaid is for clients with low incomes.

› It is federally funded.

› Individual states determine eligibility requirements.

› Private plans

» Traditional insurance reimburses for services on a fee-for-service basis.

» Managed care organizations (MCOs) – Primary care providers oversee comprehensive care for enrolled clients and focus on prevention and health promotion.

» Preferred provider organizations (PPOs) – Clients choose from a list of contracted providers. Using noncontracted providers increases the out-of-pocket costs.

» Exclusive provider organizations (EPOs) – Clients choose from a list of providers within a contracted organization.

» Long-term care insurance – This provides for long-term care expenses Medicare does not cover.

Levels of Health Care

- Preventive health care focuses on educating and equipping clients to reduce and control risk factors for disease. Examples include programs that promote immunization, stress management, and seat belt use.

- Primary health care emphasizes health promotion, and includes prenatal and well-baby care, nutrition counseling, and disease control. This level of care is a sustained partnership between clients and providers. Examples include office or clinic visits and scheduled school- or work-centered screenings (vision, hearing, obesity).

- Secondary health care includes the diagnosis and treatment of acute illness and injury. Examples include care in hospital settings (inpatient and emergency departments), diagnostic centers, and emergent care centers.

- Tertiary health care involves the provision of specialized and highly technical care. Examples include intensive care, oncology centers, and burn centers.

- Restorative health care involves intermediate follow-up care for restoring health. Examples include home health care, rehabilitation centers, and skilled nursing facilities.

- Continuing health care addresses long-term or chronic health care needs. Examples include end-of-life care, palliative care, hospice, adult day care, and in-home respite care.

Relationship Between Health Care Systems and Levels of Care

- People – The level of care depends on the needs of the client. Licensed and unlicensed health care personnel work in every level of care.

- Setting – The settings for secondary and tertiary care are usually within a hospital or specific facility. Settings for other levels of care vary.

- Regulatory agencies help ensure the quality and quantity of health care and the protection of health care consumers.

- Health care finance influences the quality and type of care by setting parameters for cost containment and reimbursement.

Safety and Quality

- In response to concerns about the safety and quality of client care in the United States, Quality and Safety Education for Nurses (QSEN) assists nursing programs in preparing nurses to provide safe, high-quality care. To draw attention to the six QSEN competencies, these icons appear throughout the review modules.

  - Safety: The minimization of risk factors that could cause injury or harm while promoting high-quality care and maintaining a secure environment for clients, self, and others.

  - Patient-Centered Care: The provision of caring and compassionate, culturally sensitive care that addresses clients' physiological, psychological, sociological, spiritual, and cultural needs, preferences, and values.

  - Evidence Based Practice: The use of current knowledge from research and other credible sources on which to base clinical judgment and client care.

  - Informatics: The use of information technology as a communication and information-gathering tool that supports clinical decision making and scientifically based nursing practice.

  - Quality Improvement: Care-related and organizational processes that involve the development and implementation of a plan to improve health care services and better meet clients' needs.

  - Teamwork and Collaboration: The delivery of client care in partnership with multidisciplinary members of the health care team to achieve continuity of care and positive client outcomes.

The Future of Health Care

- The ultimate issue in designing and delivering health care is ensuring the health and welfare of the population.

APPLICATION EXERCISES

1. A nurse is explaining the differences among the various agencies that address health care. The nurse should note that which of the following are health care regulatory agencies? (Select all that apply.)

_____ A. American Nurses Association (ANA)

_____ B. The Joint Commission

_____ C. State boards of nursing

_____ D. National League for Nursing (NLN)

_____ E. Food and Drug Administration (FDA)

2. A nurse is explaining the various types of health care coverage clients might have to a group of nursing students. The nurse should mention that which of the following health care financing mechanisms are federally funded? (Select all that apply.)

_____ A. Preferred provider organization (PPO)

_____ B. Medicare

_____ C. Long-term care insurance

_____ D. Exclusive provider organization (EPO)

_____ E. Medicaid

3. A hospital is conducting a community blood pressure screening in its lobby. This is an example of which of the following levels of care?

A. Preventive

B. Primary

C. Secondary

D. Tertiary

4. A client in a managed care organization (MCO) requires hospitalization. Which of the following parties must first approve the admission?

A. Emergency department physician

B. Utilization review committee

C. Provider

D. Managed care administrator

5. A nursing instructor is explaining the various levels of health care services to a group of nursing students. Which of the following examples of care or care settings should the nurse classify as tertiary care? (Select all that apply.)

     _____ A. Intensive care unit

     _____ B. Oncology treatment center

     _____ C. Burn center

     _____ D. Cardiac rehabilitation

     _____ E. Home health care

6. A nurse on a medical-surgical unit is acquainting a group of nurses with the Quality and Safety Education for Nurses (QSEN) initiative. Use the ATI Active Learning Template: Basic Concept to complete this item. Under Related Content, list the six QSEN competencies, along with a brief description of each.

APPLICATION EXERCISES KEY

1. A. INCORRECT: The ANA is a professional nursing organization.

    B. **CORRECT:** The Joint Commission is a health care regulatory agency.

    C. **CORRECT:** State boards of nursing are health care regulatory agencies.

    D. INCORRECT: The NLN is a professional nursing organization.

    E. **CORRECT:** The FDA is a health care regulatory agency.

    Ⓝ NCLEX® Connection: Management of Care, Information Technology

2. A. INCORRECT: PPOs are privately funded.

    B. **CORRECT:** Medicare is federally funded.

    C. INCORRECT: Long-term care insurance is privately funded.

    D. INCORRECT: EPOs are privately funded.

    E. **CORRECT:** Medicaid is federally funded.

    Ⓝ NCLEX® Connection: Management of Care, Information Technology

3. A. INCORRECT: Preventive care includes immunizations or education for minimizing risk factors for illness.

    B. **CORRECT:** A screening is an attempt to detect an undiagnosed disease at its earliest stage, and it is an example of primary care.

    C. INCORRECT: Secondary care includes hospital-based care in an emergency department or on a clinical unit.

    D. INCORRECT: Tertiary care includes specialized care located regionally, such as burn or cancer centers.

    Ⓝ NCLEX® Connection: Health Promotion and Maintenance, Health Promotion/Disease Prevention

4. A. INCORRECT: The emergency department physician may consult with the provider about a client but does not make the decision to admit the client and reimburse for the required services.

    B. INCORRECT: Utilization review committees may review the appropriateness of treatment, but they do not make admission decisions.

    C. **CORRECT:** In an MCO, the provider oversees all of the client's care including hospitalizations; therefore, the provider must approve the admission.

    D. INCORRECT: Managed care administrators may review treatment, but they do not make admission decisions.

    Ⓝ NCLEX® Connection: Management of Care, Information Technology

5. A. **CORRECT:** Tertiary health care involves the provision of specialized and highly technical care, such as the care nurses deliver in intensive care units.

    B. **CORRECT:** Tertiary health care involves the provision of specialized and highly technical care, such as the care nurses deliver in oncology treatment centers.

    C. **CORRECT:** Tertiary health care involves the provision of specialized and highly technical care, such as the care nurses deliver in burn centers.

    D. INCORRECT: This is an example of restorative care and also of tertiary prevention, but not of tertiary care.

    E. INCORRECT: This is an example of restorative care.

    Ⓝ NCLEX® Connection: Health Promotion and Maintenance, Health Promotion/Disease Prevention

6. *Using the ATI Active Learning Template: Basic Concept*
    * Related Content
        ○ Safety: Minimization of risk factors that could cause injury or harm while promoting quality care and maintaining a secure environment for clients, self, and others.
        ○ Patient-Centered Care: Provision of caring and compassionate, culturally sensitive care that addresses clients' physiological, psychological, sociological, spiritual, and cultural needs, preferences, and values.
        ○ Evidence-Based Practice: Use of current knowledge from research and other credible sources, on which to base clinical judgment and client care.
        ○ Informatics: Use of information technology as a communication and information-gathering tool that supports clinical decision-making and scientifically based nursing practice.
        ○ Quality Improvement: Care-related and organizational processes that involve the development and implementation of a plan to improve health care services and better meet clients' needs.
        ○ Teamwork and Collaboration: Delivery of client care in partnership with multidisciplinary members of the health care team, to achieve continuity of care and positive client outcomes.

    Ⓝ NCLEX® Connection: Management of Care, Information Technology

CHAPTER 2 The Interprofessional Team

Overview

- RNs and licensed practical nurses (LPNs) are integral members of the interprofessional health care team. Each discipline represented on an interprofessional team uses a set of skills that are within the scope of practice for the specific profession. In some instances, the scope of practice for one discipline overlaps with the scope of practice or set of skills for another profession. For example, the nurse and the respiratory care therapist both possess the knowledge and skill to perform chest physiotherapy (using postural drainage, percussion, and vibration to promote drainage of secretions from the lungs).

- The interprofessional health care team works collaboratively to provide holistic care to clients.

- The nurse is most often the manager of care and must understand the roles and responsibilities of other health care team members to collaborate and make appropriate referrals.

Interprofessional Personnel (Non-Nursing)

- Spiritual Support Staff

  - Provides spiritual care (pastors, rabbis, priests).

  - Example of when to refer – A client requests communion or the family asks for prayer prior to the client undergoing a procedure.

- Registered Dietitian

  - Assesses, plans for, and educates regarding nutrition needs. Designs special diets, and supervises meal preparation.

  - Example of when to refer – A client has a low albumin level and recently had an unexplained weight loss.

- Laboratory Technician

  - Obtains specimens of body fluids, and performs diagnostic tests.

  - Example of when to refer – A provider needs to see a client's complete blood count (CBC) results immediately.

- Occupational Therapist

  - Assesses and plans for clients to regain activities of daily living skills, especially motor skills of the upper extremities.

  - Example of when to refer – A client has difficulties using an eating utensil with her dominant hand following a stroke.

- Pharmacist
  - Provides and monitors medication. Supervises pharmacy technicians in states that allow this practice.
  - Example of when to refer – A client is concerned about a new medication's interactions with any of his other medications.
- Physical Therapist
  - Assesses and plans for clients to increase musculoskeletal function, especially of the lower extremities, to maintain mobility.
  - Example of when to refer – Following hip arthroplasty, a client requires assistance learning to ambulate and regain strength.
- Provider
  - Assesses, diagnoses, and treats disease and injury. Providers include medical doctors (MDs), doctors of osteopathy (DOs), advanced practice nurses (APNs), and physician assistants (PAs). State regulations vary in their requirements for supervision of APNs and PAs by a physician (MDs and DOs).
  - Example of when to refer – A client has a temperature of 39° C (102.2° F), is achy, shaking, and reports "feeling cold."
- Radiologic Technologist
  - Positions clients and performs x-rays and other imaging procedures for providers to review for diagnosis of disorders of various body parts.
  - Example of when to refer – A client reports severe pain in his hip after a fall, and the provider prescribes an x-ray of the client's hip.
- Respiratory Therapist
  - Evaluates respiratory status and provides respiratory treatments including oxygen therapy, chest physiotherapy, inhalation therapy, and mechanical ventilation.
  - Example of when to refer – A client who has respiratory disease is short of breath and requests a nebulizer treatment.
- Social Worker
  - Works with clients and families by coordinating inpatient and community resources to meet psychosocial and environmental needs that are necessary for recovery and discharge.
  - Example of when to refer – A client who has terminal cancer wishes to go home but is no longer able to perform many activities of daily living. The spouse needs medical equipment in the home to care for the client.
- Speech-Language Pathologist
  - Evaluates and makes recommendations regarding the impact of disorders or injuries on speech, language, and swallowing. Teaches techniques and exercises to improve function.
  - Example of when to refer – A client is having difficulty swallowing a regular diet after trauma to the head and neck.

 View Video: Interdisciplinary Team

FUNDAMENTALS FOR NURSING

Nursing Personnel

- The nursing team works together to advocate for and meet the needs of clients within the health care delivery system.
- The RN is the lead team member, soliciting input from all nursing team members, setting priorities, sharing information with other disciplines, and coordinating client care.

NURSING PERSONNEL BY TITLE	
EDUCATIONAL PREPARATION	**ROLES/RESPONSIBILITIES**
Registered nurse (RN)	
› Varies – Must meet the state board of nursing's requirements for licensure. › Requires completion of a diploma program, an associate degree, or a baccalaureate degree in nursing prior to taking the licensure exam (licensed).	› Function legally under state nurse practice acts. › Perform assessments; establish nursing diagnoses, goals, and interventions; and conduct ongoing client evaluations. › Participate in developing interprofessional plans for client care. › Share appropriate information among team members; initiate referrals for client assistance, including health education; and identify community resources.
Licensed practical nurse (LPN)	
› Varies – Must meet the state board of nursing's requirements. › Requires vocational or community college education prior to taking the licensure exam (licensed).	› Work under the supervision of the RN. › Collaborate within the nursing process, coordinate the plan of care, consult with other team members, and recognize the need for referrals to assist with actual or potential problems. › Possess technical knowledge and skills. › Participate in the delivery of nursing care, using the nursing process as a framework.
Unlicensed assistive personnel (UAP) including certified nursing assistants (CNAs) and certified medical assistants (CMAs), and non-nursing personnel such as dialysis technicians, monitor technicians, and phlebotomists	
› Varies – Must meet the state's formal or informal training requirements. › Requirement by most states for training and examination to attain CNA status.	› Work under the direct supervision of an RN or LPN. › Position description in the employing facility outlines specific tasks. › Tasks may include feeding clients, preparing nutritional supplements, lifting, basic care (grooming, bathing, transferring, toileting, positioning), measuring and recording vital signs, and ambulating clients.

Expanded Nursing Roles

- Advanced practice nurse (APN) – Has a great deal of autonomy. APNs usually have a minimum of a master's degree in nursing (or related field), advanced education in pharmacology and physical assessment, and certification in a specialized area of practice. Included in this role are the following:

  ○ Clinical nurse specialist (CNS) – Typically specializes in a practice setting or a clinical field.

  ○ Nurse practitioner (NP) – Collaborates with one or more providers to deliver nonemergency primary health care in a variety of settings.

  ○ Certified registered nurse anesthetist (CRNA) – Administers anesthesia and provides care during procedures under the supervision of an anesthesiologist.

  ○ Certified nurse-midwife (CNM) – Collaborates with one or more providers to deliver care to maternal-newborn clients and their families.

- Nurse educator – Teaches in schools of nursing, staff development departments in health care facilities, or client education departments.

- Nurse administrator – Provides leadership to nursing departments within a health care facility.

- Nurse researcher – Conducts research primarily to improve the quality of client care.

APPLICATION EXERCISES

1. A nurse is caring for an older adult client who lives alone and is to be discharged in 3 days. He states that it is difficult to prepare adequate nutritious meals at home for just one person. To which of the following members of the health care team should the nurse refer him?

    A. Registered dietitian

    B. Occupational therapist

    C. Physical therapist

    D. Social worker

2. A goal for a client who has difficulty with self-feeding due to rheumatoid arthritis is to use adaptive devices. The nurse caring for the client should initiate a referral with which of the following members of the interprofessional care team?

    A. Social worker

    B. Certified nursing assistant

    C. Registered dietitian

    D. Occupational therapist

3. A client who is postoperative following knee arthroplasty is concerned about the adverse effects of the medication he is receiving for pain management. Which of the following members of the interprofessional care team may assist the client in understanding the medication's effects? (Select all that apply.)

    _____ A. Provider

    _____ B. Certified nursing assistant

    _____ C. Pharmacist

    _____ D. Registered nurse

    _____ E. Respiratory therapist

4. A client who has had a cerebrovascular accident has persistent problems with dysphagia (difficulty swallowing). The nurse caring for the client should initiate a referral with which of the following members of the interprofessional care team?

    A. Social worker

    B. Certified nursing assistant

    C. Occupational therapist

    D. Speech-language pathologist

5. A nursing instructor is acquainting a group of nursing students with the roles of the various members of the health care team they will encounter on a medical-surgical unit. When she gives examples of the types of tasks certified nursing assistants (CNAs) may perform, which of the following client activities should she include? (Select all that apply.)

_____ A. Bathing

_____ B. Ambulating

_____ C. Toileting

_____ D. Determining pain level

_____ E. Measuring vital signs

6. A nurse is teaching a group of nursing students about the various nursing roles they can aspire to after they achieve mastery in basic nursing skills. Use the ATI Active Learning Template: Basic Concept to complete this item. Under Related Content, list at least five types of advance practice nursing roles along with a brief description of their primary responsibilities.

APPLICATION EXERCISES KEY

1.   A. INCORRECT: A registered dietitian usually performs the assessment of a client's nutritional status and provides teaching about the appropriate diet.

   B. INCORRECT: An occupational therapist can assist clients who have problems manipulating eating utensils.

   C. INCORRECT: A physical therapist assists clients with restoring motor function, not specifically with meal preparation.

   D. **CORRECT:** A social worker can make arrangements for a meal delivery service to provide nutritious meals daily, or recommend a congregate meal site near the client's home.

    NCLEX® Connection: Management of Care, Referrals

2.   A. INCORRECT: A social worker can coordinate community services to help the client, but not specifically with self-feeding devices.

   B. INCORRECT: A certified nursing assistant can help the client with feeding, but does not typically procure adaptive devices for the client.

   C. INCORRECT: A registered dietitian can help with educating the client about meeting nutritional needs, but cannot help with the client's physical limitations.

   D. **CORRECT:** An occupational therapist can assist clients who have physical challenges to use adaptive devices and strategies to help with self-care activities.

    NCLEX® Connection: Management of Care, Referrals

3.   A. **CORRECT:** The client's provider must be knowledgeable about any medication he prescribes for the client, including its actions, effects, and interactions.

   B. INCORRECT: It is not within the scope of a certified nursing assistant's duties to counsel the client about the medications his provider prescribes.

   C. **CORRECT:** A pharmacist must be knowledgeable about any medication she dispenses for the client, including its actions, effects, and interactions.

   D. **CORRECT:** A registered nurse must be knowledgeable about any medication she administers to the client, including its actions, effects, and interactions.

   E. INCORRECT: Although some analgesics can cause respiratory depression, requiring assistance from a respiratory therapist, it is not within this therapist's scope of practice to counsel the client about medications his provider prescribes.

    NCLEX® Connection: Management of Care, Referrals

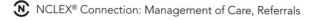

4. A. INCORRECT: A social worker can coordinate community services to help the client, but not specifically with dysphagia.

    B. INCORRECT: A certified nursing assistant can help the client with feeding, but cannot assess and treat dysphagia.

    C. INCORRECT: An occupational therapist can assist clients who have motor challenges to improve abilities with self-care and work, but cannot assess and treat dysphagia.

    D. **CORRECT:** A speech-language pathologist can initiate specific therapy for clients who have difficulty with feeding due to swallowing difficulties.

     NCLEX® Connection: Management of Care, Concepts of Management

5. A. **CORRECT:** It is within the scope of a CNA's duties to provide basic care to clients, such as bathing.

    B. **CORRECT:** It is within the scope of a CNA's duties to provide basic care to clients, such as assisting them with ambulation.

    C. **CORRECT:** It is within the scope of a CNA's duties to provide basic care to clients, such as assisting them with toileting.

    D. INCORRECT: Determining pain level is a task that requires the assessment skills of licensed personnel, such as nurses. Therefore it is outside the scope of a CNA's duties.

    E. **CORRECT:** It is within the scope of a CNA's duties to provide basic care to clients, such as measuring and recording their vital signs.

    NCLEX® Connection: Management of Care, Assignment, Delegation and Supervision

6. *Using the ATI Active Learning Template: Basic Concept*
    - Related Content
      - Clinical nurse specialist (CNS) – Typically specializes in a practice setting or a clinical field
      - Nurse practitioner (NP) – Collaborates with one or more providers to deliver nonemergency primary health care in a variety of settings
      - Certified registered nurse anesthetist (CRNA) – Administers anesthesia and provides care during procedures under the supervision of an anesthesiologist
      - Certified nurse-midwife (CNM) – Collaborates with one or more providers to deliver care to maternal-newborn clients and their families
      - Nurse educator – Teaches in schools of nursing, staff development departments in health care facilities, or client education departments
      - Nurse administrator – Provides leadership to nursing departments within a health care facility
      - Nurse researcher – Conducts research primarily to improve the quality of client care

    NCLEX® Connection: Management of Care, Concepts of Management

CHAPTER 3   Ethical Responsibilities

Overview

- Ethics is the study of conduct and character.
- Morals are the values and beliefs that guide behavior and decision making.
- Ethical theory examines principles, ideas, systems, and philosophies that affect judgments about what is right and wrong, and good and bad. Two common types of ethical theory are utilitarianism and deontology.
- Ethical principles are standards of what is right or wrong with regard to important social values and norms. Ethical principles pertaining to the treatment of clients include:
  - Autonomy – the right to make one's own personal decisions, even when those decisions might not be in that person's own best interest
  - Beneficence – positive actions to help others
  - Fidelity – agreement to keep promises
  - Justice – fairness in care delivery and use of resources
  - Nonmaleficence – avoidance of harm or injury
- Ethics committees generally address unusual or complex ethical issues.

Ethical Decision Making in Nursing

- Ethical dilemmas are problems that involve more than one choice and stem from the different values and beliefs of the decision makers. These are common in health care, and nurses must be prepared to apply ethical theory and decision making to ethical problems.
- A problem is an ethical dilemma when:
  - A review of scientific data is not enough to solve it.
  - It involves a conflict between two moral imperatives.
  - The answer will have a profound effect on the situation and the client.
- Ethical decision making is a process that requires striking a balance between science and morality. There are several steps in ethical decision making:
  - Identify whether the issue is indeed an ethical dilemma.
  - State the ethical dilemma, including all surrounding issues and individuals involved.
  - List and analyze all possible options for resolving the dilemma, and review implications of each option.
  - Select the option that is in concert with the ethical principle that applies to this situation, the decision maker's values and beliefs, and the profession's values for client care. Justify selecting that one option in light of the relevant variables.
  - Apply this decision to the dilemma, and evaluate the outcomes.

- Examples of ethical guidelines for nurses are the American Nurses Association's *Code of Ethics for Nurses with Interpretive Statements* (2001) and the International Council of Nurses' *The ICN Code of Ethics for Nurses* (2012).

- Basic principles of ethics include the following:
  - Advocacy – support of clients' health, safety, and personal rights
  - Responsibility – willingness to respect obligations and follow through on promises
  - Accountability – ability to answer for one's own actions
  - Confidentiality – protection of privacy without diminishing access to high-quality care

- Bioethics refers to the field that addresses dilemmas that arise from advancing science and technology, such as stem cell research, organ transplantation, gender reassignment, and reproductive technologies (in vitro fertilization, surrogate parenting).

THE NURSE'S ROLE IN ETHICAL DECISION MAKING	
Nurse's Role	Examples
› An agent for the client facing an ethical decision	› Caring for an adolescent client who has to decide whether to undergo an abortion even though her parents believe it is wrong › Discussing options with a parent who has to decide whether to consent to a blood transfusion for a child when his religion prohibits such treatment
› A decision maker for health care delivery	› Assigning staff nurses a higher client load than recommended because administration has cut the number of nurses per shift › Witnessing a surgeon discuss only surgical options with a client without informing the client about more conservative measures available

APPLICATION EXERCISES

1. A nurse is caring for a client who decides not to have surgery despite significant blockages in his coronary arteries. The nurse understands that this client's choice is an example of which of the following ethical principles?

    A. Fidelity

    B. Autonomy

    C. Justice

    D. Nonmaleficence

2. A nurse offers pain medication to a client who is postoperative prior to ambulation. The nurse understands that this aspect of care delivery is an example of which of the following ethical principles?

    A. Fidelity

    B. Autonomy

    C. Justice

    D. Beneficence

3. A nurse is instructing a group of nursing students about the responsibilities involved with organ donation and procurement. When the nurse explains that all clients waiting for a kidney transplant have to meet the same qualifications, the students should understand that this aspect of care delivery is an example of which of the following ethical principles?

    A. Fidelity

    B. Autonomy

    C. Justice

    D. Nonmaleficence

4. A nurse questions a medication prescription as too extreme in light of the client's advanced age and unstable status. The nurse understands that this action is an example of which of the following ethical principles?

    A. Fidelity

    B. Autonomy

    C. Justice

    D. Nonmaleficence

5. A nurse is instructing a group of nursing students about how to know and what to expect when ethical dilemmas arise. Which of the following situations should the students identify as an ethical dilemma?

    A. A nurse on a medical-surgical unit demonstrates signs of chemical impairment.

    B. A nurse overhears another nurse telling an older adult client that if he doesn't stay in bed, she will have to apply restraints.

    C. A family has conflicting feelings about the initiation of enteral tube feedings for their father, who is terminally ill.

    D. A client who is terminally ill hesitates to name her spouse on her durable power of attorney form.

6. A nurse is teaching a group of nursing students about the process of resolving ethical dilemmas. Use the ATI Active Learning Template: Basic Concept to complete this item to include the following:

    A. Underlying Principles: Define the ethical dilemma process.

    B. Nursing Interventions: List the steps of making an ethical decision.

APPLICATION EXERCISES KEY

1.   A. INCORRECT: Fidelity is an agreement to keep promises. The nurse has not made any promises; this is the client's decision.

   B. **CORRECT:** In this situation, the client is exercising his right to make his own personal decision about surgery, regardless of others' opinions of what is "best" for him. This is an example of autonomy.

   C. INCORRECT: Justice is fairness in care delivery and in the use of resources. Because the client has chosen not to use them, this principle does not apply.

   D. INCORRECT: Nonmaleficence is the avoidance of harm or injury. In this situation, harm can occur whether or not the client has surgery. However, because he chooses not to, this principle does not apply.

    NCLEX® Connection: Management of Care, Ethical Practice

2.   A. INCORRECT: Fidelity is an agreement to keep promises. Unless the nurse has specifically promised the client a pain-free recovery, which is unlikely, this principle does not apply to this action.

   B. INCORRECT: Autonomy is the right to make personal decisions, even when they are not necessarily in the person's best interest. In this situation, the nurse is delivering responsible client care. This principle does not apply.

   C. INCORRECT: Justice is fairness in care delivery and in the use of resources. Pain management is available for all clients who are postoperative, so this principle does not apply.

   D. **CORRECT:** Beneficence is taking positive actions to help others. By administering pain medication before the client attempts a potentially painful exercise like ambulation, the nurse is taking a specific and positive action to help the client.

    NCLEX® Connection: Management of Care, Ethical Practice

3.   A. INCORRECT: Fidelity is an agreement to keep promises. Because donor organs are a scarce resource compared with the numbers of potential recipients who need them, no one can promise anyone an organ. Thus, this principle does not apply.

   B. INCORRECT: Autonomy is the right to make personal decisions, even when they are not necessarily in the person's best interest. No personal decision is involved with the qualifications for organ recipients.

   C. **CORRECT:** Justice is fairness in care delivery and in the use of resources. By applying the same qualifications to all potential kidney transplant recipients, organ procurement organizations demonstrate this ethical principle in determining the allocation of these scarce resources.

   D. INCORRECT: Nonmaleficence is the avoidance of harm or injury. In this situation, harm can occur to organ donors and to recipients. The requirements of the organ procurement organizations are standard procedures and do not address avoidance of harm or injury.

    NCLEX® Connection: Management of Care, Ethical Practice

4.   A. INCORRECT: Fidelity is an agreement to keep promises. The nurse is not addressing a specific promise when she determines the appropriateness of a prescription for the client. Thus, this principle does not apply.

   B. INCORRECT: Autonomy is the right to make personal decisions, even when they are not necessarily in the person's best interest. No personal decision is involved when the nurse questions the client's prescription.

   C. INCORRECT: Justice is fairness in care delivery and in the use of resources. In this situation, the nurse is delivering responsible client care and not assessing available resources. This principle does not apply.

   D. **CORRECT:** Nonmaleficence is the avoidance of harm or injury. In this situation, administering the medication could harm the client. By questioning it, the nurse is demonstrating this ethical principle.

   (N) NCLEX® Connection: Management of Care, Ethical Practice

5.   A. INCORRECT: Delivering client care while showing signs of a substance use disorder is a legal issue, not an ethical dilemma.

   B. INCORRECT: A nurse who threatens to restrain a client has committed assault. This is a legal issue, not an ethical dilemma.

   C. **CORRECT:** Making the decision about initiating enteral tube feedings is an example of an ethical dilemma. A review of scientific data cannot resolve the issue, and it is not easy to resolve. The decision will have a profound effect on the situation and on the client.

   D. INCORRECT: The selection of a person to make health care decisions on a client's behalf is a legal decision, not an ethical dilemma.

   (N) NCLEX® Connection: Management of Care, Ethical Practice

6.   *Using the ATI Active Learning Template: Basic Concept*

   A. Underlying Principles
   • Ethical decision making: Process that requires striking a balance between science and morality.

   B. Nursing Interventions
   • Identifying whether the issue is an ethical dilemma
   • Stating the ethical dilemma, including all surrounding issues and individuals involved
   • Listing and analyzing all possible options for resolving the dilemma with implications of each option
   • Selecting the option that is in concert with the ethical principle that applies to this situation, the decision maker's values and beliefs, and the profession's values for client care
   • Justifying the selection of one option in light of relevant variables

   (N) NCLEX® Connection: Management of Care, Ethical Practice

UNIT 1	SAFE, EFFECTIVE CARE ENVIRONMENT
	SECTION: MANAGEMENT OF CARE
CHAPTER 4	Legal Responsibilities

Overview

- Understanding the laws governing nursing practice helps nurses protect clients' rights and reduce the risk of nursing liability.

- Nurses are accountable for practicing nursing within the confines of the law to

  - Shield themselves from liability

  - Advocate for clients' rights

  - Provide care that is within the nurse's scope of practice

  - Discern the responsibilities of nursing in relationship to the responsibilities of other members of the health care team

  - Provide safe, proficient care consistent with standards of care

Sources of Law

- Federal Regulations

  - Federal laws affecting nursing practice

    - Health Insurance Portability and Accountability Act (HIPAA)

    - Americans with Disabilities Act (ADA)

    - Mental Health Parity Act (MHPA)

    - Patient Self-Determination Act (PSDA)

- Criminal and Civil Laws

  - Criminal law is a subsection of public law and relates to the relationship of an individual with the government. A nurse who falsifies a record to cover up a serious mistake may be guilty of breaking a criminal law.

  - Civil laws protect individual rights. One type of civil law that relates to the provision of nursing care is tort law.

UNINTENTIONAL TORTS	EXAMPLE
Negligence	› A nurse fails to implement safety measures for a client at risk for falls.
Malpractice (professional negligence)	› A nurse administers a large dose of medication due to a calculation error. The client has a cardiac arrest and dies.

QUASI-INTENTIONAL TORTS	EXAMPLE
Breach of confidentiality	› A nurse releases a client's medical diagnosis to a member of the press.
Defamation of character	› A nurse tells a coworker that she believes the client has been unfaithful to her spouse.

INTENTIONAL TORTS	EXAMPLE
Assault – the conduct of one person makes another person fearful and apprehensive	› A nurse threatens to place an NG tube in a client who is refusing to eat.
Battery – intentional and wrongful physical contact with a person that involves an injury or offensive contact	› A nurse restrains a client and administers an injection against her wishes.
False imprisonment – a person is confined or restrained against his will	› A nurse uses restraints on a competent client to prevent his leaving the health care facility.

- State Laws
  - Each state has enacted statutes that define the parameters of nursing practice and gives the authority to regulate the practice of nursing to its state board of nursing.
  - In turn, the boards of nursing have the authority to adopt rules and regulations that further regulate nursing practice. Although the practice of nursing is similar among states, it is critical that nurses know the laws and rules governing nursing in the state in which they practice.
  - Boards of nursing have the authority to issue and revoke a nursing license.
  - Boards also set standards for nursing programs and further delineate the scope of practice for RNs, licensed practical nurses, and advanced practice nurses.
- Licensure
  - In general, nurses must have a current license in every state in which they practice. The states (about half of them) that have adopted the nurse licensure compact are exceptions. This model allows licensed nurses who reside in a compact state to practice in other compact states under a multistate license. Within the compact, nurses must practice in accordance with the statues and rules of the state in which they provide care.

Professional Negligence

- Professional negligence is the failure of a person who has professional training to act in a reasonable and prudent manner. The terms "reasonable and prudent" generally describe a person who has the average judgment, intelligence, foresight, and skill that a person with similar training and experience would have.
- Negligence issues that prompt most malpractice suits include failure to
  - Follow professional and facility-established standards of care
  - Use equipment in a responsible and knowledgeable manner
  - Communicate effectively and thoroughly with clients
  - Document care the nurse provided

- Nursing students face liability if they harm clients as a result of their direct actions or inaction. They should not perform tasks for which they are not prepared and should have supervision as they learn new procedures. If they harm a client, they, the instructor, and the facility share liability for the wrong action or inaction.

THE FIVE ELEMENTS NECESSARY TO PROVE NEGLIGENCE		
Element of Liability	Explanation	Example: Client Who is a Fall Risk
1. Duty to provide care as defined by a standard	› Care a nurse should give or what a reasonably prudent nurse would do	› The nurse should complete a fall risk assessment for all clients during admission.
2. Breach of duty by failure to meet standard	› Failure to give the standard of care	› The nurse does not perform a fall risk assessment during admission.
3. Foreseeability of harm	› Knowledge that failing to give the proper standard of care could harm the client	› The nurse should know that failure to take fall risk precautions could endanger a client at risk for falls.
4. Breach of duty has potential to cause harm (combines elements 2 and 3)	› Failure to meet the standard had potential to cause harm – relationship must be provable	› Without a fall risk assessment, the nurse does not know the client's risk for falls and does not take the proper precautions.
5. Harm occurs	› Actual harm to the client occurs	› The client falls out of bed and fractures his hip.

- Nurses can avoid liability for negligence by
  - Following standards of care
  - Giving competent care
  - Communicating with other health team members
  - Developing a caring rapport with clients
  - Fully documenting assessments, interventions, and evaluations

---

CLIENTS' RIGHTS

Overview

- Nurses are accountable for protecting the rights of clients. Examples include informed consent, refusal of treatment, advance directives, confidentiality, and information security.
  - Clients' rights are legal privileges or powers clients have when they receive health care services.
  - Clients using the services of a health care institution retain their rights as individuals and citizens.
  - The American Hospital Association identifies patients' rights in health care settings. See "The Patient Care Partnership" at www.aha.org.
  - Nursing facilities that participate in Medicare programs also follow "Resident Rights" statutes that govern their operation.

Nursing Role in Clients' Rights

- Nurses must ensure that clients understand their rights and protect their clients' rights.

- Regardless of the age of the client, the client's nursing needs, or the health care setting, the basic tenets are the same. The client has the right to

  - Understand the aspects of care to be active in the decision-making process

  - Accept, refuse, or request modification of the plan of care

  - Receive care from competent individuals who treat the client with respect

---

INFORMED CONSENT

Overview

- Informed consent is a legal process by which a client has given written permission for a procedure or treatment. Consent is informed when a provider explains and the client understands:

  - The reason the client needs the treatment or procedure

  - How the treatment or procedure will benefit the client

  - The risks involved if the client chooses to receive the treatment or procedure

  - Other options to treat the problem, including not treating the problem

- The nurse's role in the informed consent process is to witness the client's signature on the informed consent form and to ensure that the provider obtained informed consent appropriately.

 View Video: Informed Consent

Informed Consent Guidelines

- Clients must consent to all care they receive in a health care facility. For most aspects of nursing care, "implied consent" is adequate. Clients provide implied consent when they adhere to the instructions the nurse provides. For example, the nurse is preparing to perform a tuberculosis skin test, and the client holds out his arm for the nurse.

- For an invasive procedure or surgery, the client must provide written consent.

- State laws prescribe who is able to give informed consent. Laws vary regarding age limitations and emergencies. Nurses are responsible for knowing the laws in the state(s) in which they practice.

- A competent adult must sign the form for informed consent. The person who signs the form must be capable of understanding the information from the health care professional who will perform the service, such as a surgical procedure, and the person must be able to communicate with the health care professional. When the person giving the informed consent is unable to communicate due to a language barrier or a hearing impairment, a trained medical interpreter must intervene. Many health care facilities contract with professional interpreters who have additional skills in medical terminology to assist with providing information.

- Individuals who may grant consent for another person include the following:
  - Parent of a minor
  - Legal guardian
  - Court-specified representative
  - An individual who has durable power of attorney authority for health care
  - Emancipated minors (minors who are independent from their parents, such as a married minor) for themselves
- The nurse must verify that consent is "informed" and witness the client signing the consent form.

RESPONSIBILITIES FOR INFORMED CONSENT		
Provider	**Client**	**Nurse**
› Obtains informed consent. › To do so, the provider must give the client » The purpose of the procedure. » A complete description of the procedure. » A description of the professionals who will perform and participate in the procedure. » A description of the potential harm, pain, or discomfort that might occur. » Options for other treatments. » The option to refuse treatment and the consequences of doing so.	› Gives informed consent. › To give informed consent, the client must » Give it voluntarily (no coercion involved). » Be competent and of legal age or be an emancipated minor. When the client is unable to provide consent, another authorized person must give consent. » Receive enough information to make a decision based on an understanding of what to expect.	› Witnesses informed consent. › This means the nurse must » Ensure that the provider gave the client the necessary information. » Ensure that the client understood the information and is competent to give informed consent. » Have the client sign the informed consent document. » Notify the provider if the client has more questions or appears not to understand any of the information. The provider is then responsible for giving clarification. » Document questions the client has, notification of the provider, reinforcement of teaching, and use of an interpreter.

Refusal of Treatment

- The Patient Self-Determination Act (PSDA) stipulates that staff must inform clients they admit to a health care facility of their right to accept or refuse care. Competent adults have the right to refuse treatment, including the right to leave a health care facility without a discharge prescription from the provider.
- If the client refuses a treatment or procedure, the client signs a document indicating that he understands the risk involved with refusing the treatment or procedure and that he has chosen to refuse it.
- When a client decides to leave the facility against medical advice (without a discharge prescription), the nurse notifies the provider and discusses with the client the risks to expect when leaving the facility prior to discharge.
- The nurse asks the client to sign an "Against Medical Advice" form and documents the incident.

Standards of Care (Practice)

- Nurses base practice on established standards of care or legal guidelines for care, such as the following:

  - The nurse practice act of each state.

  - Published standards of nursing practice from professional organizations and specialty groups, including the American Nurses Association (ANA), the American Association of Critical Care Nurses (AACN), and the American Association of Occupational Health Nurses (AAOHN).

  - Health care facilities' policies and procedures, which establish the standard of practice for employees of that facility. They provide detailed information about how the nurse should respond to or provide care in specific situations and while performing client care procedures.

- Standards of care define and direct the level of care nurses should give, and they implicate nurses who did not follow these standards in malpractice lawsuits.

- Nurses should refuse to practice beyond the legal scope of practice or outside of their areas of competence regardless of reason (staffing shortage, lack of appropriate personnel).

- Nurses should use the formal chain of command to verbalize concerns related to assignment in light of current legal scope of practice, job description, and area of competence.

Impaired Coworkers

- Impaired health care providers pose a significant risk to client safety.

- A nurse who suspects a coworker of any behavior that jeopardizes client care or could indicate a substance use disorder has a duty to report the coworker to the appropriate manager.

- Many facilities' policies provide access to assistance programs that facilitate entry into a treatment program.

- Each state has laws and regulations that govern the disposition of nurses who have substance use disorders. Criminal charges could apply.

Advance Directives

- The purpose of advance directives is to communicate a client's wishes regarding end-of-life care should the client become unable to do so.

- The Patient Self-Determination Act (PSDA) requires asking all clients on admission to a health care facility whether they have advance directives.

  - Staff should give clients without advance directives written information that outlines their rights related to health care decisions and how to formulate advance directives.

  - A health care representative should be available to help with this process.

Types of Advance Directives

- Living Will
  - A living will is a legal document that expresses the client's wishes regarding medical treatment in the event the client becomes incapacitated and is facing end-of-life issues.
  - Most state laws include provisions that protect health care providers who follow a living will from liability.
- Durable Power of Attorney for Health Care
  - A durable power of attorney for health care is a document in which clients designate a health care proxy to make health care decisions for them if they are unable to do so. The proxy may be any competent adult the client chooses.
- Provider's Orders
  - Unless a provider writes a "do not resuscitate" (DNR) or "allow natural death" (AND) prescription in the client's medical record, the nurse initiates cardiopulmonary resuscitation (CPR) when the client has no pulse or respirations. The provider consults the client and the family prior to administering a DNR or AND.

Nursing Role in Advance Directives

- Nursing responsibilities include the following:
  - Provide written information about advance directives.
  - Document the client's advance directives status.

  - Ensure that the advance directives reflect the client's current decisions.
  - Inform all members of the health care team of the client's advance directives.

Mandatory Reporting

- Health care providers have a legal obligation to report their findings in accordance with state law in the following situations:
  - Abuse
    - Nurses must report any suspicion of abuse (child or elder abuse, domestic violence) following facility policy.
  - Communicable Diseases
    - Nurses must report communicable disease diagnoses to the local or state health department.
    - For a complete list of reportable diseases and a description of the reporting system, go to the Centers for Disease Control and Prevention's website, www.cdc.gov. Each state mandates which diseases to report in that state. Reporting allows officials to:
      - Ensure appropriate medical treatment of diseases (tuberculosis).
      - Monitor for common-source outbreaks (foodborne, hepatitis A).
      - Plan and evaluate control and prevention plans (immunizations).
      - Identify outbreaks and epidemics.
      - Determine public health priorities based on trends.

APPLICATION EXERCISES

1. A nurse observes an assistive personnel (AP) reprimanding a client for not using the urinal properly. The AP tells him she will put a diaper on him if he does not use the urinal more carefully next time. Which of the following torts is the AP committing?

    A. Assault

    B. Battery

    C. False imprisonment

    D. Invasion of privacy

2. An adult client who is competent tells the nurse that he is thinking about leaving the hospital against medical advice. The nurse believes that this is not in the client's best interest, so she administers a PRN sedative medication the client has not requested along with his usual medication. Which of the following types of tort has the nurse committed?

    A. Assault

    B. False imprisonment

    C. Negligence

    D. Breach of confidentiality

3. A client who will undergo neurosurgery the following week tells the nurse in the surgeon's office that he will prepare his advance directives before he goes to the hospital. Which of the following statements by the client indicates to the nurse that he understands advance directives?

    A. "I'd rather have my brother make decisions for me, but I know it has to be my wife."

    B. "I know they won't go ahead with the surgery unless I prepare these forms."

    C. "I plan to write that I don't want them to keep me on a breathing machine."

    D. "I will get my regular doctor to approve my plan before I hand it in at the hospital."

4. A client is about to undergo an elective surgical procedure. Which of the following actions are appropriate for the nurse who is providing preoperative care regarding informed consent? (Select all that apply.)

_____ A. Make sure the surgeon obtained the client's consent.

_____ B. Witness the client's signature on the consent form.

_____ C. Explain the risks and benefits of the procedure.

_____ D. Describe the consequences of choosing not to have the surgery.

_____ E. Tell the client about alternatives to having the surgery.

5. A nurse has noticed several occasions in the past week when another nurse on the unit seemed drowsy and unable to focus on the issue at hand. Today, she found the nurse asleep in a chair in the break room when she was not on a break. Which of the following actions should the nurse take?

A. Remind the nurse that safe client care is a priority on the unit.

B. Ask others on the team whether they have observed the same behavior.

C. Report her observations to the nurse manager on the unit.

D. Conclude that her coworker's fatigue is not her problem to solve.

6. A nurse is teaching a group of nursing students about avoiding liability for negligence. Use the ATI Active Learning Template: Basic Concept to complete this item to include the following:

A. Underlying Principles: List the five elements necessary to prove negligence.

B. Nursing Interventions: List at least four ways nurses can avoid liability for negligence.

APPLICATION EXERCISES KEY

1. A. **CORRECT:** By threatening the client, the AP is committing assault. Her threats could make the client become fearful and apprehensive.

    B. INCORRECT: Battery is actual physical contact without the client's consent. Because the AP has only verbally threatened the client, battery has not occurred.

    C. INCORRECT: Unless the AP restrains the client, there is no false imprisonment involved.

    D. INCORRECT: Invasion of privacy most often involves disclosing information about a client to an unauthorized individual.

     NCLEX® Connection: Management of Care, Legal Rights and Responsibilities

2. A. INCORRECT: Assault is an action that threatens harmful contact without the client's consent. The nurse has made no threats in this situation.

    B. **CORRECT:** The nurse gave the medication as a chemical restraint to keep the client from leaving the facility against medical advice. This is false imprisonment because the client neither requested nor consented to receiving the sedative.

    C. INCORRECT: Negligence is a breach of duty that results in harm to the client. It is unlikely that the medication the nurse administered without his consent actually harmed the client.

    D. INCORRECT: The nurse has not disclosed any protected health information, so there is no breach of confidentiality involved in this situation.

     NCLEX® Connection: Management of Care, Legal Rights and Responsibilities

3. A. INCORRECT: The client may designate any competent adult to be his health care proxy. It does not have to be his spouse.

    B. INCORRECT: Although the hospital staff must ask the client whether he has prepared advance directives and provide written information about them if he hasn't, they may not refuse care based on the lack of advance directives.

    C. **CORRECT:** The client has the right to decide and specify which medical procedures he wants when a life-threatening situation arises.

    D. INCORRECT: The client does not need his provider's approval to submit his advance directives. However, he should give his primary care provider a copy of the document for his records.

    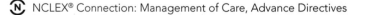 NCLEX® Connection: Management of Care, Advance Directives

4.   A. **CORRECT:** It is the nurse's responsibility to verify that the surgeon obtained the client's consent and that he understands the information the surgeon gave him.

   B. **CORRECT:** It is the nurse's responsibility to witness the client's signing of the consent form, and to verify that he is consenting voluntarily and appears to be competent to do so. The nurse also should verify that he understands the information the surgeon gave him.

   C. INCORRECT: It is the surgeon's responsibility, not the nurse's, to explain the risks and benefits of the procedure.

   D. INCORRECT: It is the surgeon's responsibility, not the nurse's, to describe the consequences of choosing not to have the surgery.

   E. INCORRECT: It is the surgeon's responsibility, not the nurse's, to tell the client about any available alternatives to having the surgery.

    NCLEX® Connection: Management of Care, Informed Consent

5.   A. INCORRECT: Confronting the coworker might cause her to respond defensively and does nothing to resolve the problem.

   B. INCORRECT: Finding out whether others have noticed the problem is immaterial and should not affect the nurse's course of action.

   C. **CORRECT:** Any nurse who notices behavior that could jeopardize client care or could indicate a substance use disorder has a duty to report the situation immediately to the nurse manager.

   D. INCORRECT: The nurse may not be responsible for solving the problem, but she does have a duty to take action since she has observed the problem.

    NCLEX® Connection: Management of Care, Legal Rights and Responsibilities

6.   *Using the ATI Active Learning Template: Basic Concept*

   A. Underlying Principles
   - Duty to provide care as defined by a standard
   - Breach of duty by failure to meet standard
   - Foreseeability of harm
   - Breach of duty has potential to cause harm
   - Harm occurs

   B. Nursing Interventions
   - Following standards of care
   - Giving competent care
   - Communicating with other health team members
   - Developing a caring rapport with clients
   - Fully documenting assessments, interventions, and evaluations

    NCLEX® Connection: Management of Care, Legal Rights and Responsibilities

Overview

- The chart or medical record is the legal record of care.

- The medical record is a confidential, permanent, and legal document that is admissible in court. Nurses are legally and ethically responsible for ensuring confidentiality. Only those health care providers who are involved directly in a client's care may access that client's medical record.

 View Video: Confidentiality

- Nurses document the care they provide as documentation or charting, and it should reflect the nursing process.

- There is a rapidly growing trend for maintaining medical records electronically, which creates challenges in protecting the privacy and safety of health information.

- Information to document

  - Assessments

  - Medication administration

  - Treatments and responses

  - Client education

- Documentation is a standard for many accrediting agencies, including The Joint Commission (formerly JCAHO). The Joint Commission mandates the use of computerized databases to expedite the accreditation process. Health care facilities use the computerized data for budget management, quality improvement programs, research, and many other endeavors.

- Purposes for medical records include communication, legal documentation, financial billing, education, research, and auditing.

- The purpose of reporting is to provide continuity of care among all team members who provide care to the same clients.

- Nurses should conduct reporting in a confidential manner.

Documentation

- Factual – Subjective and objective data

  - Nurses should document subjective data as direct quotes, within quotation marks, or summarize and identify the information as the client's statement.

  - Objective data should be descriptive and should include what the nurse sees, hears, feels, and smells. Document without derogatory words, judgments, or opinions. Document the client's behavior accurately. Instead of writing "client is agitated," write "client pacing back and forth in his room, yelling loudly."

- Accurate and concise – Document facts and information precisely – what the nurse sees, hears, feels, smells – without any interpretations of the situation. Only those abbreviations and symbols The Joint Commission and the facility approve are acceptable.

- Complete and current – Document information that is comprehensive and timely. Never pre-chart an assessment, intervention, or evaluation.

- Organized – Communicate information in a logical sequence.

Legal Guidelines

- Begin each entry with the date and time.

- Record entries legibly, in nonerasable black ink, and do not leave blank spaces in the nurses' notes.

- Do not use correction fluid, erase, scratch out, or blacken out errors in the medical record. Make corrections promptly, following the facility's procedure for error correction.

- Sign all documentation as the facility requires, generally with name and title.

- Documentation should reflect assessments, interventions, and evaluations, not personal opinions or criticism of others' care.

Documentation Formats

- Flow charts show trends in vital signs, blood glucose levels, pain level, and other frequent assessments.

- Narrative documentation records information as a sequence of events in a storylike manner.

- Charting by exception uses standardized forms that identify norms and allows selective documentation of deviations from those norms.

- Problem-oriented medical records consist of a database, problem list, care plan, and progress notes. Examples (of which there are multiple variations) include the following:

  - SOAP

    - S – Subjective data

    - O – Objective data

    - A – Assessment (includes a nursing diagnosis based on the assessment)

    - P – Plan

- ○ PIE
  - ▪ P – Problem
  - ▪ I – Intervention
  - ▪ E – Evaluation
- ○ DAR (focus charting)
  - ▪ D – Data
  - ▪ A – Action
  - ▪ R – Response
- Electronic health records are replacing manual formats in many settings.
  - ○ Advantages include standardization, accuracy, confidentiality, easy access for multiple users, and rapid acquisition and transfer of clients' information.
  - ○ Challenges include learning the system, knowing how to correct errors, and maintaining security.
  - ○ Documentation rules and formats are similar to those for paper charting.

Reporting Formats

- Change-of-Shift Report
  - ○ Nurses give this report at the conclusion of each shift to the nurse assuming responsibility for the clients.
  - ○ Formats include face to face, audiotaping, or presentation during walking rounds in each client's room (unless the client has a roommate or visitors are present).
  - ○ An effective report should:
    - ▪ Include significant objective information about the client's health problems.
    - ▪ Proceed in a logical sequence.
    - ▪ Include no gossip or personal opinion.
    - ▪ Relate recent changes in medications, treatments, procedures, and the discharge plan.
- Telephone reports are useful when contacting the provider or other members of the interprofessional team.
  - ○ It is important to:
    - ▪ Have all the data ready prior to contacting any member of the interprofessional team.
    - ▪ Use a professional demeanor.
    - ▪ Use exact, relevant, and accurate information.
    - ▪ Document the name of the person, the time, content of the message, and the instructions or information received during the report.

- Telephone or Verbal Prescriptions
  - It is best to avoid these, but they are sometimes necessary during emergencies and at unusual times.
  - Have a second nurse listen to a telephone prescription.
  - Repeat it back, making sure to include the medication's name (spell if necessary), dosage, time, and route.
  - Question any prescription that may seem inappropriate for the client.
  - Make sure the provider signs the prescription in person within the time frame the facility specifies, typically 24 hr.
- Transfer Reports
  - These should include demographic information, medical diagnosis, providers, an overview of health status (physical, psychosocial), plan of care, recent progress, any alterations that might become an urgent or emergent situation, directives for any assessments or client care essential within the next few hours, most recent vital signs, medications and last doses, allergies, diet, activity, special equipment or adaptive devices (oxygen, suction, wheelchair), advance directives and resuscitation status, and family involvement in care and health care proxy.
- Incident Reports (Unusual Occurrences)
  - Incident/variance reports are an important part of a facility's quality improvement plan.
  - An incident is the occurrence of an accident or an unusual event. Examples of incidents are medication errors, falls, and needlesticks.
  - Nurses must document the facts without judgment or opinion.
  - Nurses must not refer to an incident report in the client's medical record.
  - Incident reports contribute to changes that help improve health care quality.

Information Security

- Mandatory adherence with the Health Insurance Portability and Accountability Act of 1996 (HIPAA) began in 2003 to help ensure the confidentiality of health information.
- A major component of HIPAA, the Privacy Rule, promotes the use of standard methods of maintaining the privacy of protected health information (PHI) among health care agencies.
- It is essential for nurses to be aware of clients' rights to privacy and confidentiality. Facilities' policies and procedures help ensure adherence with HIPAA regulations.
- The Privacy Rule requires that nurses protect all written and verbal communication about clients. Components of the privacy rule include the following:
  - Only health care team members directly responsible for a client's care may access that client's record. Nurses may not share information with other clients or staff not caring for the client.
  - Clients have a right to read and obtain a copy of their medical record.
  - Nurses may not photocopy any part of a medical record except for authorized exchange of documents between facilities and providers.

○ Staff must keep medical records in a secure area to prevent inappropriate access to the information. They may not use public display boards to list client names and diagnoses.

○ Electronic records are password protected. The public may not view them.

▪ Staff must use only their own passwords to access information.

○ Nurses must not disclose clients' information to unauthorized individuals or family members who request it in person or by telephone or e-mail.

▪ Many hospitals use a code system to identify those individuals who may receive information about a client.

▪ Nurses should ask any individual inquiring about a client's status for the code and disclose information only when the individual can give the code.

○ Communication about a client should only take place in a private setting where unauthorized individuals cannot overhear it.

○ To adhere to HIPAA regulations, each health care facility has specific policies and procedures to monitor staff adherence, technical protocols, computer privacy, and data safety.

○ Information security protocols include the following:

▪ Log off from the computer before leaving the workstation to ensure that others cannot view protected health information on the monitor.

▪ Never share a user ID or password with anyone.

▪ Never leave a medical record or other printed or written PHI where others can access it.

▪ Shred any printed or written client information for reporting or client care after use.

○ Social media precautions include the following:

▪ Know the implications of HIPAA before using social networking sites for school or work-related communication.

▪ Become familiar with your facility's or school's policies or about using social networking.

▪ Do not use or view social networking media in clinical settings.

▪ Do not post information about your school, clinical sites, clinical experiences, clients, and other health care staff on social networking sites.

APPLICATION EXERCISES

1. A nurse is preparing information for change-of-shift report. Which of the following information should the nurse include in the report?

    A. The client's input and output for the shift

    B. The client's blood pressure from the previous day

    C. A bone scan that is scheduled for today

    D. The medication routine from the medication administration record

2. A nurse enters a client's room and finds him sitting in his chair. He states, "I fell in the shower, but I got myself back up and into my chair." How should the nurse document this in the client's chart?

    A. The client fell in the shower.

    B. The client states he fell in the shower and was able to get himself back into his chair.

    C. The nurse should not document this information in the chart because she did not witness the fall.

    D. The client fell in the shower but is now resting comfortably.

3. A nursing instructor is reviewing documentation with a group of nursing students. Which of the following legal guidelines should they follow when documenting in a client's record? (Select all that apply.)

    _____ A. Cover errors with correction fluid, and write in the correct information.

    _____ B. Put the date and time on all entries.

    _____ C. Document objective data, leaving out opinions.

    _____ D. Use as many abbreviations as possible.

    _____ E. Wait until the end of the shift to document.

4. The skin barrier covering a client's intestinal fistula keeps falling off when she stands up to ambulate. The nurse has reapplied it twice during the current shift, but it remains intact only when the client is supine in bed. The nurse telephoned the physical therapist about the difficulties containing the drainage from the fistula, so the therapist did not ambulate the client today. The client sat in a chair during lunch with an absorbent pad over the fistula. The client ate all the food on her tray. The wound care nurse confirmed that she will see the client later today. The client states she feels frustrated at not having physical therapy, but the nurse thinks the client welcomed having a day to rest. Which of the following information should the nurse include in the change-of-shift report? (Select all that apply.)

_____ A. The physical therapist did not ambulate the client today.

_____ B. The skin barrier's seal stays on in bed but loosens when the client stands.

_____ C. The client seemed to welcome having a "day off" from physical therapy.

_____ D. The wound care nurse will see the client later today.

_____ E. The client ate all the food on her lunch tray.

5. A nurse is receiving a provider's prescription by telephone for morphine for a client who is reporting moderate to severe pain. Which of the following nursing actions are appropriate? (Select all that apply.)

_____ A. Repeat the details of the prescription back to the provider.

_____ B. Have another nurse listen to the telephone prescription.

_____ C. Obtain the prescriber's signature on the prescription within 24 hr.

_____ D. Decline the verbal prescription because it is not an emergency situation.

_____ E. Tell the charge nurse that the provider has prescribed morphine by telephone.

6. A nurse is introducing a group of nursing students to the various approaches to problem-oriented documentation. Use the ATI Active Learning Template: Basic Concept to complete this item. Under Underlying Principles, list three common methods of problem-oriented charting with definitions of their acronyms.

APPLICATION EXERCISES KEY

1. A. INCORRECT: Unless there is a significant change in the client's intake and output, the oncoming nurse can read that information in the chart.

   B. INCORRECT: Unless there is a significant change since the client's blood pressure measurements the previous day, the oncoming nurse can read that information in the chart.

   C. **CORRECT:** The bone scan is important because the nurse might have to modify the client's care to accommodate leaving the unit.

   D. INCORRECT: Unless there is a significant change in the client's medication routine, the oncoming nurse can read that information in the chart.

   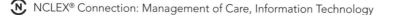 NCLEX® Connection: Management of Care, Continuity of Care

2. A. INCORRECT: Because the nurse did not witness the fall, she cannot document it as objective data.

   B. **CORRECT:** By writing what the client states, the information is subjective data.

   C. INCORRECT: The nurse did not witness the fall, but it is important information to include in the chart.

   D. INCORRECT: Because the nurse did not witness the fall, she cannot document it as objective data.

   NCLEX® Connection: Safety and Infection Control, Reporting of Incident/Event/Irregular Occurrence Variance

3. A. INCORRECT: Correction fluid implies that the nurse might have tried to hide the previous documentation or deface the medical record.

   B. **CORRECT:** The day and time confirm the recording of the correct sequence of events.

   C. **CORRECT:** Documentation must be factual, descriptive, and objective, without opinions or criticism.

   D. INCORRECT: Too many abbreviations can make the entry difficult to understand. Nurses should minimize their use, and use only those the facility approves.

   E. INCORRECT: Documentation should be current. Waiting until the end of the shift may result in data omission.

   NCLEX® Connection: Management of Care, Information Technology

4.   A. **CORRECT:** The oncoming nurse needs to know about any changes in or deviations from the client's plan of care, such as missing a physical therapy session.

   B. **CORRECT:** The current problem about the adhesion of the skin barrier is important information the oncoming nurse needs to know and address.

   C. INCORRECT: This is the nurse's opinion about the client's reaction to missing physical therapy. This does not belong in the change-of-shift report.

   D. **CORRECT:** The oncoming nurse needs to know about any consultations that will take place during the shift.

   E. INCORRECT: Unless this is a change from the client's usual intake, it is not necessary to report routine tasks and procedures.

   Ⓝ NCLEX® Connection: Management of Care, Continuity of Care

5.   A. **CORRECT:** The nurse should repeat the medication's name, dosage, time or interval, route, and any other pertinent information back to the provider and receive and document confirmation.

   B. **CORRECT:** Having another nurse listen to the telephone prescription is a safety precaution that helps prevent medication errors due to miscommunication.

   C. **CORRECT:** The provider must sign the prescription within the time frame the facility specifies in its policies (generally 24 hr).

   D. INCORRECT: Unrelieved pain can become an emergency situation without the appropriate pain management interventions.

   E. INCORRECT: There is no need to inform the charge nurse every time a nurse receives a medication prescription, whether by telephone, verbally, or in the medical record.

   Ⓝ NCLEX® Connection: Safety and Infection Control, Accident/Error/Injury Prevention

6.   *Using the ATI Active Learning Template: Basic Concept*
   • Underlying Principles
      ○ SOAP
         ▪ S – Subjective data
         ▪ O – Objective data
         ▪ A – Assessment (includes a nursing diagnosis based on the assessment)
         ▪ P – Plan
      ○ PIE
         ▪ P – Problem
         ▪ I – Intervention
         ▪ E – Evaluation
      ○ DAR (focus charting)
         ▪ D – Data
         ▪ A – Action
         ▪ R – Response

   Ⓝ NCLEX® Connection: Management of Care, Information Technology

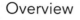

UNIT 1   SAFE, EFFECTIVE CARE ENVIRONMENT
         SECTION: MANAGEMENT OF CARE

CHAPTER 6 **Delegation and Supervision**

Overview

- Delegating is the process of transferring the authority and responsibility to another member of the health care team to complete a task while retaining the accountability.

- Supervising is the process of directing, monitoring, and evaluating the performance of tasks by another member of the health care team. RNs are responsible for the supervision of client care tasks delegated to assistive personnel (AP) and licensed practical nurses (LPNs).

  - Licensed personnel are nurses who have completed a course of study and successfully passed either an LPN or RN examination.

  - Unlicensed personnel are individuals who have had training to function in an assistive role to licensed nurses in the provision of client care.

    - These individuals may be nursing personnel, such as certified nursing assistants (CNAs) or certified medication assistants (CMAs), or they may be non-nursing personnel, such as dialysis technicians, monitor technicians, or phlebotomists.

    - Some health care entities may differentiate between nurse and non-nurse assistive personnel or APs by using the acronym NAP for nursing assistive personnel.

Delegating and Supervising

- A licensed nurse is responsible for providing clear directions when delegating a task initially and for periodic reassessment and evaluation of the outcome of the task.

  - RNs may delegate to other RNs, LPNs, and AP.

    - RNs must be knowledgeable about the applicable state nurse practice act and regulations regarding the use of LPNs and AP.

    - RNs must delegate tasks so that they can complete higher-level tasks that only RNs can perform. This allows more efficient use of all members of the health care team.

  - LPNs may delegate to other LPNs and AP.

- Delegation Factors

  - Nurses can delegate only tasks appropriate for the skill and education level of the nurse who is receiving the assignment.

  - RNs cannot delegate the nursing process, client education, or tasks that require nursing judgment to LPNs or AP.

- Task factors – Prior to delegating client care, the nurse should consider the following:
  - Predictability of outcome
    - Will the completion of the task have a predictable outcome?
    - Is it a routine treatment?
    - Is it a new treatment?
  - Potential for harm
    - Is there a chance that something negative may happen to the client (risk for bleeding, risk for aspiration)?
    - Is the client unstable?
  - Complexity of care
    - Are complex tasks required as a part of the client's care?
    - Is the delegatee legally able to perform the task, and does she have the necessary skills?
  - Need for problem solving and innovation
    - Is judgment essential while performing the task?
    - Does it require nursing assessment skills?
  - Level of interaction with the client
    - Is there a need to provide psychosocial support or education during the performance of the task?
- Delegatee factors – Considerations for selection of an appropriate delegatee
  - Education, training, and experience
  - Knowledge and skill to perform the task
  - Level of critical thinking required to complete the task
  - Ability to communicate with others as it pertains to the task
  - Demonstrated competence
  - Facility policies and procedures
  - Licensing legislation (state nurse practice acts)

EXAMPLES OF TASKS NURSES MAY DELEGATE TO LPNS AND AP (PROVIDED FACILITY POLICY AND STATE PRACTICE GUIDELINES PERMIT)		
To LPNs		
› Monitoring findings (as input to the RN's ongoing assessment) › Reinforcing client teaching from a standard care plan › Performing tracheostomy care	› Suctioning › Checking nasogastric tube patency › Administrating enteral feedings	› Inserting a urinary catheter › Administrating medication (excluding IV medications in some states)
To AP		
› Activities of daily living (ADLs) › Bathing › Grooming › Dressing › Toileting	› Ambulating › Feeding (without swallowing precautions) › Positioning	› Bed making › Specimen collection › Intake and output (I&O) › Vital signs (for stable clients)

- Delegation and Supervision Guidelines
  - Use the five rights of delegation to decide:
    - Tasks to delegate (right task)
    - Under what circumstances (right circumstance)
    - To whom (right person)
    - What information to communicate (right direction/communication)
    - How to supervise/evaluate (right supervision/evaluation)

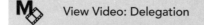 View Video: Delegation

  - Use professional judgment and critical thinking skills when delegating.
  - Right task
    - Identify what tasks are appropriate to delegate for each specific client.
      - A right task is repetitive, requires little supervision, and is relatively noninvasive for a certain client.
    - Delegate activities to appropriate levels of team members (LPN, AP) according to professional standards of practice, legal and facility guidelines, and available resources.

RIGHT TASK	WRONG TASK
› Delegate an AP to assist a client who has pneumonia to use a bedpan.	› Delegate an AP to administer a nebulizer treatment to a client who has pneumonia.

  - Right circumstance
    - Assess the health status and complexity of care the client requires.
    - Match the complexity of care demands to the skill level of the team member.
    - Consider the workload of the team member.

RIGHT CIRCUMSTANCE	WRONG CIRCUMSTANCE
› Delegate an AP to assist in measuring vital signs of a client who is postoperative and stable.	› Delegate an AP to assist in measuring vital signs of a client who is postoperative and required naloxone (Narcan) for depressed respirations.

  - Right person
    - Assess and verify the competence of the team member.
      - The task must be within the team member's scope of practice.
      - The team member must have the necessary competence and training.
    - Continually review the performance of the team member, and determine care competence.
    - Assess the team member's performance according to standards, and when necessary, take steps to remediate any failure to meet standards.

RIGHT PERSON	WRONG PERSON
› Delegate an LPN to administer enteral feedings to a client who has a head injury.	› Delegate an AP to administer enteral feedings to a client who has a head injury.

○ Right direction/communication – Communicate in writing, orally, or both

- Data to collect

- Method and timeline for reporting, including when to report concerns and assessment findings

- Specific task(s) to perform; client-specific instructions

- Expected results, timelines, and expectations for follow-up communication

RIGHT DIRECTION/COMMUNICATION	WRONG DIRECTION/COMMUNICATION
› Delegate an AP to assist the client in room 312 with a shower before 0900.	› Delegate an AP to assist the client in room 312 with morning hygiene.

○ Right supervision/evaluation – The delegating nurse must do the following:

- Provide supervision, either directly or indirectly (assigning supervision to another licensed nurse).

- Provide clear directions and understandable expectations of the task(s) to perform (time frames, what to report).

- Monitor performance.

- Provide feedback.

- Intervene if necessary (unsafe clinical practice).

- Evaluate the client, and determine client outcome status.

- Evaluate client care tasks, and identify needs for performance improvement activities and additional resources.

RIGHT SUPERVISION	WRONG SUPERVISION
› Delegate an AP to assist in ambulating a client after completing the admission assessment.	› Delegate an AP to assist in ambulating a client prior to performing an admission assessment.

- Supervision

  ○ Occurs after delegation

  ○ Oversees staff's performance of delegated activities

  ○ Determines whether

    - Completion of tasks is on schedule.

    - Performance was at a satisfactory level.

    - Delegatee documented and reported unexpected findings.

    - Delegatee needed assistance to complete assigned tasks in a timely manner.

    - Supervising nurse should reevaluate and possibly change the assignment.

APPLICATION EXERCISES

1. A nurse on a medical-surgical unit has received change-of-shift report and will care for four clients. Which of the following client's needs may the nurse assign to an assistive personnel (AP)?

    A. Feeding a client who was admitted 24 hr ago with aspiration pneumonia

    B. Reinforcing teaching with a client who is learning to walk using a quad cane

    C. Reapplying a condom catheter for a client who has urinary incontinence

    D. Applying a sterile dressing to a pressure ulcer

2. A nurse is delegating the ambulation of a client who had knee arthroplasty 5 days ago to an AP. Which of the following information should the nurse share with the AP? (Select all that apply.)

    _____ A. The roommate is up independently.

    _____ B. The client ambulates with his slippers on over his antiembolic stockings.

    _____ C. The client uses a front-wheeled walker when ambulating.

    _____ D. The client had pain medication 30 min ago.

    _____ E. The client is allergic to codeine.

    _____ F. The client ate 50% of his breakfast this morning.

3. An RN is making assignments for client care to a licensed practical nurse (LPN) at the beginning of the shift. Which of the following assignments should the LPN question?

    A. Assisting a client who is 24 hr postoperative to use an incentive spirometer

    B. Collecting a clean-catch urine specimen from a client who was admitted on the previous shift

    C. Providing nasopharyngeal suctioning for a client who has pneumonia

    D. Replacing the cartridge and tubing on a patient-controlled analgesia (PCA) pump

4. A nurse is preparing an in-service program about delegation. Which of the following elements should she identify when presenting the five rights of delegation? (Select all that apply.)

    _____ A. Right client

    _____ B. Right supervision/evaluation

    _____ C. Right direction/communication

    _____ D. Right time

    _____ E. Right circumstances

5. A nurse manager of a medical-surgical unit is assigning care responsibilities for the oncoming shift. A client is awaiting transfer back to the unit from the PACU following thoracic surgery. To which staff member should the nurse assign to this client?

    A. Charge nurse

    B. RN

    C. Licensed practical nurse (LPN)

    D. Assistive personnel (AP)

6. A nurse manager is reviewing the responsibilities of delegation with a group of nurses on a medical unit. Use the ATI Active Learning Template: Basic Concept to complete this item. Under Nursing Interventions, list at least five tasks the delegating nurse must perform when supervising and evaluating a delegatee.

APPLICATION EXERCISES KEY

1. A. INCORRECT: It would be inappropriate to delegate the feeding of a client who has aspiration pneumonia because the client is at risk for further aspiration.

    B. INCORRECT: Either an RN or an LPN, not an AP, may reinforce teaching.

    C. **CORRECT:** The application of a condom catheter is a noninvasive, routine procedure that the nurse may delegate to an AP.

    D. INCORRECT: Either an RN or an LPN, not an AP, may apply a sterile dressing.

     NCLEX® Connection: Management of Care, Assignment, Delegation and Supervision

2. A. INCORRECT: The AP does not need to know the status of the client's roommate to complete this assignment.

    B. **CORRECT:** To complete this assignment safely, the AP should make sure the client wears stockings and slippers.

    C. **CORRECT:** To complete this assignment safely, the AP should make sure the client uses a front-wheeled walker.

    D. **CORRECT:** To complete this assignment safely, the AP should know that the client should be feeling the effects of the pain medication.

    E. INCORRECT: The AP does not need to know the client's allergy status to complete this assignment.

    F. INCORRECT: The AP does not need to know the client's food intake to complete this assignment.

     NCLEX® Connection: Management of Care, Confidentiality/ Information Security

3. A. INCORRECT: Assisting a client to use an incentive spirometer is within the scope of practice of the LPN.

    B. INCORRECT: Collecting a clean-catch urine specimen is within the scope of practice of the LPN.

    C. INCORRECT: Providing nasopharyngeal suctioning is within the scope of practice of the LPN.

    D. **CORRECT:** The RN is responsible for maintaining the PCA pump.

     NCLEX® Connection: Management of Care, Concepts of Management

4. A. INCORRECT: The right client is one of the rights of medication administration, not of delegation.

    B. **CORRECT:** The right supervision/evaluation is one of the five rights of delegation. They also include the right task and the right person.

    C. **CORRECT:** Right direction/communication is one of the five rights of delegation. They also include the right task and the right person.

    D. INCORRECT: Although the delegatee needs to know whether there is a time frame or a specific time to perform the task, the right time is not one of the five rights of delegation. It is one of the rights of medication administration.

    E. **CORRECT:** The right circumstances is one of the five rights of delegation. They also include the right task and the right person.

     NCLEX® Connection: Management of Care, Assignment, Delegation and Supervision

5. A. INCORRECT: Although the charge nurse can provide all the care this client requires in the immediate postoperative period, administrative responsibilities might prevent the close monitoring and assessment this client needs.

    B. **CORRECT:** A client returning from surgery requires assessment and establishment of a plan of care. RNs are responsible for assessment (especially when a client is potentially unstable), initiation of an individualized plan of care, and identification of expected client outcomes. An RN is the appropriate choice.

    C. INCORRECT: Although LPNs can perform some of the tasks crucial in the immediate postoperative period, they cannot provide the comprehensive care this client needs at this time.

    D. INCORRECT: Although an AP can perform some of the tasks crucial in the immediate postoperative period, they cannot provide the comprehensive care this client needs at this time, particularly assessment.

     NCLEX® Connection: Management of Care, Assignment, Delegation and Supervision

6. *Using the ATI Active Learning Template: Basic Concept*
    - Nursing Interventions
      ○ Provide supervision, either directly or indirectly.

      ○ Provide clear directions and understandable expectations of the task(s) to perform (time frames, what to report).

      ○ Monitor performance.

      ○ Provide feedback.

      ○ Intervene if necessary (unsafe clinical practice).

      ○ Evaluate the client, and determine client outcomes status.

      ○ Evaluate client care tasks, and identify needs for performance improvement activities and additional resources.

     NCLEX® Connection: Management of Care, Assignment, Delegation and Supervision

chapter 7

Overview

- The Nursing Process

  - Is a cyclical, critical thinking process that consists of five steps to follow in a purposeful, goal-directed, systematic way to achieve optimal client outcomes. The nursing process is a variation of scientific reasoning that helps nurses organize nursing care and apply the optimal available evidence to care delivery.

  - Is a dynamic, continuous, client-centered, problem-solving, and decision-making framework that is foundational to nursing practice.

  - Provides a framework throughout which nurses can apply knowledge, experience, judgment, and skills, as well as established standards of nursing practice to the formulation of a plan of nursing care. This plan is applicable to any client system, including individuals, families, groups, and communities.

  - Includes five sequential but overlapping steps – Assessment/data collection, analysis/data collection, planning, implementation, and evaluation. Each step of the nursing process depends on the satisfactory completion of the preceding step(s). The accuracy and thoroughness of assessment/analysis/data collection and planning have a direct impact on implementation and evaluation. Use of the nursing process results in a comprehensive, individualized, client-centered plan of nursing care that nurses can deliver in a timely and reasonable manner.

  - Helps nurses integrate critical thinking creatively to base nursing judgments on reason.

  - Promotes the professionalism of nursing while differentiating the practice of nursing from the practice of medicine and that of other health care professionals.

Assessment (RN)/Data Collection (PN)

- Assessment/Data collection involves the systematic collection of information about clients' present health status to identify needs and additional data to collect based on findings. Nurses can collect data during an initial assessment (baseline data), a focused assessment, and ongoing assessments.

- Methods of data collection include observation, interviews with clients and families, medical history, a comprehensive or focused physical examination, diagnostic and laboratory reports, and collaboration.

- To collect data effectively, nurses must ask clients appropriate questions, listen carefully to responses, and have excellent head-to-toe physical assessment skills. Nurses also must employ clinical judgment and critical thinking in accurately recognizing when to collect assessment data. They also must recognize the need to collect assessment data prior to interventions.

- Nurses collect subjective data (symptoms) during a nursing history. They include clients' feelings, perceptions, and descriptions of health status. Clients are the only ones who can describe and verify their own symptoms.

- Nurses observe and measure objective data (signs) during a physical examination. They feel, see, hear, and smell objective data through observation or physical assessment of the client.

SOURCES OF DATA	SUBJECTIVE	OBJECTIVE
Primary sources of data	› What the client tells the nurse: "My shoulder is really, really sore."	› Data the nurse obtains through observation and examination: › Client grimaces when attempting to brush her hair with her left arm.
Secondary sources of data	› What others tell the nurse based on what the client has told them: "She told me that her shoulder is sore every morning."	› Data the nurse collects from other sources (family, friends, caregivers, health care professionals, literature review, medical records): › Physical therapy note in chart indicates client has decreased range of motion of left shoulder.

- During this assessment/data collection, the nurse validates, interprets, and clusters data.

- Documentation of the assessment data must be thorough, concise, and accurate.

Analysis (RN)/Data Collection (PN)

- Nurses use critical thinking skills (a diagnostic reasoning process) to identify clients' health status or problem(s), interpret or monitor the collected database, reach an appropriate nursing judgment about health status and coping mechanisms, and provide direction for nursing care.

- Analysis/Data collection requires nurses to look at the data and

  ○ Recognize patterns or trends

  ○ Compare the data with expected standards or reference ranges

  ○ Arrive at conclusions to guide nursing care

- RNs make multiple analyses based on their interpretations of collected data. They decide, using reasoning and judgment, which data account for clients' health status or problems. At times, this requires further data collection and analysis. As nurses again cluster the collected data, a specific finding might serve as an alert to a specific problem that requires planning and intervention.

- As with the assessment/data collection step, complete and accurate documentation is essential. Documentation should focus on facts and should be highly descriptive.

Planning

- When planning client care (RN) or contributing to a client's plan of care (PN), nurses must establish priorities and optimal outcomes of care they can readily measure and evaluate. These established priorities and outcomes of client care then direct nurses in selecting interventions to include in a plan of care to promote, maintain, or restore health.

- Nurses do three types of planning. Initially, they develop a comprehensive plan of care for clients based on comprehensive assessments they complete, for example, on admission to a health care facility or to a home health organization.

- Nurses do ongoing planning throughout the provision of care. While obtaining new information and evaluating responses to care, they modify and individualize the initial plan of care.

- Discharge planning is a process of anticipating and planning for clients' needs after discharge. To be effective, discharge planning must begin as soon as clients are admitted.

- Throughout the planning process, nurses set priorities, determine client outcomes, and select specific nursing interventions.

- Nurses participate in priority setting when they identify a preferential order of problems. This guides the delivery of nursing care. They can use guidelines to set priorities, such as Maslow's hierarchy of basic needs.

 View Image: Maslow's Hierarchy

- Nurses work with clients to identify goals and outcomes.
  - ○ Goals identify optimal status, whereas outcomes identify the observable criterion that will determine success or failure of the goal.
  - ○ Often these terms are interchangeable. With any format, the goal/outcome must be client-centered, singular, observable, measurable, time-limited, mutually agreeable, and reasonable.
  - ○ Concise, measurable goals help nurses and clients evaluate progress toward the planned outcome and the effectiveness of nursing care.

- Nurses identify actions and interventions that help achieve optimal outcomes.
  - ○ Scientific principles provide the rationale for nursing interventions, which include the following:
    - ▪ Nurse-initiated/independent interventions – Nurses use evidence and scientific rationale to take autonomous actions to benefit clients. They base these actions on identified problems and health care needs, and make sure they are within their scope of practice. Nurses perform or delegate the interventions and are accountable for them. An example is repositioning a client at least every 2 hr to prevent skin breakdown.
    - ▪ Provider-initiated/dependent interventions – Interventions nurses initiate as a result of a provider's prescription (written, standing, or verbal) or the facility's protocol, such as blood administration procedures.
    - ▪ Collaborative interventions – Interventions nurses carry out in collaboration with other health care team professionals, such as ensuring that a client receives and eats his evening snack.

- The nursing care plan (NCP) is the end product of the planning step. Nurses organize the NCP for quick identification of problems, outcomes, and interventions to implement.

Implementation

- In this step of the nursing process, nurses base the care they provide on assessment data, analyses, and the plan of care they developed in the previous steps of the nursing process. In this step, they must use problem-solving, clinical judgment, and critical thinking to select and implement appropriate therapeutic interventions using nursing knowledge, priorities of care, and planned goals or outcomes to promote, maintain, or restore health. Nurses also use interpersonal skills (therapeutic communication) and technical skills (psychomotor performance) when implementing nursing interventions.

- Therapeutic interventions also include measures nurses take to minimize risk and to respond to unplanned events, such as an observation of unsafe practice, a change in a status, or the emergence of a life-threatening situation.

- Nurses use evidence-based rationale for the selection and implementation of all therapeutic interventions. Additionally, caring and professional behavior should be at the center of all therapeutic nursing interventions.

- During implementation, nurses perform nursing actions, delegate tasks, supervise other health care staff, and document the care and clients' responses.

Evaluation

- In this step of the nursing process, nurses evaluate clients' responses to nursing interventions and form a clinical judgment about the extent to which clients have met the goals and outcomes.

- The evaluation of progress toward achievement of client outcomes is what determines whether or not to modify the plan of care.

- Nurses determine the effectiveness of the nursing care plan. They collect data based on the outcome criteria then compare what actually happened with the planned outcomes. This helps determine what further actions to take.

- Questions to consider
  - "Did the client meet the planned outcomes?"
  - "Were the nursing interventions appropriate and effective?"
  - "Should I modify the outcomes or interventions?"

- Client outcomes in specific, measurable terms are easier to evaluate.

- Factors that can lead to lack of goal achievement
  - An incomplete database
  - Unrealistic client outcomes
  - Nonspecific nursing interventions
  - Inadequate time for the client to achieve the outcomes

APPLICATION EXERCISES

1. By the second postoperative day, a client has not achieved satisfactory pain relief. Based on this evaluation, what should the nurse do next according to the nursing process?

    A. Reassess the client to determine the reasons for unsatisfactory pain relief.

    B. See whether the pain lessens during the next 24 hr.

    C. Change the plan to ensure that the client achieves adequate pain relief.

    D. Teach the client about the plan of care for managing his pain.

2. A nursing instructor is reviewing the steps of the nursing process with a group of nursing students. The students should identify which of the following data as objective? (Select all that apply.)

    _____ A. Respiratory rate of 22/min with even, unlabored respirations

    _____ B. "I can only walk three blocks before my legs start to hurt."

    _____ C. Pain level 3 on a scale of 0 to 10

    _____ D. Skin pink, warm, and dry

    _____ E. Urine output of 300 mL/8 hr

    _____ F. Dressing clean, dry, and intact

3. A nursing instructor is reviewing which actions nurses can initiate without a provider's prescription with a group of nursing students. The students should identify which of the following interventions as nurse-initiated? (Select all that apply.)

    _____ A. Give morphine sulfate 1 to 2 mg IV every 1 hr as needed for pain.

    _____ B. Insert an NG tube to relieve a client's gastric distention.

    _____ C. Show a client how to use progressive muscle relaxation.

    _____ D. Perform a daily bath after the evening meal.

    _____ E. Reposition a client every 2 hr to reduce pressure ulcer risk.

4. During evaluation, the nurse must gather information about the client to

    A. identify whether the client outcomes have been met.

    B. organize resources to proceed with implementing interventions.

    C. establish client-centered outcomes that are measurable and realistic.

    D. determine the priority of care and appropriate interventions.

5. A nursing student is reporting to the clinical instructor about the care she gave to a client. She states: "The client said his leg pain was back, so I checked his medical record, and he last received his pain medication 6 hr ago. The prescription reads every 4 hr PRN for pain, so I decided he needs it. I asked the unit nurse to observe me preparing and administering it. I checked with the client 40 min later, and he said his pain is going away." The instructor should inform the student that she left out which of the following steps of the nursing process?

    A. Assessment

    B. Planning

    C. Intervention

    D. Evaluation

6. A nurse educator is reviewing with a group of nursing students the actions and thought processes nurses use during the steps of the nursing process. Use the ATI Active Learning Template: Basic Concept to complete this item to include the following:

    A. Nursing Interventions:
- List at three actions to take during the analysis or data collection step.
- List four factors to consider during the evaluation step when clients have not achieved their goals.

APPLICATION EXERCISES KEY

1. A. **CORRECT:** The nurse should reassess the client to determine why he has not achieved satisfactory pain relief. Various factors may be influencing the lack of pain relief.

    B. INCORRECT: Although it is important to observe a gradual lessening of postoperative pain, which the nurse should expect, there is another essential action to take before this observation.

    C. INCORRECT: Changing the plan may be necessary, but there is another action the nurse should take before altering the plan.

    D. INCORRECT: The current plan is not working, so teaching the client about this plan is providing false reassurance and does not address the client's current pain.

    Ⓝ NCLEX® Connection: Reduction of Risk Potential, System Specific Assessments

2. A. **CORRECT:** Objective data are those nurses observe and measure.

    B. INCORRECT: Subjective data are those clients report. This is an example of subjective data.

    C. INCORRECT: Subjective data are those clients report. This is an example of subjective data.

    D. **CORRECT:** Objective data are those nurses observe and measure.

    E. **CORRECT:** Objective data are those nurses observe and measure.

    F. **CORRECT:** Objective data are those nurses observe and measure.

    Ⓝ NCLEX® Connection: Management of Care, Legal Rights and Responsibilities

3. A. INCORRECT: Although nurses have flexibility in when to administer a PRN medication, the provider must first prescribe it in those terms.

    B. INCORRECT: Clients require a provider's prescription for the insertion of an NG tube. This is a provider-initiated intervention.

    C. **CORRECT:** This is an appropriate nurse-initiated intervention for stress relief. Unless it is a contraindication for a specific client, the nurse may use this technique with clients without a provider's prescription.

    D. **CORRECT:** This is a routine nursing care procedure. Unless it is a contraindication for a specific client, the nurse may determine when bathing is optimal for a client without a provider's prescription.

    E. **CORRECT:** This is an appropriate nurse-initiated intervention for clients who are at risk for developing pressure ulcers. Unless it is a contraindication for a specific client, the nurse may use this strategy without a provider's prescription.

    Ⓝ NCLEX® Connection: Health Promotion and Maintenance, Techniques of Physical Assessment

4. A. **CORRECT:** Evaluation involves gathering information about the client to determine whether client outcomes have been met.

   B. INCORRECT: Organizing resources takes place during the implementation step.

   C. INCORRECT: Establishing client-centered outcomes takes place in the planning step.

   D. INCORRECT: Establishing priorities of care takes place in the planning step.

   N NCLEX® Connection: Management of Care, Legal Rights and Responsibilities

5. A. **CORRECT:** The nursing student should have used the assessment step of the nursing process by asking the client to evaluate the severity of his pain on a 0 to 10 scale. She also should have asked about the characteristics of his pain and assessed for any changes that might have contributed to worsening of the pain.

   B. INCORRECT: The nursing student used the planning step of the nursing process when she decided that it was appropriate to administer the medication and, recognizing her level of experience in administering pain medication, prepared the dose under supervision from the unit staff.

   C. INCORRECT: The nursing student used the implementation step of the nursing process when she administered the medication.

   D. INCORRECT: The nursing student used the evaluation step of the nursing process when she checked the effectiveness of the pain medication in relieving the client's pain.

   N NCLEX® Connection: Health Promotion and Maintenance, Techniques of Physical Assessment

6. *Using ATI Active Learning Template: Basic Concept*

   A. Nursing Interventions
   - Analysis/data collection
     - Recognize patterns or trends.
     - Compare the data with expected standards or reference ranges.
     - Arrive at conclusions to guide nursing care.
   - Factors to consider during evaluation for unmet goals
     - An incomplete database
     - Unrealistic client outcomes
     - Nonspecific nursing interventions
     - Inadequate time for the client to achieve the outcomes

   N NCLEX® Connection: Health Promotion and Maintenance, Techniques of Physical Assessment

CHAPTER 8   Critical Thinking and Clinical Judgment

Overview

- Nursing practice requires the application of knowledge from biological, social, and physical sciences; knowledge of pathophysiology; and knowledge of nursing procedures and skills. Nurses also must use multiple thinking skills—including critical thinking skills such as interpretation, analysis, evaluation, inference, and explanation—to make clinical judgments about problems in nursing practice. A nursing knowledge base with foundational thinking skills, including recall and comprehension, is a prerequisite to critical thinking in nursing.

- In nursing, critical thinking is an active, orderly, well thought-out reasoning process that guides a nurse in various approaches to making a nursing judgment by applying knowledge and experience, problem-solving, logic, reasoning, and decision-making. A critical thinker prioritizes, explores various courses of action, keeps ethics in mind, and determines appropriate outcomes.

- To have a positive impact on a client's health status, a nurse must be able to think critically, correctly identify problems, and both devise and implement the best solutions (interventions). Critical thinking discourages quick judgments that lead to single-focused solutions.

- Critical thinking requires lifelong learning and the ability to acquire relevant experiences that can be reflected on continuously to improve nursing judgment.

- The components of critical thinking include knowledge, experience, critical thinking competencies, attitudes, and intellectual and professional standards.

- Critical thinking incorporates reflection, language, and intuition, and it evolves through three distinct levels as a nurse gains knowledge and experience while maturing into a competent nursing professional.

  - Reflection – Purposefully thinking back or recalling a situation to discover its meaning and gain insight into the event. A nurse should reflect on the following:
    - "Why did I say that or do this?"
    - "Did the original plan of care achieve optimal client outcomes?"
      - If so – "Which interventions were successful?"
      - If not – "Which interventions were unsuccessful?"

  - Language – Precise, clear language demonstrating focused thinking and communicating unambiguous messages and expectations to clients and other health care team members. A nurse should ask the following:
    - "Did I use language appropriate for the client?"
    - "Did I communicate the message clearly to the provider?"

  - Intuition – An inner sensing that facts do not currently support something. Intuition should spark the nurse to search the data to confirm or disprove the feeling. The nurse should ask the following:
    - "Did the vital signs reflect any changes that account for the client's present status?"
    - "When the client's status changed in this way last month, there was a specific reason for it. Is that what is happening here?"

Levels of Critical Thinking

- Basic Critical Thinking
  - A nurse trusts the experts and thinks concretely based on the rules.
  - Basic critical thinking results from limited nursing knowledge and experience, as well as inadequate critical thinking experience.
    - Example – A client reports pain 1 hr after receiving a pain medication. Instead of reassessing the client's pain, the nurse tells the client he must wait 2 more hours before he can receive another dose.
- Complex Critical Thinking
  - The nurse begins to express autonomy by analyzing and examining data to determine the best alternative.
  - Complex critical thinking results from an increase in nursing knowledge, experience, intuition, and more flexible attitudes.
    - Example – A nurse realizes that a client is not ambulating as often as prescribed because of a fear of missing her daughter's phone call. The nurse assures the client that the staff will listen for and answer her phone when she is out of her room.
- Commitment
  - The nurse expects to make choices without help from others and fully assumes the responsibility for those choices.
  - Commitment results from an expert level of knowledge, experience, developed intuition, and reflective, flexible attitudes.
    - Example – A nurse increases the rate of an IV fluid infusion when a client's blood pressure indicates hypovolemic shock 24 hr after surgery.

Components of Critical Thinking

- Knowledge – Information that's specific to nursing and comes from:
  - Basic nursing education.
  - Continuing education courses.
  - Advanced degrees and certifications.
- Experience – Decision-making ability derived from opportunities to observe, sense, and interact with clients followed by active reflection. A nurse:
  - Demonstrates an understanding of clinical situations.
  - Recognizes and analyzes cues for relevance.
  - Incorporates experience into intuition.

- Competence – Cognitive processes a nurse uses to make nursing judgments.
  - General critical thinking
    - Scientific method
    - Problem solving
    - Decision making
    - Diagnostic reasoning and inference
    - Clinical decision-making – collaboration

  View Video: Priority Setting

  - Specific critical thinking in nursing
    - The nursing process

THE NURSING PROCESS	CRITICAL THINKING SKILLS
› Assessment/Data Collection – Collect information about a client's present health status to identify needs, and to identify additional data to collect based on findings.	› Observe. › Use correct techniques for collecting data. › Differentiate between relevant and irrelevant data, and between important and unimportant data. › Organize, categorize, and validate data. › Interpret assessment data and draw a conclusion.
› Analysis/Data Collection – Interpret or monitor the collected database, reach an appropriate nursing judgment about a client's health status and coping mechanisms, and provide direction for nursing care.	› Identify clusters and cues. › Detect inferences. › Recognize an actual or potential problem or risk. › Avoid making judgments.
› Planning – Establish priorities and optimal outcomes of care to measure and evaluate. Then, select the nursing interventions to include in a client's plan of care to promote, maintain, or restore health.	› Identify goals and outcomes for client care. › Set priorities. › Determine appropriate strategies and interventions for inclusion on a client's plan of care or teaching plan. › Take knowledge and apply it to more than one situation. › Create outcome criteria. › Theorize. › Consider the consequences of implementation.
› Implementation – Provide care based on assessment data, analyses, and the plan of care.	› Use knowledge base. › Use appropriate skills and teaching strategies. › Test theories. › Delegate and supervise nursing care. › Communicate appropriately in response to a situation.
› Evaluation – Examine a client's response to nursing interventions and form a clinical judgment about meeting goals and outcomes.	› Determine accuracy of theories. › Evaluate outcomes based on specific criteria. › Determine understanding of teaching.

- Attitudes – Mindsets that affect how a nurse approaches a problem. Attitudes of critical thinkers include:
  - Confidence – Feels sure of abilities.
  - Independence – Analyzes ideas for logical reasoning.
  - Fairness – Is objective, nonjudgmental.
  - Responsibility – Adheres to standards of practice.
  - Risk taking – Takes calculated chances in finding better solutions to problems.
  - Discipline – Develops a systematic approach to thinking.
  - Perseverance – Continues to work at a problem until there's a resolution.
  - Creativity – Uses imagination to find solutions to unique client problems.
  - Curiosity – Requires more information about clients and problems.
  - Integrity – Practices truthfully and ethically.
  - Humility – Acknowledges weaknesses.
- Standards – Model for comparing care to determine acceptability, excellence, and appropriateness.
  - Intellectual standards ensure the thorough application of critical thinking.
  - Professional standards
    - Nursing judgment based on ethical criteria
    - Evaluation that relies on evidence-based practice
    - Demonstration of professional responsibility

FUNDAMENTALS FOR NURSING

APPLICATION EXERCISES

1. A nurse is caring for a client who is 24 hr postoperative following an inguinal hernia repair. The client is tolerating clear liquids well, has active bowel sounds, and is expressing a desire for "real food." The nurse tells the client that she will call the surgeon and ask. The surgeon hears the nurse's report and prescribes a full liquid diet. The nurse used which of the following levels of critical thinking?

    A. Basic

    B. Commitment

    C. Complex

    D. Integrity

2. A nurse is caring for a client who is 24 hr postoperative following abdominal surgery. The nurse suspects the client's pain management is inadequate. Which of the following data reinforce this suspicion? (Select all that apply.)

    A. The client seems easily agitated.

    B. The client is nonadherent with coughing, deep breathing, and dangling.

    C. The client may have pain medication every 4 to 6 hr but accepts it every 6 to 7 hr.

    D. The client reports tenderness in his right lower leg.

    E. The client's vital signs are heart rate 110/min, respiratory rate 20/min, temperature 37° C (98.6° F), and blood pressure 136/80 mm Hg.

3. A nurse is caring for a client who has a new prescription for antihypertensive medication. Prior to administering the medication, the nurse uses an electronic database to gather information about the medication and the effects it might have on this client. Which of the following components of critical thinking is the nurse using when he reviews the medication information?

    A. Knowledge

    B. Experience

    C. Intuition

    D. Competence

4. A nurse receives a prescription for an antibiotic for a client who has cellulitis. The nurse checks the client's medical record, discovers that she is allergic to the antibiotic, and calls the provider to request a prescription for a different antibiotic. Which of the following critical thinking attitudes did the nurse demonstrate?

    A. Fairness

    B. Responsibility

    C. Risk taking

    D. Creativity

5. A nurse uses a head-to-toe approach to conduct a physical assessment of a client who will undergo surgery the following week. Which of the following critical thinking attitudes did the nurse demonstrate?

    A. Confidence

    B. Perseverance

    C. Integrity

    D. Discipline

6. A nurse educator is reviewing with a group of nursing students the critical thinking skills nurses use during each of the steps of the nursing process. Use the ATI Active Learning Template: Basic Concept to complete this item. Under Nursing Interventions, list at three critical thinking skills for each of the five steps of the nursing process.

APPLICATION EXERCISES KEY

1. A. **CORRECT:** At the basic level, thinking is concrete and based on a set of rules, such as obtaining the prescription for diet progression.

    B. INCORRECT: At the commitment level, the nurse expects to have to make choices without help from others and fully assumes the responsibility for those choices. However, postoperative protocols generally involve obtaining a prescription for diet progression.

    C. INCORRECT: Advanced experience and knowledge at the complex level will prompt the nurse to request diet progression to full liquids based on active bowel sounds and the client's tolerance of clear liquid, not solely on the client's request.

    D. INCORRECT: Integrity is a critical thinking attitude that comes into play when the nurse's opinion differs from that of the client. The nurse must then review her own position and decide how to proceed to help achieve outcomes satisfactory to all parties.

     NCLEX® Connection: Management of Care, Advocacy

2. A. INCORRECT: Without more data, this finding alone does not suggest that the client has unrelieved pain. It might be his usual disposition, a result of hospitalization and surgery, or many other factors.

    B. **CORRECT:** Refusal to perform interventions that could increase his pain level (coughing, deep breathing) supports that the client has unrelieved pain.

    C. **CORRECT:** Acceptance of pain medication only at or beyond the maximum interval suggests that the client has pain between the time the effects of the previous dose subside and the new dose takes effect.

    D. INCORRECT: Sudden tenderness or swelling in a lower extremity is more likely to suggest a new problem, such as deep-vein thrombosis.

    E. **CORRECT:** Elevated blood pressure and pulse rate without elevated temperature or other signs of distress support that the client has unrelieved pain.

    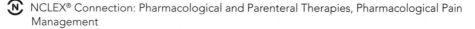 NCLEX® Connection: Pharmacological and Parenteral Therapies, Pharmacological Pain Management

3. A. **CORRECT:** By using the electronic database, the nurse takes the initiative to increase his knowledge base, which is the first component of critical thinking.

    B. INCORRECT: The nurse has had no prior experience with administering this medication to this client.

    C. INCORRECT: Intuition requires experience, which the nurse lacks in administering this medication to this client.

    D. INCORRECT: Competence involves making judgments, but no one can make a judgment about how the nurse handles researching and administering this medication to this client until he performs those tasks.

     NCLEX® Connection: Pharmacological and Parenteral Therapies, Medication Administration

4. A. INCORRECT: Fairness is using a nonjudgmental, objective approach in looking at clients and situations. This attitude does not apply here.

    B. **CORRECT:** The nurse is responsible for administering medications in a safe manner and according to standards of practice. Checking the medical record for allergies helps ensure safety.

    C. INCORRECT: Risk taking is a calculated approach to solving a problem that is not responding to traditional methods. This attitude does not apply here.

    D. INCORRECT: Creativity is an approach that uses imagination to find solutions to unique client problems. This problem is not unique, and it requires a straightforward solution.

     NCLEX® Connection: Safety and Infection Control, Accident/Error/Injury Prevention

5. A. INCORRECT: Confidence is feeling sure of one's own abilities. The nurse may feel confident of her physical assessment skills, but choosing a particular method or sequence requires another attitude.

    B. INCORRECT: Perseverance is continuing to work at a problem until the nurse resolves it. This attitude does not apply here.

    C. INCORRECT: Integrity is a practicing truthfully and ethically. This specific attitude does not apply here.

    D. **CORRECT:** Discipline is developing a systematic approach to thinking. Proceeding head to toe is a systematic approach to collecting the data a physical assessment yields.

     NCLEX® Connection: Health Promotion and Maintenance, Techniques of Physical Assessment

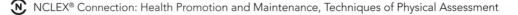

6.   *Using the ATI Active Learning Template: Basic Concept*

-   Nursing Interventions
    -   Assessment/Data collection
        -   Observe.
        -   Use correct techniques for collecting data.
        -   Differentiate between relevant and irrelevant data and between important and unimportant data.
        -   Organize, categorize, and validate data.
        -   Interpret assessment data and draw a conclusion.
    -   Analysis/Data Collection
        -   Identify clusters and cues.
        -   Detect inferences.
        -   Recognize an actual or potential problem or risk.
        -   Avoid making judgments.
    -   Planning
        -   Identify goals and outcomes for client care.
        -   Set priorities.
        -   Determine appropriate strategies and interventions for inclusion on a plan of care or teaching plan.
        -   Take knowledge and apply it to more than one situation.
        -   Create outcome criteria.
        -   Theorize.
        -   Consider the consequences of implementation.
    -   Implementation
        -   Use knowledge base.
        -   Use appropriate skills and teaching strategies.
        -   Test theories.
        -   Delegate and supervise nursing care.
        -   Communicate appropriately in response to a situation.
    -   Evaluation
        -   Determine accuracy of theories.
        -   Evaluate outcomes based on specific criteria.
        -   Determine understanding of teaching.

    NCLEX® Connection: Management of Care, Legal Rights and Responsibilities

chapter 9

Overview

- Responsibilities of nurses include ensuring continuity of care and information sharing throughout the processes of admission, transfers, and discharge.

- The admission assessment provides baseline data to use in the development of the nursing care plan. Comparisons with future assessments help monitor client status and response to treatment.

- Many clients experience anxiety, fear of the unknown, and loss of independence and self-identity at the time of admission to the hospital or health care facility. Children may experience separation anxiety if parents are not present during the hospitalization. When nurses recognize clients' concerns and provide respectful, culturally sensitive care, the clients' experiences will be more positive.

- Discharge planning is an interprofessional process that starts at admission. Nurses conduct discharge planning with clients and families for optimal results.

- Nurses establish the ability of clients to participate in the admission assessment. Clients in distress or with mental status changes may need to have a family member provide necessary information.

- Nurses begin establishing the therapeutic relationship with clients and families during the admission process.

- Nurses promote professional communication between health care providers.

- Nurses use the nursing process as a guide to plan teaching and interventions for clients during discharge.

- Nurses use standard handoff communication tools, such as Introduction, Situation, Background, Assessment, Recommendation (I-SBAR) to facilitate transfers and discharges.

Admission Process

- Equipment
  - Prior to arrival of the client, bring necessary equipment into the room. This should include appropriate documentation forms, equipment to measure vital signs, a pulse oximeter, and hospital attire for the client.

- Procedure
  - Introduce yourself.
  - Explain the roles of other care delivery staff.
  - If in a semiprivate room, introduce the client to his roommate.
  - Provide hospital attire and assist as necessary.
  - Position the client comfortably.
  - Apply the identification bracelet and allergy band, if needed.
  - Provide facility-specific brochures and informational material.

- ○ Provide information about advance directives.
- ○ Document the client's advance directives status in the medical record. Place a copy in the medical record if it is available.
- ○ Assess/collect the following data.
  - ▪ Baseline data – Vital signs, height, weight, allergy status, medications
  - ▪ Biographical information
  - ▪ The client's reason for seeking health care
  - ▪ Present illness and symptoms
  - ▪ Health history
    - □ Current illness
    - □ Current medications (prescription and over-the-counter)
    - □ Prior illnesses, chronic diseases
    - □ Surgeries
    - □ Previous hospitalizations
    - □ Other relevant data
  - ▪ Family history (hypertension, cancer, heart disease, diabetes mellitus)
  - ▪ Psychosocial assessment
    - □ Alcohol, tobacco, drug, and caffeine use
    - □ History of mental illness
    - □ History of abuse or homelessness
    - □ Home situation/significant others
  - ▪ Nutrition
    - □ Current diet, any chewing or swallowing problems
    - □ Recent weight gain/loss
  - ▪ Spiritual health/quality-of-life concerns
    - □ Religion
    - □ Advance directives, living will
  - ▪ Review of systems
  - ▪ Safety assessments
    - □ History of falls
    - □ Sensory deficits (vision, hearing)
    - □ Use of assistive devices (walker, cane, crutches, wheelchair)
  - ▪ Discharge information
    - □ Family members in the home
    - □ Transportation for discharge
    - □ Any relevant phone numbers
    - □ Medical equipment needs at home

- ○ Inventory any personal items.
  - ▪ Examples are clothing, jewelry, money, credit cards, assistive devices (hearing aids, cane, dentures), medications, and religious articles.
  - ▪ Document leaving items at the bedside, storing items in the room closet, sending items home with family, and locking up valuables in the facility's safe. Discourage keeping valuables at the bedside.
- ○ Orient the client and family to the room and the facility. Share information, including the following:
  - ▪ Call light operation
  - ▪ Electric bed operation
  - ▪ Telephone services/television controls
  - ▪ Overhead lighting operation
  - ▪ Smoking policy
  - ▪ Restroom locations
  - ▪ Waiting areas
  - ▪ Meal times
  - ▪ Usual time for providers' visits
  - ▪ Dining/vending services
  - ▪ Visiting policies

Transfer and Discharge Process

- Indications for Transfer and Discharge
  - ○ The level of care has changed. For example, health status has improved so a client no longer needs intensive care.
  - ○ Another setting is required to provide necessary care, for example, a transfer from the medical unit to the surgical suite.
  - ○ The facility does not offer the type of care a client now requires. For example, after the acute phase of a stroke, the client now requires care in a skilled facility.
  - ○ The client no longer needs inpatient care and is ready to return home.
- Discharge Planning
  - ○ This should begin on admission, unless it is long-term care.
  - ○ Assess whether or not the client will be able to return to his previous residence.
  - ○ Determine whether or not the client will need and/or have someone to assist him at home.
  - ○ Assess the residence to see if the client will need adaptations or specific equipment.
  - ○ Make a referral to the social worker to arrange for community services.
  - ○ Communicate health status and needs to community service providers.
  - ○ The provider documents that the client may be discharged. However, a client who is legally competent has the right to leave the facility at any time. The nurse notifies the client's provider, has the client sign the proper forms if possible, and provides discharge teaching.

- Discharge Education
  - The nurse discusses the discharge instructions with the client and provides a printed copy.
  - Instructions should use clear, concise language that the client will understand.

 View Video: Discharge Teaching

  - Standards for discharge education
    - Identifying safety concerns at home
    - Reviewing signs and symptoms of potential complications and when to contact either emergency care or the provider
    - Providing the phone number of the provider
    - Providing names and phone numbers of community resources that give care at the client's residence
    - Step-by-step instructions for performing continuing treatments, such as dressing changes
    - Dietary restrictions and guidelines, including those that pertain to medication administration
    - Amount and frequency of therapies to perform to support continued independence at home
    - Directions on how to take medications and explanations for why adherence is important
- Equipment
  - Items to transfer/discharge with the client
    - Personal belongings at the bedside (flowers, books, clothing, personal care items)
    - Valuables from the safe (if leaving the facility)
    - Medications (especially those belonging to the client or those that cannot be returned to the pharmacy for credit)
    - Assistive devices
    - Medical records or a transfer form
- Procedure
  - Responsibilities of the nurse

TRANSFERRING/DISCHARGING A CLIENT	RECEIVING A TRANSFERRED CLIENT
› On the day and time of transfer, confirm that the receiving facility or unit is expecting the client, and that the room or bed is available.	› Have any specialized equipment ready.
› Communicate the time the client will transfer to the receiving facility or unit.	› If appropriate, inform the client's roommate of the impending admission or transfer.
› Complete documentation (medical records, transfer form).	› Inform other health care team members of the client's arrival and needs.
› Give a verbal transfer report in person or via telephone.	› Meet with the client and family on arrival to complete the admission process and orient the client and family to the new facility or unit.
› Confirm the mode of transportation the client will use to complete the transfer or discharge (car, wheelchair, ambulance).	› Assess how the client tolerates the transfer.
› Make sure the client is dressed appropriately if going outside the facility.	› Review transfer documentation.
› Account for all of the client's valuables.	› Implement appropriate nursing interventions in a timely manner.

- ○ Transfer documentation
    - Medical diagnosis and care providers
    - Demographic information
    - Overview of health status, plan of care, and recent progress
    - Any alterations that may precipitate an immediate concern
    - Notification of any assessments or care essential within the next few hours
    - Most recent vital signs and medications, including PRN
    - Allergies
    - Diet and activity orders
    - Special equipment or adaptive devices (oxygen, suction, wheelchair)
    - Advance directives and emergency code status
    - Family involvement in care and health care proxy, if applicable
- ○ Discharge documentation
    - Type of discharge (provider prescription or against medical advice [AMA])
    - Date and time of discharge, who went with the client, and transportation (wheelchair to car, gurney to ambulance)
    - Where the client went (home, long-term care facility)
    - A summary of the client's condition at discharge (steady gait, ambulating independently, in no apparent distress)
    - A description of any unresolved difficulties and procedures for follow up
    - Disposition of valuables, medications brought from home, and prescriptions
    - Discharge instructions
- ○ Discharge instructions
    - Step-by-step instructions for procedures at home
    - Precautions to take when performing procedures or administering medications
    - Signs and symptoms of complications to report
    - Names and numbers of health care providers and community services to contact
    - Plans for follow-up care and therapies

APPLICATION EXERCISES

1. A nurse is performing an admission assessment for an older adult client. After gathering the assessment data and performing the review of systems, which of the following actions is a priority for the nurse?

    A. Orient the client to his room.

    B. Conduct a client care conference.

    C. Review the client's medical orders.

    D. Develop a plan of care.

2. A nurse is admitting a client who has acute cholecystitis to a medical-surgical unit. Which of the following actions are essential steps of the admission procedure? (Select all that apply.)

    _____ A. Explain the roles of other care delivery staff.

    _____ B. Begin discharge planning.

    _____ C. Provide information about advance directives.

    _____ D. Document the client's wishes about organ donation.

    _____ E. Introduce the client to his roommate.

3. A nurse is transferring a client from an acute-care hospital to a rehabilitation facility. Which of the following information about the client should the nurse include in the transfer report? (Select all that apply.)

    _____ A. Alert and oriented

    _____ B. Refuses to eat spinach

    _____ C. Has a shellfish allergy

    _____ D. Requests morphine every 4 hr

    _____ E. Misses the two cats he has at home

4. A nurse is preparing the discharge summary for a client who has had knee arthroplasty and is going home. Which of the following information about the client should the nurse include in the discharge summary? (Select all that apply.)

_____ A. Advance directives status

_____ B. Where to go for follow-up care

_____ C. Instructions for diet and medications

_____ D. Most recent vital sign data

_____ E. Contact information for the home health care agency

5. As part of the admission process, a nurse at a long-term care facility is gathering a nutrition history for a client who has dementia. Which of the following components of the nutrition evaluation is the priority for the nurse to determine from the client's family?

A. Body mass index

B. Usual times for meals and snacks

C. Favorite foods

D. Any difficulty swallowing

6. A nurse educator is reviewing with a group of nursing students the essential components of an admission assessment or data collection. Use the ATI Active Learning Template: Basic Concept to complete this item. Under Nursing Interventions, list at least three aspects of the health history the nurse must gather and document, as well as at least three aspects of the psychosocial evaluation the nurse must gather and document.

APPLICATION EXERCISES KEY

1. A. **CORRECT:** The greatest risk to this client is injury from unfamiliar surroundings. Therefore, the priority action is to orient the client to the room. Before the nurse leaves the room, the client should know how to use the call light and other equipment at the bedside.

   B. INCORRECT: Conducting a client care conference is important, but it is not the priority action at this time.

   C. INCORRECT: Reviewing the client's medical prescriptions in the medical record is essential, but it is not the priority action at this time.

   D. INCORRECT: Developing a plan of care is essential, but it is not the priority action at this time.

   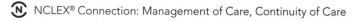 NCLEX® Connection: Management of Care, Continuity of Care

2. A. **CORRECT:** The client's hospitalization is likely to be more positive if the client understands who can perform which care activities for her.

   B. **CORRECT:** Unless the client is entering a long-term care facility, discharge planning should begin on admission.

   C. **CORRECT:** The Patient Self-Determination Act requires asking clients if they have advance directives and providing information about them.

   D. INCORRECT: Asking about organ donation at the point of admission could instill fear unnecessarily.

   E. **CORRECT:** Any action that can reduce the stress of hospitalization is therapeutic. Introductions to other clients and staff can encourage communication and psychological comfort.

   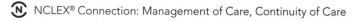 NCLEX® Connection: Management of Care, Continuity of Care

3. A. **CORRECT:** The client's level of consciousness is relevant for evaluating health status and maintaining safety and comfort.

   B. INCORRECT: Although it is important to convey the client's dietary prescription, incorporating personal dietary preferences is not a priority in the transfer report.

   C. **CORRECT:** Information about the client's allergy is essential for maintaining his safety and comfort.

   D. **CORRECT:** It is essential to convey any information about medications or other therapies the client will need within the next few hours.

   E. INCORRECT: Although it is important to convey psychological issues that might require prompt intervention, missing pets is an expected consequence of hospitalization and is not a priority in the transfer report.

   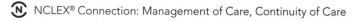 NCLEX® Connection: Management of Care, Continuity of Care

4. A. INCORRECT: Advance directives status is important in transfer documentation, when other care providers will take over a client's care. They are not an essential component of a discharge summary for a client who is returning to his home.

    B. **CORRECT:** It is essential to include the names and contact information of health care providers and community resources the client will need after he returns home.

    C. **CORRECT:** The client will need written information detailing his medication and dietary therapy at home. A client who has had knee arthroscopy typically requires analgesics, possibly anticoagulants, and dietary instructions for avoiding postoperative complications such as constipation.

    D. INCORRECT: Vital sign measurements are important in transfer documentation, when other care providers will take over a client's care. They are not an essential component of a discharge summary for a client who is returning to his home.

    E. **CORRECT:** It is essential to include the names and contact information of health care providers and community resources the client will need after he returns home. For example, a client who has had knee arthroplasty might require physical therapy at home until he can travel to a physical therapy department or facility.

     NCLEX® Connection: Management of Care, Continuity of Care

5. A. INCORRECT: It is important to calculate the client's body mass index to help determine the appropriateness of the client's weight status and related risks. However, there is a higher priority among these options.

    B. INCORRECT: It is important for the nurse to know and try to follow the meal schedule the client follows at home. However, there is a higher priority among these options.

    C. INCORRECT: It is important for the nurse to know which foods are the client's favorites in case it becomes difficult to get the client to consume adequate nutrients. However, there is a higher priority among these options.

    D. **CORRECT:** The greatest risk to a client related to a nutrition-related evaluation is from difficulty swallowing, or dysphagia. It puts the client at risk for aspiration, which can be life-threatening.

     NCLEX® Connection: Basic Care and Comfort, Nutrition and Oral Hydration

6. *Using the ATI Active Learning Template: Basic Concept*
    - Nursing Interventions
      ○ Health history
        ▪ Current illness
        ▪ Current medications (prescription and over the counter)
        ▪ Prior illnesses, chronic diseases
        ▪ Surgeries
        ▪ Previous hospitalizations
      ○ Psychosocial assessment
        ▪ Alcohol, tobacco, drug, and caffeine use
        ▪ History of mental illness
        ▪ History of abuse or homelessness
        ▪ Home situation/significant others

     NCLEX® Connection: Management of Care, Continuity of Care

UNIT 1   Safe, Effective Care Environment

SECTION: SAFETY AND INFECTION CONTROL

› Medical and Surgical Asepsis
› Infection Control
› Client Safety
› Home Safety
› Ergonomic Principles
› Security and Disaster Plans

NCLEX® CONNECTIONS

When reviewing the chapters in this unit, keep in mind the relevant sections of the NCLEX® outline, in particular:

Client Needs: Safety and Infection Control

› Relevant topics/tasks include:
  » Accident/Injury Prevention
    › Identify deficits that may impede client safety.
  » Ergonomic Principles
    › Assess the client's ability to balance, transfer, and use assistive devices prior to planning care.
  » Reporting of Incident/Event/Irregular Occurrence/Variance
    › Acknowledge and document practice errors.
  » Safe Use of Equipment
    › Facilitate appropriate and safe use of equipment.
  » Standard Precautions/Transmission-Based Precautions/Surgical Asepsis
    › Apply principles of infection control.

chapter 10

Overview

- Asepsis – The absence of illness-producing micro-organisms. Hand hygiene is the primary behavior.

    - Medical asepsis – The use of precise practices to reduce the number, growth, and spread of micro-organisms ("clean technique"). It applies to administering oral medication, managing nasogastric tubes, providing personal hygiene, and performing many other common nursing tasks.

    - Surgical asepsis – The use of precise practices to eliminate all micro-organisms from an object or area and prevent contamination ("sterile technique"). It applies to parenteral medication administration, insertion of urinary catheters, surgical procedures, sterile dressing changes, and many other common nursing procedures.

- Before beginning any task or procedure that requires aseptic technique, health care team members must check for latex allergies. If the client or any member of the team has a latex allergy, the team must use latex-free gloves, equipment, and supplies.

Practices That Promote Medical Asepsis

- Always use hand hygiene: handwashing with an antimicrobial or plain soap and water; using alcohol-based products such as gels, foams, and rinses; or performing a surgical scrub.

    - The three essential components of handwashing are the following:

        - Soap

        - Running water

        - Friction

    - All health care personnel must perform hand hygiene, either with an alcohol-based product or with soap and water, before and after every client contact, after removing gloves, after contact with body fluids, before eating, and after using the restroom. When hands are visibly soiled, wash them with soap and water. It is also important for clients and visitors to practice hand hygiene.

    - Perform hand hygiene using recommended antiseptic solutions when caring for clients who are immunocompromised or have infections with multidrug-resistant or extremely virulent micro-organisms.

    - Perform hand hygiene after contact with anything in clients' rooms and after touching any contaminated items, whether or not gloves were worn, and before putting gloves on and after taking them off. Performing hand hygiene may be necessary between tasks and procedures on the same client to prevent cross-contamination of different body sites.

○ Wash hands with soap and warm water. Rub hands together vigorously, and rinse under running water. Wash for at least 15 seconds to remove transient flora and up to 2 min when hands are more soiled. After washing, dry hands with a clean paper towel before turning off the faucet. If the sink does not have foot or knee pedals for turning off the water, use a clean, dry paper towel to turn off the faucet(s).

○ For hand hygiene with an alcohol-based product, dispense the manufacturer's recommended amount (usually 3 to 5 mL) in the palm of the hand. Rub vigorously, remembering to cover all surfaces of both hands and fingers. Continue to rub until both hands are completely dry.

- Additional examples of practices that reduce the growth and spread of micro-organisms are changing linens daily, cleaning floors and bedside stands, and separating clean from contaminated materials.

- Use masks, gloves, gowns, and protective eyewear to help control the contact and spread of micro-organisms to staff and clients.

- Do not place items on the floor (even soiled laundry). The floor is grossly contaminated.

- Emphasize the importance of covering the mouth and nose when coughing or sneezing, using and disposing of facial tissues, and performing hand hygiene to prevent spraying and spreading droplet infections. Encourage clients and visitors to practice respiratory hygiene/cough etiquette. Ensure spatial separation of 3 ft from those with a cough, or have them wear a mask.

- Do not shake linens because doing so can spread micro-organisms in the air. Keep soiled items from touching clothing.

- Clean the least soiled areas first to prevent moving more contaminants into the cleaner areas.

- Use plastic bags for moist, soiled items, following facility protocol for bag selection, to prevent further contamination of items or of individuals handling the soiled items. Put all soiled items directly into the appropriate receptacle to avoid handling soiled items more than once.

- Place all laboratory specimens in biohazard containers or bags for transport or disposal.

- Pour any liquids used for client care directly into the drain, and avoid splattering to prevent spreading droplets. Empty body fluids at water level of toilet to avoid splashing.

- Wash hair frequently, and keep it short or pulled back to prevent contamination of the care area or the clients.

- Keep natural nails short and clean (no artificial nails). The area around and under the nails can harbor micro-organisms.

- Remove jewelry from hands and wrists to facilitate hand disinfection.

Practices that Maintain a Sterile Field

- Prolonged exposure to airborne micro-organisms can make sterile items nonsterile.

  ○ Avoid coughing, sneezing, and talking directly over a sterile field.

  ○ Advise clients to avoid sudden movements, refrain from touching supplies, and avoid coughing, sneezing, or talking over a sterile field.

- Only sterile items may be in a sterile field.

  ○ The outer wrappings and 1-inch edges of packaging that contains sterile items are not sterile. The inner surface of the sterile drape or kit, except for that 1-inch border around the edges, is the sterile field to which other sterile items may be added. To position the field on the table surface, grasp the 1-inch border before donning sterile gloves. Discard any object that comes into contact with the 1-inch border.

  ○ Touch sterile materials only with sterile gloves.

  ○ Consider any object held below the waist or above the chest contaminated.

  ○ Sterile materials may touch other sterile surfaces or materials; however, contact with nonsterile materials at any time contaminates a sterile area, no matter how short the contact.

- Microbes can move by gravity from a nonsterile item to a sterile item.

  ○ Do not reach across or above a sterile field.

  ○ Do not turn your back on a sterile field.

  ○ Hold items to add to a sterile field at a minimum of 6 inches above the field.

- Any sterile, nonwaterproof wrapper that comes in contact with moisture becomes nonsterile by a wicking action that allows microbes to travel rapidly from a nonsterile surface to the sterile surface.

  ○ Keep all surfaces dry.

  ○ Discard any sterile packages that are torn, punctured, or wet.

Nursing Interventions

- Equipment

  ○ Select a clean area above waist level in the client's environment (a bedside stand) to set up the sterile field.

  ○ Check that all sterile packages (additional dressings, sterile bowl, sterile gloves, and solution) are dry and have a future expiration date. Any chemical tape must show the appropriate color change.

  ○ Make sure an appropriate waste receptacle is nearby.

- Procedure

  ○ Perform hand hygiene.

  ○ Open the covering of the package per the manufacturer's directions, slipping the package onto the center of the workspace with the top flap of the wrapper opening away from the body.

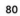

  ○ Grasp the tip of the top flap of the package, and with arm positioned away from the sterile field, unfold the top flap away from body.

  ○ Next, open the side flaps, using the right hand for the right flap and the left hand for the left flap.

- ○ Grasp the last flap, and turn it down toward the body.
- ○ Additional sterile packages
  - ▪ Open next to the sterile field by holding the bottom edge with one hand and pulling back on the top flap with the other hand. Place the packages that will be used last furthest from the sterile field, and open these first.
  - ▪ Add them directly to the sterile field. Lift the package from the dry surface, holding it 15 cm (6 in) above the sterile field, pulling the two surfaces apart, and dropping it onto the sterile field.
- ○ Pour sterile solutions by:
  - ▪ Removing the bottle cap.
  - ▪ Placing the bottle cap face up on a clean (nonsterile) surface.
  - ▪ Holding the bottle with the label in the palm of the hand so that the solution does not run down the label.
  - ▪ First pouring a small amount (1 to 2 mL) of the solution into an available receptacle.
  - ▪ Pouring the solution (without splashing) onto the dressing or site without touching the bottle to the site.
- ○ Once the sterile field is set up, don sterile gloves.
- ○ Sterile gloving includes opening the wrapper and handling only the outside of the wrapper. Don gloves by using the following steps.
  - ▪ With the cuff side pointing toward the body, use the nondominant hand and pick up the dominant-hand glove by grasping the folded bottom edge of the cuff and lifting it up and away from the wrapper.
  - ▪ While picking up the edge of the cuff, pull the dominant glove onto the hand.
  - ▪ With the sterile dominant-gloved hand, place the fingers of the dominant hand inside the cuff of the nondominant glove, lifting it off the wrapper, and put the nondominant hand into it.
  - ▪ When both hands are gloved, adjust the fingers.
  - ▪ During that time, only a sterile gloved hand may touch the other sterile gloved hand.
  - ▪ At the close of the sterile procedure, or if the gloves tear, remove the gloves. Take them off by grasping the outer part of one glove at the wrist, pulling the glove down over the fingers and into the hand that is still gloved. Then, place the ungloved hand inside the soiled glove and pull the glove off so that it is inside out and only the clean inside part is exposed. Discard into an appropriate receptacle.

APPLICATION EXERCISES

1. When entering a client's room to change a surgical dressing, a nurse notes that the client is coughing and sneezing. When preparing the sterile field, it is important that the nurse

    A. keep the sterile field at least 6 ft away from the client's bedside.

    B. instruct the client to refrain from coughing and sneezing during the dressing change.

    C. place a mask on the client to limit the spread of micro-organisms into the surgical wound.

    D. keep a box of facial tissues nearby for the client to use during the dressing change.

2. A nurse is wearing sterile gloves in preparation for performing a sterile procedure. Which of the following objects may the nurse touch without breaching sterile technique? (Select all that apply.)

    _____ A. A bottle containing a sterile solution

    _____ B. The edge of the sterile drape at the base of the field

    _____ C. The inner wrapping of an item on the sterile field

    _____ D. An irrigation syringe on the sterile field

    _____ E. One gloved hand with the other gloved hand

3. A nurse has removed a sterile pack from its outside cover and placed it on a clean work surface in preparation for an invasive procedure. Which of the following flaps should the nurse unfold first?

    A. The flap closest to the body

    B. The right side flap

    C. The left side flap

    D. The flap farthest from the body

4. A nurse is reviewing hand hygiene techniques with a group of assistive personnel (AP). Which of the following instructions should the nurse include when discussing handwashing? (Select all that apply.)

    _____ A. Apply 3 to 5 mL of liquid soap to dry hands.

    _____ B. Wash the hands with soap and water for at least 15 seconds.

    _____ C. Rinse the hands with hot water.

    _____ D. Use a clean paper towel to turn off hand faucets.

    _____ E. Allow the hands to air dry after washing.

5. A nurse has prepared a sterile field for assisting a provider with a chest tube insertion. Which of the following events should the nurse recognize as contaminating the sterile field? (Select all that apply.)

_____ A. The provider drops a sterile instrument onto the near side of the sterile field.

_____ B. The nurse moistens a cotton ball with sterile normal saline and places it on the sterile field.

_____ C. The procedure is delayed 1 hr because the provider receives an emergency call.

_____ D. The nurse turns to speak to someone who enters through the door behind the nurse.

_____ E. The client's hand brushes against the outer edge of the sterile field.

6. A nursing instructor is reviewing with a group of nursing students the procedure for putting on sterile gloves. Use the ATI Active Learning Template: Nursing Skill to complete this item. Under Nursing Actions, list the steps involved in putting on a pair of sterile gloves.

APPLICATION EXERCISES KEY

1. A. INCORRECT: It would be difficult for the nurse to maintain a sterile field away from the bedside. But more important, this might not have any effect on the transmission of some micro-organisms.

   B. INCORRECT: The client may be unable to refrain from coughing and sneezing during the dressing change.

   C. **CORRECT:** Placing a mask on the client prevents contamination of the surgical wound during the dressing change.

   D. INCORRECT: Keeping tissues close by for the client to use still allows contamination of the surgical wound.

    NCLEX® Connection: Safety and Infection Control, Standard Precautions/Transmission-Based Precautions/Surgical Asepsis

2. A. INCORRECT: A bottle of sterile solution is sterile on the inside and nonsterile on the outside. The nurse must prepare the sterile container of solution on the field before putting on sterile gloves.

   B. INCORRECT: The 1-inch border at the outer edge of the sterile field is not sterile. The nurse may not touch it with sterile gloves.

   C. **CORRECT:** The inner wrappings of any objects the nurse dropped onto the sterile field are sterile. The nurse may touch them with sterile gloves.

   D. **CORRECT:** Any objects the nurse dropped onto the sterile field during the setup are sterile. The nurse may touch the syringe with sterile gloves.

   E. **CORRECT:** One sterile gloved hand may touch the other sterile gloved hand because both are sterile.

    NCLEX® Connection: Safety and Infection Control, Standard Precautions/Transmission-Based Precautions/Surgical Asepsis

3. A. INCORRECT: The flap closest to the nurse's body is the innermost flap and the last one to unfold.

   B. INCORRECT: The nurse should unfold the side flap that is closest to the top of the package before the one underneath it; however, there is another flap the nurse should unfold first.

   C. INCORRECT: The nurse should unfold the side flap that is closest to the top of the package before the one underneath it; however, there is another flap the nurse should unfold first.

   D. **CORRECT:** The priority goal in setting up a sterile field is to maintain sterility and thus reduce the risk to the client's safety. Unless the nurse pulls the top flap (the one furthest from her body) away from her body first, she risks touching part of the inner surface of the wrap and thus contaminating it.

    NCLEX® Connection: Safety and Infection Control, Standard Precautions/Transmission-Based Precautions/Surgical Asepsis

4. A. INCORRECT: The APs should apply alcohol rubs to dry hands, and wet the hands first before applying soap for handwashing.

   B. **CORRECT:** This is the amount of time it takes to remove transient flora from the hands. For soiled hands, the recommendation is 2 min.

   C. INCORRECT: The APs should use warm water to minimize the removal of protective skin oils.

   D. **CORRECT:** If the sink does not have foot or knee pedals, the APs should turn off the water with a clean paper towel and not with their hands.

   E. INCORRECT: The APs should dry their hands with a clean paper towel. This helps prevent chapped skin.

    NCLEX® Connection: Safety and Infection Control, Standard Precautions/Transmission-Based Precautions/Surgical Asepsis

5. A. INCORRECT: As long as the provider has not reached over the sterile field, such as by placing the instrument on a near portion of the field, the field remains sterile.

   B. **CORRECT:** Fluid permeation of the sterile drape or barrier contaminates the field.

   C. **CORRECT:** Prolonged exposure to air contaminates a sterile field.

   D. **CORRECT:** Turning away from a sterile field contaminates the field because the nurse cannot see if a piece of clothing or hair made contact with the field.

   E. INCORRECT: The 1-inch border at the outer edge of the sterile field is not sterile. Unless the client reached further into the field, the field remains sterile.

    NCLEX® Connection: Safety and Infection Control, Standard Precautions/Transmission-Based Precautions/Surgical Asepsis

6. *Using the ATI Active Learning Template: Nursing Skill*
   - Nursing Actions
     ○ With the cuff side pointing toward the body, use the nondominant hand to pick up the dominant-hand glove by grasping the folded bottom edge of the cuff and lifting it up and away from the wrapper.
     ○ While picking up the edge of the cuff, pull the dominant glove onto the hand.
     ○ With the sterile dominant-gloved hand, place the fingers of the dominant hand inside the cuff of the nondominant glove, lifting it off the wrapper, and put the nondominant hand into it.
     ○ Adjust the fingers.

    NCLEX® Connection: Safety and Infection Control, Standard Precautions/Transmission-Based Precautions/Surgical Asepsis

chapter 11

Overview

- An infection occurs when the presence of a pathogen leads to a chain of events. All components of the chain must be present and intact for the infection to occur. A nurse uses infection control practices (medical asepsis, surgical asepsis, standard precautions) to break the chain and thus stop the spread of infection.

Types of Pathogen

- Pathogens are the micro-organisms or microbes that cause infections.
  - ○ Bacteria (*Staphylococcus aureus*, *Escherichia coli*, *Mycobacterium tuberculosis*)
  - ○ Viruses – Organisms that use the host's genetic machinery to reproduce (HIV, hepatitis, herpes zoster, herpes simplex)
  - ○ Fungi – Molds and yeasts (*Candida albicans*, Aspergillus)
  - ○ Prions – Protein particles (new variant Creutzfeldt-Jakob disease)
  - ○ Parasites – Protozoa (malaria, toxoplasmosis) and helminths (worms [flatworms, roundworms], flukes [Schistosoma])
- Virulence is the ability of a pathogen to invade and injure a host.
- Herpes zoster is a common viral infection that erupts years after exposure to chickenpox and invades a specific nerve tract.

Immune Defenses

- Nonspecific innate – Native immunity restricts entry or immediately responds to a foreign organism (antigen) through the activation of phagocytic cells, complement, and inflammation. This occurs with all micro-organisms, regardless of previous exposure.
  - ○ Temporary immunity that does not have memory of past exposures
  - ○ Intact skin, the body's first line of defense
  - ○ Mucous membranes, secretions, enzymes, phagocytic cells, and protective proteins
  - ○ Inflammatory response with phagocytic cells, the complement system, and interferons localize the invasion and prevent its spread
- Specific adaptive immunity allows the body to make antibodies in response to a foreign organism (antigen). This reaction directs against an identifiable micro-organism.
  - ○ Requires time to react to antigens
  - ○ Provides permanent immunity
  - ○ Involves B- and T-lymphocytes
  - ○ Produces specific antibodies against specific antigens (immunoglobulins [IgA, IgD, IgE, IgG, IgM])

Infection Process

- The infection process (chain of infection)

 View Image: Chain of Infection

- ○ Causative agent (bacteria, virus, fungus, prion, parasite)
- ○ Reservoir (human, animal, water, soil, insects)
- ○ Portal of exit from (means for leaving) the host
  - Respiratory tract (droplet, airborne)
    - □ *Mycobacterium tuberculosis* and *Streptococcus pneumoniae*
  - Gastrointestinal tract
    - □ Shigella, *Salmonella enteritidis*, *Salmonella typhi*, hepatitis A
  - Genitourinary tract
    - □ *Escherichia coli*, hepatitis A, herpes simplex virus (type 1), HIV
  - Skin/mucous membranes
    - □ Herpes simplex virus and varicella
  - Blood/body fluids
    - □ HIV and hepatitis B and C
- ○ Mode of transmission
  - Contact
    - □ Direct physical contact – Person to person
    - □ Indirect contact with an inanimate object – Object to person
    - □ Fecal-oral transmission – Handling food after using a restroom and failing to wash hands
  - Droplet
    - □ Sneezing, coughing, and talking
  - Airborne
    - □ Sneezing and coughing
  - Vector borne
    - □ Animals or insects as intermediaries (ticks transmit Lyme disease; mosquitoes transmit West Nile and malaria)
- ○ Portal of entry to the host
  - May be the same as the portal of exit
- ○ Susceptible host
  - Compromised defense mechanisms (immunocompromised, breaks in skin) leave the host more susceptible to infections

- Stages of an infection
  - Incubation – interval between the pathogen entering the body and the presentation of the first symptom.
  - Prodromal stage – interval from onset of general symptoms to more distinct symptoms. During this time, the pathogen is multiplying.
  - Illness stage – interval when symptoms specific to the infection occur.
  - Convalescence – interval when acute symptoms disappear. Total recovery could take days to months.

Risks of Infection

- A nurse should assess each client for the risks of infection specific to the client, the disease or injury, and the environment. The most common risks include:
  - Inadequate hand hygiene (client and caregivers).
  - Individuals who have compromised health or defenses against infection, which include:
    - Those who are immunocompromised.
    - Those who have had surgery.
    - Those with indwelling devices.
    - A break in the skin (the body's best protection against infection).
    - Those with poor oxygenation.
    - Those with impaired circulation.
    - Those who have chronic or acute disease such as diabetes mellitus, adrenal insufficiency, renal failure, hepatic failure, or chronic lung disease.
  - Caregivers using medical or surgical asepsis that does not follow the established standards.
  - Clients who have poor personal hygiene or poor nutrition, smoke, or consume excessive amounts of alcohol, and those experiencing stress.
  - Clients who live in a very crowded environment.
  - Older adult clients.
    - Older adults have a slowed response to antibiotic therapy, slowed immune response, loss of subcutaneous tissue and thinning of the skin, decreased vascularity and slowed wound healing, decreased cough and gag reflexes, chronic illnesses, decreased gastric acid production, decreased mobility, bowel and bladder incontinence, dementia, and greater incidence of invasive devices such as a urinary catheter or feeding tube.
  - Individuals who make poor lifestyle choices that put them at risk, which include:
    - Clients who use IV drugs and share needles.
    - Clients who engage in unprotected sex.
  - Clients who have recently been exposed to:
    - Poor sanitation.
    - Mosquito-borne or parasitic diseases
    - Diseases endemic to the area visited, but not in the client's home country.

Types of Infections

- Health Care-Associated Infections (HAIs)

    - These are infections that a client acquires while receiving care in a health care setting. Formerly called nosocomial infections, these can come from an exogenous source (from outside the client) or an endogenous source (inside the client when part of the client's flora is altered).

    - The most common setting for HAIs is the intensive care unit.

    - The best way to prevent HAIs is through frequent and effective hand hygiene.

    - The most common site of HAIs is the urinary tract. The most common causative agents are *Escherichia coli*, *Staphylococcus aureus*, and enterococci.

        - Other sites of HAIs are surgical wounds, respiratory tract, and bloodstream.

    - An iatrogenic infection is a type of HAI resulting from a diagnostic or therapeutic procedure.

    - HAIs are not always preventable and are not always iatrogenic.

    - Use current evidence-based practice guidelines to prevent HAIs due to multidrug-resistant organisms.

Assessment/Data Collection

- The signs and symptoms, identifiable in the nursing assessment, of generalized or systemic infection

    - Fever

    - Presence of chills, which occur when temperature is rising, and diaphoresis, which occurs when temperature is decreasing

    - Increased pulse and respiratory rate (in response to the high fever)

    - Malaise

    - Fatigue

    - Anorexia, nausea, and vomiting

    - Abdominal cramping and diarrhea

    - Enlarged lymph nodes (repositories for "waste")

- Older adults have a reduced inflammatory and immune response, and thus may have an advanced infection before it is identified. Atypical symptoms such as agitation, confusion, or incontinence may be the only symptom.

    - Other symptoms may vary depending on the site of the infection (dyspnea, cough, purulent sputum, and crackles in lung fields, dysuria, urinary frequency, hematuria and pyuria, rash, skin lesions, purulent wound drainage, erythema and odynophagia, dysphagia, hyperemia, enlarged tonsils, change in level of consciousness, nuchal rigidity, photophobia, headache)

- Inflammation is the body's local response to injury or infection. The inflammatory response has three stages. Signs and symptoms during the first stage of the inflammatory response (local infection)

    - Redness (from dilation of arterioles bringing blood to the area)

    - Warmth of the area on palpation

    - Edema

    - Pain or tenderness

- ○ Loss of use of the affected part

- ○ In the second stage, the micro-organisms have been are killed. Fluid containing dead tissue cells and WBCs accumulates and exudate appears at the site of infection. The exudate leaves the body by draining into the lymph system. The types of exudate are:

  - Serous (clear).

  - Sanguineous (contains red blood cells).

  - Purulent (contains leukocytes and bacteria).

- ○ In the third stage, damaged tissue is replaced by scar tissue. Gradually, the new cells take on characteristics that are similar in structure and function to the old cells.

- In addition to the items found on physical assessment, laboratory and diagnostic results indicating infection include:

  - ○ Leukocytosis (WBCs greater than 10,000/μL).

  - ○ Increases in the specific types of WBCs on differential (left shift = an increase in neutrophils).

  - ○ Elevated erythrocyte sedimentation rate (ESR) over 20 mm/hr. An increase indicates an active inflammatory process or infection.

  - ○ Presence of micro-organisms on culture of the specific fluid/area.

- Diagnostic Procedures

  - ○ Gallium scan – Nuclear scan that uses a radioactive substance to identify hot spots of WBCs

  - ○ Radioactive gallium citrate – Injected by IV and accumulates in area of inflammation

  - ○ X-rays, CT scan, magnetic resonance imaging (MRI), and biopsies to determine the presence of infection, abscesses, and lesions

Nursing Interventions

- General Guidelines

  - ○ Use frequent and effective hand hygiene before and after care.

  - ○ Educate the client about the required and recommended immunizations and where to obtain them. The target groups include children, older adults, those with chronic disease, and those who are immunocompromised and their families and contacts.

  - ○ Educate the client and ask for a return demonstration of good oral hygiene. Good oral hygiene decreases the protein (which attracts micro-organisms) in the oral cavity, which thereby decreases the growth of micro-organisms that can migrate through breaks in the oral mucosa.

  - ○ Encourage the client to consume an adequate amount of fluids. Adequate fluid intake prevents the stasis of urine by flushing the urinary tract and decreasing the growth of micro-organisms. Adequate hydration also keeps the skin from breaking down. Intact skin prevents micro-organisms from entering the body.

  - ○ For immobile clients, ensure that pulmonary hygiene (turning, coughing, deep breathing, incentive spirometry) is done every 2 hr, or as prescribed. Good pulmonary hygiene decreases the growth of micro-organisms and the development of pneumonia by preventing stasis of pulmonary excretions, stimulating ciliary movement and clearance, and expanding the lungs.

- ○ Use of aseptic technique and proper personal protective equipment (such as gloves, masks, gowns, and goggles) in the provision of care to all clients prevents unnecessary exposure to micro-organisms.

- ○ Teach and use respiratory hygiene/cough etiquette. It applies to anyone entering a health care setting: clients, visitors, and staff with signs or symptoms of illness, whether diagnosed or undiagnosed. This includes cough, congestion, rhinorrhea, or an increase in the production of respiratory secretions. The components of respiratory hygiene and cough etiquette include:

  - ▪ Covering the mouth and nose when coughing and sneezing.

  - ▪ Using facial tissues to contain respiratory secretions, and disposing of them promptly into a hands-free receptacle.

  - ▪ Wearing a surgical mask when coughing to minimize contamination of the surrounding environment.

  - ▪ Turning the head when coughing and staying a minimum of 3 ft away from others, especially in common waiting areas.

  - ▪ Performing hand hygiene after contact with respiratory secretions.

- • Isolation Guidelines

  - ○ Isolation guidelines are a group of actions that include hand hygiene and the use of barrier precautions, which intend to reduce the transmission of infectious organisms.

  - ○ The precautions apply to every client, regardless of the diagnosis, and implementation of them must occur whenever there's anticipation of coming into contact with a potentially infectious material.

  - ○ Change personal protective equipment after contact with each client, and between procedures with the same client if in contact with large amounts of blood and body fluids.

  - ○ Clients in isolation are at a higher risk for depression and loneliness. Assist the client and their family to understand the reason for isolation and provide sensory stimulation.

 View Video: Precautions

- ○ Standard Precautions (Tier One)

  - ▪ This tier of standard precautions applies to all body fluids (except sweat), nonintact skin, and mucous membranes. A nurse should implement for all clients.

  - ▪ Hand hygiene using an alcohol-based waterless product is recommended after contact with the client, body fluids, and contaminated equipment and articles, and after removal of gloves.

  - ▪ Alcohol-based waterless antiseptic is preferred unless the hands are visibly dirty, because the alcohol-based product is more effective in removing micro-organisms.

  - ▪ Clean gloves are worn when touching all body fluids, nonintact skin, mucous membranes, and contaminated equipment and articles.

  - ▪ Remove gloves and complete hand hygiene between each client.

  - ▪ Masks, eye protection, and face shields are required when care may cause splashing or spraying of body fluids.

  - ▪ Gloves are worn when touching anything that has the potential to contaminate the hands of the nurse. This includes body secretions, excretions, blood and body fluids, nonintact, skin mucous membranes, and contaminated items.

- Hand hygiene is required after removal of the gown. Use a sturdy moisture-resistant bag should for soiled items, and tie the bag securely in a knot at the top.

- Properly clean all equipment for client care; dispose of one-time use items according to facility policy.

- Bag and handle contaminated laundry to prevent leaking or contamination of clothing or skin.

- Enable safety devices on all equipment and supplies after use; dispose of all sharps in a puncture-resistant container.

- A client does not need a private room unless he is is unable to maintain appropriate hygienic practices.

  ○ Transmission Precautions (Tier Two)

    - Use airborne precautions to protect against droplet infections smaller than 5 mcg (measles, varicella, pulmonary or laryngeal tuberculosis). Airborne precautions require:

      □ A private room.

      □ Masks and respiratory protection devices for caregivers and visitors.

        ▸ Use an N95 or high-efficiency particulate air (HEPA) respirator if the client is known or suspected to have tuberculosis.

      □ Negative pressure airflow exchange in the room of at least six to 12 exchanges per hour, depending on the age of the structure.

        ▸ If splashing or spraying is a possibility, wear full face (eyes, nose, mouth) protection.

    - Droplet precautions protect against droplets larger than 5 mcg and travel 3 to 6 ft from the client (streptococcal pharyngitis or pneumonia, Haemophilus influenzae type B, scarlet fever, rubella, pertussis, mumps, mycoplasma pneumonia, meningococcal pneumonia and sepsis, pneumonic plague). Droplet precautions require:

      □ A private room or a room with other clients with the same infectious disease, ensuring that each client have their own equipment.

      □ Masks for providers and visitors.

    - Contact precautions protect visitors and caregivers when they are within 3 ft of the client against direct client and environmental contact infections (respiratory syncytial virus, shigella, enteric diseases caused by micro-organisms, wound infections, herpes simplex, impetigo, scabies, multidrug-resistant organisms). Contact precautions require:

      □ A private room or a room with other clients with the same infection.

      □ Gloves and gowns worn by the caregivers and visitors.

      □ Disposal of infectious dressing material into a single, nonporous bag without touching the outside of the bag.

- Medications

  ○ Antipyretics

    - Antipyretics (acetaminophen and aspirin) are used for fever and discomfort as prescribed.

    - Nursing Considerations

      □ Monitor fever to determine effectiveness of medication.

      □ Graph the client's temperature fluctuations on the medical record for trending.

- ○ Antimicrobial therapy
    - ▪ Antimicrobial therapy kills or inhibits the growth of micro-organisms (bacteria, fungi, viruses, protozoans). Antimicrobial medications either kill pathogens or prevent their growth. Give anthelmintics for worm infestations. There are currently no treatments for prions.
    - ▪ Nursing Considerations
        - □ Administer antimicrobial therapy as prescribed.
        - □ Monitor for medication effectiveness (reduced fever, and increase in the level of comfort, decreasing WBC count).
        - □ Maintain a medication schedule to assure consistent therapeutic blood levels of the antibiotic.

- • Care After Discharge
    - ○ Client Education
        - ▪ Teach the client about:
            - □ Any infection control measures at home.
            - □ Self-administration of medication therapy.
            - □ Complications that need to he needs to immediately.

- • Multidrug-resistant infection
    - ○ Antimicrobials are becoming less effective for some strains of pathogens due to the pathogen's ability to adapt and become resistant to previously sensitive antibiotics. This significantly limits the number of antibiotics that are effective against the pathogen. Use of antibiotics, especially broad-spectrum antibiotics, has significantly decreased to prevent new strains from evolving. Taking the measures below can ensure an antimicrobial is necessary and therapy has been effective.
    - ○ Methicillin-resistant *Staphylococcus aureus* (MRSA) is a strain of *Staphylococcus aureus* that is resistant to all antibiotics, except vancomycin. Vancomycin-resistant *Staphylococcus aureus* (VRSA) is a strain of *Staphylococcus aureus* that is resistant to vancomycin, but so far is sensitive to other antibiotics specific to a client's strain.
    - ○ Nursing Actions
        - ▪ Obtain specimens for culture and sensitivity prior to initiation of antimicrobial therapy.
        - ▪ Monitor antimicrobial levels and ensure that therapeutic levels are maintained.
    - ○ Client Education
        - ▪ Complete the full course of antimicrobial therapy.
        - ▪ Avoid overuse of antimicrobials.

- • Transporting a Client
    - ○ If movement of the client to another area of the facility is unavoidable, the nurse takes precautions to ensure that the environment is not contaminated. For example, a surgical mask is placed on the client with an airborne or droplet infection, and a draining wound is well covered.

- • Guidelines for Cleaning Contaminated Equipment
    - ○ Always wear gloves and protective eyewear.
    - ○ Rinse first in running cold water. Hot water coagulates proteins, making them adhere.
    - ○ Wash the article in warm water with soap.

- ○ Use a brush or abrasive to clean corners or hard-to-reach areas.
- ○ Rinse well in warm water.
- ○ Dry the article – It is considered clean at this point.
- ○ Clean the equipment used in cleaning and the sink (still dirty unless a disinfectant is used).
- ○ If indicated, follow facility policy for recommended disinfection or sterilization.
- ○ Remove gloves and perform hand hygiene.
- Reporting Communicable Diseases
  - ○ A complete list of reportable diseases and the reporting system are available through the Centers for Disease Control and Prevention's website (www.cdc.gov). There are more than 60 communicable diseases that must be reported to the public health departments to allow for officials to:
    - Ensure appropriate medical treatment of diseases (tuberculosis).
    - Monitor for common-source outbreaks (foodborne – hepatitis A).
    - Plan and evaluate control and prevention plans (immunizations for preventable diseases).
    - Identify outbreaks and epidemics.
    - Determine public health priorities based on trends.

Herpes Zoster (Shingles)

- Herpes zoster is a viral infection. It initially produces chickenpox, after which the virus lies dormant in the dorsal root ganglia of the sensory cranial and spinal nerves. It is then reactivated as shingles later in life.
  - ○ Shingles is usually preceded by a prodromal period of several days, during which pain, tingling, or burning may occur along the involved dermatome.
  - ○ Shingles can be very painful and debilitating.
- Assessment
  - ○ Risk Factors
    - Concurrent illness
    - Stress
    - Compromise to the immune system
    - Fatigue
    - Poor nutritional status
    - Older adult clients are more susceptible to herpes zoster infection. The immune function of older adults may also be compromised, so assess them carefully for local or systemic signs of infection.
  - ○ Subjective Data
    - Paresthesia
    - Pain that is unilateral and extends horizontally along a dermatome

- ○ Objective Data
  - ▪ Physical Assessment Findings
    - □ Vesicular, unilateral rash (the rash and lesions occur on the skin area innervated by the infected nerve)
    - □ Rash that is erythematous, vesicular, pustular, or crusting (depending on the stage)
    - □ Rash that usually resolves in 14 to 21 days
    - □ Low-grade fever
  - ▪ Laboratory Tests
    - □ Cultures provide a definitive diagnosis. But, the virus grows so slowly that cultures are often of minimal diagnostic use.
    - □ Occasionally, an immunofluorescence assay can be done.
- • Patient-Centered Care
  - ○ Nursing Care
    - ▪ Assess/Monitor:
      - □ Pain.
      - □ Condition of the lesions.
      - □ Presence of fever.
      - □ Neurologic complications.
      - □ Signs of infection.
    - ▪ Use an air mattress or bed cradle for pain prevention and control of affected areas.
    - ▪ Isolate the client until the vesicles have crusted over.
    - ▪ Maintain strict wound care precautions.
    - ▪ Avoid exposing the client to infants, pregnant women who have not had chickenpox, and clients who are immunocompromised, although anyone who has not had chickenpox and has not been vaccinated is at risk.
    - ▪ Moisten dressings with cool tap water or 5% aluminum acetate (Burow's solution) and apply to the affected skin for 30 to 60 min, four to six times per day as prescribed.
    - ▪ Use lotions to help relieve itching and discomfort.
    - ▪ Administer medications as prescribed.
  - ○ Medications
    - ▪ Analgesics (NSAIDs, narcotics) enhance client comfort.
    - ▪ Antiviral agents, such as acyclovir (Zovirax), may shorten the clinical course.
- • Complications
  - ○ Postherpetic neuralgia
    - ▪ Characterized by pain that persists for longer than 1 month following resolution of the vesicular rash
    - ▪ Tricyclic antidepressants may be prescribed
    - ▪ Postherpetic neuralgia is common in adults older than 60 years of age

APPLICATION EXERCISES

1. A nurse is caring for a client diagnosed with severe acute respiratory syndrome (SARS). The nurse is aware that health care professionals are required to report communicable and infectious diseases. Which of the following illustrate the rationale for reporting? (Select all that apply.)

_____ A. Planning and evaluating control and prevention strategies

_____ B. Determining public health priorities

_____ C. Ensuring proper medical treatment

_____ D. Identifying endemic disease

_____ E. Monitoring for common-source outbreaks

2. A nurse is contributing to the plan of care for a client who is being admitted to the facility with a suspected diagnosis of pertussis. Which of the following should the nurse include in the plan of care? (Select all that apply.)

_____ A. Place the client in a room that has negative air pressure of at least six exchanges per hour.

_____ B. Wear a mask when providing care within 3 ft of the client.

_____ C. Place a surgical mask on the client if transportation to another department is unavoidable.

_____ D. Use sterile gloves when handling soiled linens.

_____ E. Wear a gown when performing care that may result in contamination from secretions.

3. A nurse is caring for a client who presents with linear clusters of fluid-containing vesicles with some crustings. Which of the following should the nurse suspect?

A. Allergic reaction

B. Ringworm

C. Systemic lupus erythematosus

D. Herpes zoster

4. A nurse is caring for a client who reports a severe sore throat, pain when swallowing, and swollen lymph nodes. The client is experiencing which of the following stages of infection?

    A. Prodromal

    B. Incubation

    C. Convalescence

    D. Illness

5. A nurse educator is reviewing with a newly hired nurse the difference in clinical manifestations of a localized versus a systemic infection. The nurse indicates understanding when she states that which of the following are clinical manifestations of a systemic infection? (Select all that apply.)

    _____ A. Fever

    _____ B. Malaise

    _____ C. Edema

    _____ D. Pain or tenderness

    _____ E. Increase in pulse and respiratory rate

6. A nurse educator is teaching a module on the chain of infection during nursing orientation to a group of newly licensed nurses. Use the ATI Active Learning Template: Basic Concept to complete this item. Under Related Content, list the six links in the chain of infection that must be present for an infection to occur.

APPLICATION EXERCISES KEY

1.   A. **CORRECT:** Reporting of communicable and infectious diseases assists with planning and evaluating control and prevention strategies.

   B. **CORRECT:** Reporting of communicable and infectious diseases assists with determining public health policies.

   C. **CORRECT:** Reporting of communicable and infectious diseases assists with ensuring proper medical treatment is available.

   D. INCORRECT: Endemic disease is already prevalent within a population, so reporting is not necessary.

   E. **CORRECT:** Reporting of communicable and infectious diseases assists with monitoring for common-source outbreaks.

    NCLEX® Connection: Physiological Adaptations, Illness Management

2.   A. INCORRECT: A nurse should place a client in a private room and initiate droplet precautions if he has pertussis. The client's room does not need to have negative air pressure.

   B. **CORRECT:** The nurse should wear a mask when within 3 ft of the client.

   C. **CORRECT:** The nurse should place a surgical mask on the client during transport to another area of the facility.

   D. INCORRECT: The nurse should wear a gown when performing care that may result in contamination from body fluids.

   E. **CORRECT:** A gown should be worn if the nurse's clothing or skin may be contaminated with body secretions or excretions.

    NCLEX® Connection: Safety and Infection Control, Standard Precautions/Transmission-Based Precautions/Surgical Asepsis

3.   A. INCORRECT: A pink body rash can indicate an allergic reaction.

   B. INCORRECT: Red circles with white centers occur with ringworm.

   C. INCORRECT: A red edematous rash bilaterally on the cheeks can indicate systemic lupus erythematosus.

   D. **CORRECT:** Vesicles that follow along a unilateral dermatome can indicate herpes zoster.

    NCLEX® Connection: Physiological Adaptations, Pathophysiology

4. A. **INCORRECT:** The prodromal stage consists of nonspecific clinical manifestations of the infection.

    B. **INCORRECT:** The incubation period consists of the time when the pathogen first enters the body prior to the appearance of any symptoms of infection.

    C. **INCORRECT:** Convalescence is when acute symptoms of the infection fade.

    D. **CORRECT:** The illness stage is when the client experiences signs and symptoms specific to the infection.

     NCLEX® Connection: Physiological Adaptations, Pathophysiology

5. A. **CORRECT:** A fever indicates that the infection is affecting the whole body, and therefore systemic.

    B. **CORRECT:** Malaise indicates that the infection is affecting the whole body, and therefore systemic.

    C. **INCORRECT:** Edema is a localized symptom indicating a localized, not systemic, infection.

    D. **INCORRECT:** Pain and tenderness is a localized symptom indicating a localized, not systemic, infection.

    E. **CORRECT:** An increase in pulse and respiratory rate indicates that the infection is affecting the whole body, and therefore systemic.

     NCLEX® Connection: Physiological Adaptations, Pathophysiology

6. *Using the ATI Active Learning Template: Basic Concept*
    - Related Content
      - The infection process (chain of infection)
        - Causative agent
        - Reservoir
        - Portal of exit (means of leaving) from the host
        - Mode of transmission
        - Portal of entry to the host
        - Susceptible host

     NCLEX® Connection: Safety and Infection Control, Standard Precautions/Transmission-Based Precautions/Surgical Asepsis

chapter 12

Overview

- Providing for safety and preventing injury are major nursing responsibilities. Many factors affect the client's ability to protect himself. Those factors include the client's:
  - Age, with the young and old at greater risk
  - Mobility
  - Cognitive and sensory awareness
  - Emotional state
  - Ability to communicate
  - Lifestyle and safety awareness
- All health care workers must be aware of:
  - Knowing how to assess clients and their environment for safety using risk assessment tools
  - Encouraging clients to speak up and be involved or take an active role in their health care and prevention of errors
  - Creating a culture of checks and balances to avoid errors when working under stress
  - Communicating risk factors and plan of care with clients, family, and other health care workers via a dry erase board in the client's room or other means per facility protocol
  - Protocols for responding to dangerous situations
  - Quality care priorities established by the National Quality Forum, including Never Events.
  - Using the current evidence to promote a culture of safety, with the National Patient Safety Goals as a guide
  - Knowing the disaster plan of the facility; understanding the chain of command and roles; using common terminology when communicating with the team
  - Identifying and documenting the incidents and responses per health care agency policy. These reports will help to identify trends, patterns, and the root cause of an event.
  - Knowing the location of material safety data sheets (MSDS) and hazardous chemicals in the environment.
- It is the provider's responsibility to assess, report, and document client allergies and to provide client care that avoids exposure to allergens.
- Equipment should be used by the nurse only after a safety inspection and adequate instruction.

Falls

Ⓖ
- Older adult clients may be at an increased risk for falls due to decreased strength, impaired mobility and balance, and endurance limitations combined with decreased sensory perception.

- Other clients at increased risk include those with decreased visual acuity, generalized weakness, urinary frequency, gait and balance problems (cerebral palsy, injury, multiple sclerosis) and cognitive dysfunction. Side effects of medications (orthostatic hypotension, drowsiness) also can increase the client's risk for falls.

- Clients are at greater risk for falls when more than one of the risk factors are present.

- Prevention of client falls is a major nursing priority. All clients admitted to health care institutions should be assessed for risk factors related to falls, and based on the assessment, preventative measures should be implemented.

- Prevention of Falls

  ○ Complete a fall-risk assessment upon admission and at regular intervals on the client.

  ○ The plan for each client is individualized based on the fall-risk assessment.

    ■ For example, if the client has orthostatic hypotension, instruct the client to avoid getting up too quickly, to sit on the side of the bed for a few seconds prior to standing, and to stand at the side of the bed for a few seconds prior to walking.

    ■ General measures to prevent falls include the following:

      □ Be sure the client knows how to use the call light, that it is in reach, and encourage its use.

      □ Respond to call lights in a timely manner.

      □ Use fall-risk alerts, such as ID wristbands per facility protocol.

      □ Provide regular toileting and orientation of confused clients as needed.

      □ Ensure adequate lighting.

      □ Orient the client to the setting (grab bars, call light) to ensure he knows how to use all assistive devices and can locate necessary items.

      □ Place clients at risk for falls near the nursing station.

      □ Ensure that bedside tables and overbed tables and frequently used items (telephone, water, tissues) are within the client's reach.

      □ Maintain the bed in the low position.

      □ For clients who are sedated, unconscious, or otherwise compromised, the bed rails are kept up, and the bed is kept in the low position.

      □ Avoid the use of full side bed rails for clients who get out of bed or attempt to get out of bed without assistance.

      □ Provide the client with nonskid footwear and nonskid bath mats for use in tubs and showers.

      □ Use gait belts and additional safety equipment, as needed, when moving clients.

      □ Keep the floor free from clutter with a clear path to the bathroom (no scatter rugs, cords, furniture).

- Keep assistive devices nearby after validation of safe use by the client and family (glasses, walkers, transfer devices).

- Educate the client and family/caregivers on identified risks and the plan of care. Clients and family who are aware of risks are more likely to call for assistance.

- Lock wheels on beds, wheelchairs, and carts to prevent the device from rolling during transfers or stops.

- Use chair or bed sensors for clients at risk for getting up unattended to alert staff of independent ambulation.

  - Report and document all incidents per the health care facility's policy. This provides valuable information that may be helpful in preventing similar incidents.

Seizure Precautions

- A seizure is a sudden surge of electrical activity in the brain. It may occur at any time during a person's life and may be due to epilepsy, fever, or a variety of medical conditions. Partial seizures (also called focal seizures) are due to electrical surges in one part of the brain, and generalized seizures involve the entire brain.

- Seizure precautions (measures to protect the client from injury should a seizure occur) are taken for clients who have a history of seizures that involve the entire body and/or result in unconsciousness.

  - Ensure rescue equipment is at the bedside, including oxygen, an oral airway, and suction equipment and padding for the side rails of the bed. A saline lock may be inserted for intravenous access if the client is at high risk for experiencing a generalized seizure.

  - Inspect the client's environment for items that may cause injury in the event of a seizure, and remove items that are not necessary for current treatment.

  - Assist the client at risk for a seizure with ambulation and transferring to reduce the risk of injury.

  - Advise all caregivers and family not to put anything in the client's mouth (except in status epilepticus, where an airway is needed) in the event of a seizure.

  - Advise all caregivers and family not to restrain the client in the event of a seizure, ensure the client's safety by lowering him to the floor or bed, protect his head, remove nearby furniture, provide privacy, put the client on his side with his head flexed slightly forward if possible, and loosen clothing to prevent injury.

- In the event of a seizure

  - Stay with the client, and call for help.

  - Administer medications as prescribed.

  - Note the duration of the seizure and the sequence and type of movement.

  - After a seizure, assess mental status, oxygenation saturation, and vital signs of the client. Explain what happened to the client, and provide comfort, understanding, and a quiet environment for the client to recover.

  - Document the seizure in the client's record with any precipitating behaviors and a description of the event (movements, any injuries, length of seizure, aura, postictal state), and report it to the provider.

Seclusion and Restraints

- Nurses must know and follow federal/state/facility policies that govern the use of restraints.

- Use of seclusion rooms and/or restraints may be authorized for clients in some cases.

- In general, seclusion and/or restraints should be ordered for the shortest duration necessary and only if less restrictive measures are not sufficient. It is for the physical protection of the client or the protection of other clients or staff.

- A client may voluntarily request temporary seclusion in cases in which the environment is disturbing or seems too stimulating.

- Restraints can be either physical or chemical, such as sedatives and neuroleptic or psychotropic medications to calm the client.

- Seclusion and/or restraint must never be used for the following:

  ○ Convenience of the staff

  ○ Punishment for the client

  ○ Clients who are extremely physically or mentally unstable

  ○ Clients who cannot tolerate the decreased stimulation of a seclusion room

- Restraints should

  ○ Never interfere with treatment

  ○ Restrict movement as little as is necessary to ensure safety

  ○ Fit properly and be as discreet as possible

  ○ Be easily removed or changed to decrease the chance of injury and to provide for the greatest level of dignity

- When all other less restrictive means have been tried to prevent a client from harming self or others, the following must occur in order for seclusion or restraint to be used:

  ○ The treatment must be prescribed by the provider in writing, based on a face-to-face assessment of the client.

    ▪ In an emergency situation in which there is immediate risk to the client or others, the nurse may place a client in restraints. The nurse must obtain a prescription from the provider as soon as possible in accordance with agency policy (usually within 1 hr).

  ○ The prescription must include the reason for the restraint, the type of restraint, the location of the restraint, how long the restraint may be used, and the type of behaviors demonstrated by the client that warrant use of the restraint.

  ○ The prescription and the renewal are limited to 4 hr for an adult, 2 hr for clients ages 9 to 17, and 1 hr for clients younger than 9 years of age. Prescriptions may be renewed, if needed, with a maximum of 24 consecutive hours.

  ○ PRN prescriptions for restraints are not allowed.

- ○ Nursing responsibilities
  - ▪ Assess skin integrity, and provide skin care per facility protocol, usually every 2 hr.
  - ▪ Offer food and fluid.
  - ▪ Provide with means for hygiene and elimination.
  - ▪ Monitor for vital signs.
  - ▪ Offer range of motion of extremities.
- ○ Always explain the need for the restraint to the client and family, emphasizing that the restraint is needed to ensure the safety of the client and will be used only as long as it is necessary.
- ○ Obtain signed consent from client or guardian, if required.
- ○ Review the manufacturer's instructions for correct application.
- ○ Remove or replace restraints frequently to ensure good circulation to the area and allow for full range of motion to the limb that has been restricted.
- ○ Pad bony prominences.
- ○ Use a quick-release knot to tie the restraint to the bed frame (loose knots that are easily removed) where it will not tighten when the bed is raised or lowered.
- ○ Ensure that the restraint is loose enough for range of motion and with enough room to fit two fingers between the device and the client to prevent injury.
- ○ Regularly assess the need for continued use of the restraints to allow for discontinuation of the restraint or limiting the restraint at the earliest possible time while ensuring the client's safety.
- ○ Never leave the client unattended without the restraint.
- ○ Document
  - ▪ Precipitating events and behavior of the client prior to seclusion or restraint
  - ▪ Alternative actions taken to avoid seclusion or restraint
  - ▪ The time restraints were applied and removed (if discontinued)
  - ▪ Type of restraint used and location
  - ▪ Client's behavior while restrained
  - ▪ Type and frequency of care (range of motion, neurosensory checks, removal, integumentary checks)
  - ▪ Condition of the body part being restrained
  - ▪ Client's response when the restraint is removed
  - ▪ Medication administration
- ○ An emergency situation must be present for the nurse to use seclusion or restraints without first obtaining a provider's written prescription. If this treatment is initiated, the nurse must obtain the written prescription within a specified period of time (usually within 1 hr).

Fire Safety

- Fires in health care facilities are usually due to problems related to electrical or anesthetic equipment. Unauthorized smoking also may be the cause of a fire.
- All staff must be instructed in fire response procedures, which includes the following:
  - Knowing the location of exits, alarms, fire extinguishers, and oxygen turn-off valves
  - Ensuring fire doors are not blocked with equipment
  - Knowing the evacuation plan for the unit and facility
- The fire response in the health care setting always follows this sequence (RACE):
  - R – Rescue: Rescue and protect clients in close proximity to the fire by evacuating them to a safer location. Ambulatory clients can walk unattended to a safe location.
  - A – Alarm: Activate the facility alarm system, and then report fire details and location per facility protocol.
  - C – Contain: Contain the fire by closing doors and windows as well as turning off any sources of oxygen and electrical devices. Clients who are on life support are ventilated with a bag-valve mask.
  - E – Extinguish: Extinguish the fire if possible using an appropriate fire extinguisher.
    - There are three classes of fire extinguisher:
      - Class A is for paper, wood, upholstery, rags, or other types of trash fires.
      - Class B is for flammable liquids and gas fires.
      - Class C is for electrical fires.
    - To use a fire extinguisher, use the PASS sequence:
      - P – Pull the pin.
      - A – Aim at the base of the fire.
      - S – Squeeze the levers.
      - S – Sweep the extinguisher from side to side, covering the area of the fire.

APPLICATION EXERCISES

1. A nurse is caring for a client who was just admitted to the unit after falling at a nursing home. This client is oriented to person, place, and time and can follow directions. Which of the following actions by the nurse are appropriate to decrease the risk of a fall? (Select all that apply.)

_____ A. Place a belt restraint on the client when he is sitting on the bedside commode.

_____ B. Keep the bed in low position with full side rails up.

_____ C. Ensure that the client's call light is within reach.

_____ D. Provide the client with nonskid footwear.

_____ E. Complete a fall-risk assessment.

2. A nurse manager is reviewing care of a client who has had a seizure with nurses on the unit. Which of the following statements by a nurse requires further instruction?

A. "I will place the client on his side."

B. "I will go to the nurses' station for assistance."

C. "I will administer medications as prescribed."

D. "I will be prepared to insert an airway."

3. A nurse observes smoke coming from under the door of the staff lounge. Which of the following is the priority action by the nurse?

A. Extinguish the fire.

B. Pull the fire alarm.

C. Evacuate the clients.

D. Close all open doors on the unit.

4. A charge nurse is designating room assignments for clients who will be admitted to the unit. Based on the nurse's knowledge of fall prevention, which of the following clients should be assigned to the room closest to the nurses' station?

A. A 43-year-old client who is postoperative following a laparoscopic cholecystectomy

B. A 61-year-old client being admitted for telemetry to rule out a myocardial infarction

C. A 50-year-old client who is postoperative following an open reduction internal fixation of the ankle

D. A 79-year-old client who is postoperative following a below-the-knee amputation

5. A nurse is caring for a newly admitted client who has a documented history of falls. Which of the following is the priority action by the nurse?

     A. Complete a fall-risk assessment.

     B. Educate the client and family on fall risks.

     C. Complete a physical assessment.

     D. Survey the client's belongings.

6. A nurse educator is teaching about the safe use of seclusion and restraints to a group of newly licensed nurses. What should be included in the teaching? Use the ATI Active Learning Template: Basic Concept to complete this item. Under Nursing Interventions, describe six nursing responsibilities when caring for a client in either seclusion or restraints.

APPLICATION EXERCISES KEY

1. A. INCORRECT: It is inappropriate to restrain this client and could be considered false imprisonment.

    B. INCORRECT: Full side rails for this client may put the client at greater risk for a fall because he may attempt to climb over the bed rails to get out of bed.

    C. **CORRECT:** Ensuring that the call light is within reach enables the client to contact the nursing staff to ask for assistance and prevents the client from falling out of bed while reaching for the call light.

    D. **CORRECT:** Nonskid footwear may keep the client from slipping.

    E. **CORRECT:** A fall-risk assessment serves as the basis for an individualized plan of care.

    N NCLEX® Connection: Safety and Infection Control, Accident/Error/Injury Prevention

2. A. INCORRECT: When a seizure occurs, the client should be placed in a side-lying position to allow for drainage of secretions and to prevent the tongue from occluding the airway.

    B. **CORRECT:** During a seizure, the client should not be left alone. The nurse remains with the client and calls for assistance using the call light.

    C. INCORRECT: Administering medications is an appropriate action by the nurse.

    D. INCORRECT: Nothing should be placed in the client's mouth except an airway, if needed. A tongue blade can cause injury and airway obstruction.

    N NCLEX® Connection: Physiological Adaptations, Alterations in Body Systems

3. A. INCORRECT: Although extinguishing the fire is part of the fire response, it is not the priority action.

    B. INCORRECT: Although pulling the fire alarm is part of the fire response, it is not the priority action.

    C. **CORRECT:** Rescue is the first action in the fire response. Protecting and evacuating clients in close proximity to the fire is the priority action.

    D. INCORRECT: Although containing the fire by closing doors is part of the fire response, it is not the priority action.

    N NCLEX® Connection: Safety and Infection Control, Accident/Error/Injury Prevention

4. A. INCORRECT: Although this client just had surgery, risk factors for falls are low based on the client's age and type of surgery.

    B. INCORRECT: Although this client is on telemetry, this client does not display as many risk factors as another client who is to be admitted.

    C. INCORRECT: Although this client just had surgery, this client does not display as many risk factors as another client who is to be admitted.

    D. **CORRECT:** This client should be assigned to a room near the nurses' station due to risk factors that include client's age, mobility, and balance issues related to the surgery, and potential side effects, such as drowsiness, as a result of analgesic medication.

    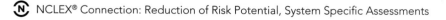 NCLEX® Connection: Reduction of Risk Potential, System Specific Assessments

5. A. **CORRECT:** The greatest risk to this client is injury due to a fall. Therefore, the priority action is to determine the client's fall risk. This will guide the nurse in implementing appropriate safety measures.

    B. INCORRECT: It is important for family members to be aware of the client's risk for falls. Providing instruction to the client and family is an appropriate nursing action, but this is not the priority action.

    C. INCORRECT: Completing a physical assessment will help to identify further risk for injury and provide baseline physical data, but this is not the priority action.

    D. INCORRECT: Surveying the client's belongings (glasses, medications, hearing aids, canes, walkers) may provide clues to potential fall risks. However, this is not the priority action.

    NCLEX® Connection: Safety and Infection Control, Accident/Error/Injury Prevention

6.   *Using the ATI Active Learning Template: Basic Concept*

- Nursing Interventions
  - Nursing responsibilities include knowing how often the client should be
    - Assessed – Including neurosensory checks of affected extremities (circulation, sensation, mobility). These checks are usually done at least every 2 hr.
    - Offered food and fluid.
    - Provided with means for hygiene and elimination.
    - Monitored for vital signs.
    - Offered range of motion of extremities.
  - Frequency of client assessments in regard to food, fluids, comfort, and safety should be performed and documented every 15 to 30 min.
  - Other responsibilities include the following:
    - Explaining the need for the restraint to the client and family, emphasizing that the restraint is needed to ensure the safety of the client and will be used only as long as it is necessary.
    - Obtaining signed consent from client or guardian, if required.
    - Reviewing the manufacturer's instructions for correct application.
    - Removing or replacing restraints frequently to ensure adequate circulation to the area and allowing for full range of motion to the restricted limb.
    - Padding bony prominences.
    - Using a quick-release knot to tie the restraint to the bed frame where it will not tighten when the bed is raised or lowered.
    - Ensuring that the restraint is loose enough for range of motion and with enough room to fit two fingers between the device and the client to prevent injury.
    - Regularly assessing the need for continued use of the restraints to allow for discontinuation of the restraint or limiting the restraint at the earliest possible time.
    - Never leaving the client unattended without the restraint.
    - Completing documentation to include the following:
      - Precipitating events and behavior of the client prior to seclusion or restraint
      - Alternative actions taken to avoid seclusion or restraint
      - The time restraints were applied and removed (if discontinued)
      - Type of restraint used and location
      - Client's behavior while restrained
      - Type and frequency of care (range of motion, neurosensory checks, removal, integumentary checks)
      - Condition of the body part being restrained
      - Client's response when the restraint is removed
      - Medication administration

Ⓝ NCLEX® Connection: Safety and Infection Control, Use of Restraints/Safety Devices

chapter 13

Overview

- In addition to taking measures to prevent injury of clients in a health care setting, nurses play a pivotal role in promoting safety in the client's home and community. Nurses often collaborate with the client, family, and members of the interprofessional team (social workers, occupational therapists, and physical therapists) to promote the safety of the client.

- A number of factors contribute to the client's risk for injury.

  - Age and developmental status

  - Mobility and balance

  - Knowledge about safety hazards

  - Sensory and cognitive awareness

  - Communication skills

  - Home and work environment

  - Community in which the client lives

- To initiate a plan of care, the nurse must identify risk factors using a risk assessment tool and complete a nursing history, a physical examination, and a home hazard appraisal.

- In the plan of care for safety preparedness, include emergency nursing principles.

  - Basic first aid

  - CPR

Safety Risks Based on Age and Developmental Status

- The age and developmental status of the client creates specific safety risks. Some of the accident prevention measures for specific age groups are found below:

INFANTS AND TODDLERS	
RISK	**PREVENTION EDUCATION**
Aspiration	› Keep all small objects out of reach. › Check toys and objects for loose or small parts and sharp edges. › Do not feed the infant hard candy, peanuts, popcorn, or whole or sliced pieces of hot dog. › Do not place the infant in the supine position while feeding or prop the infant's bottle. › A pacifier (if used) should be constructed of one piece and never placed on string or ribbon around the neck.
Suffocation	› Teach "back to sleep" mnemonic and always place infants on back to rest. › Keep plastic bags out of reach. › Make sure crib mattress fits snugly and that crib slats are no more than 2 ⅜ inches apart. › Never leave an infant or toddler alone in the bathtub. › Do not place anything in crib with infant. › Remove crib toys, such as mobiles, from over the bed as soon as the infant begins to push up. › Keep latex balloons away from infants and toddlers. › Fence swimming pools and use a locked gate. › Begin swimming lessons when the child's developmental status allows for protective responses such as closing her mouth under water. › Teach caregivers CPR and Heimlich maneuver. › Keep toilet lids down and bathroom doors closed.
Poisoning	› Keep house plants and cleaning agents out of reach. › Inspect and remove sources of lead, such as paint chips, and provide parents with information about prevention of lead poisoning. › Place poisons, paint, and gasoline in locked cabinet. › Keep medications in child-proof containers and locked up. › Dispose of medications which are not longer used or are out of date.
Falls	› Keep crib and playpen rails up. › Never leave the infant unattended on a changing table or other high surface. › Use gates on stairs, and ensure windows have screens. › Restrain according to manufacturer's recommendations and supervise when in high chair, swing, stroller, etc. › Place in a low bed when toddler starts to climb.
Motor vehicle/ Injury	› Place infants and toddlers in an a rear-facing car seat until 2 years of age or until they exceed the height and weight limit of the car seat. They can then sit in a forward-facing car seat. › Use a car seat with a five-point harness for infants and children. › All car seats should be federally approved and be placed in the back seat.
Burns	› Test the temperature of formula and bath water. › Place pots on back burner and turn handle away from front of stove. › Supervise the use of faucets. › Keep matches and lighters out of reach.

PRESCHOOLERS AND SCHOOL-AGE CHILDREN	
RISK	**PREVENTION EDUCATION**
Drowning	› Be sure child has learned to swim and knows rules of water safety. › Place locked fences around home and neighborhood pools. › Provide supervision near pools or water.
Motor vehicle/ Injury	› Use booster seats for children who are less than 4 feet 9 inches tall and weigh less than 40 lb (usually 4 to 8 years old). The child should be able to sit with his back against the car seat, and his legs should dangle over the seat. › If car has a passenger air bag, place children under 12 years in the back seat. › Use seat belts properly after booster seats are no longer necessary. › Use protective equipment when participating in sports, riding a bike, or riding as a passenger on a bike. › Supervise and teach safe use of equipment. › Teach the child to play in safe areas and never to run after a ball or toy that goes into a road. › Teach child safety rules of the road. › Teach child what to do if approached by stranger. › Begin sex education for school-age child.
Firearms	› Keep firearms unloaded, locked up, and out of reach. › Teach to never touch a gun or stay at a friend's house where a gun is accessible. › Store bullets in a different location from guns.
Play injury	› Teach to not run with candy or objects in mouth. › Remove doors from refrigerators or other potentially confining structures. › Teach playground safety. › Teach to play in safe areas, and avoid heavy machinery, railroad tracks, areas of excavation, quarries, trunks, and vacant buildings. › Teach to never swim alone and to wear a life jacket in boats. › Wear protective helmets and knee and elbow pads, when needed. › Teach to avoid strangers and keep parents informed of strangers.
Burns	› Reduce setting on water heater to no higher than 120° F. › Teach dangers of playing with matches, fireworks, and firearms. › Teach school-age child how to properly use microwave and other cooking instruments.
Poison	› Teach child about the hazards of alcohol, cigarettes, and prescription, non-prescription, and illegal drugs. › Keep potentially dangerous substances out of reach.

ADOLESCENTS	
RISK	PREVENTION EDUCATION
Motor vehicle/ Injury	› Ensure the teen has completed a driver's education course. › Set rules on the number of people allowed to ride in cars, seat belt use, and to call for a ride home if a driver is impaired. › Reinforce teaching on proper use of protective equipment when participating in sports. › Be alert to signs of depression. › Teach about the hazards of firearms and safety precautions with firearms. › Teach water safety. › Teach to check water depth before diving. › Educate on the hazards of smoking, alcohol, legal and illegal drugs, and unprotected sex.
Burns	› Teach to use sunblock and protective clothing. › Teach the dangers of sunbathing and tanning beds.

- Safety Risks and Prevention Measures for Young and Middle-Age Adults

  ○ Motor vehicle crashes are the most common cause of death and injury to the adult. Occupational injuries contribute to the injury and death rate of the adult. High consumption of alcohol and suicide are also major concerns for adults.

  ○ Nurses can promote client safety for young and middle age adults by:

    ▪ Reminding clients to drive defensively and to not drive after drinking alcohol.

    ▪ Reinforcing teaching about the long-term effects related to high alcohol consumption.

    ▪ Ensuring home safety with smoke and carbon monoxide detectors, fire alarms, well-lit and uncluttered staircases.

    ▪ Being attuned to behaviors that suggest the presence of depression and/or thoughts of suicide and referring clients as appropriate and encouraging counseling.

    ▪ Teaching diving and water safety.

    ▪ Encouraging clients to become proactive about safety in the work place and in the home.

    ▪ Discussing dangers of social networking and the Internet.

    ▪ Ensuring that clients understand the hazards of excessive sun exposure and the need to protect the skin with the use of sun-blocking agents and protective clothing.

  ○ Safety Risks and Prevention Measures for Older Adults

    ▪ The rate at which age-related changes occur varies greatly among older adults.

    ▪ Many older adults are able to maintain a lifestyle that promotes independence and the ability to protect themselves from safety hazards.

    ▪ Risk factors for falls in older adults include:

      □ Physical, cognitive, and sensory changes.

      □ Changes in the musculoskeletal and neurological systems.

      □ Impaired vision and/or hearing.

      □ Frequent trips to the bathroom at night because of nocturia and incontinence.

    ▪ A decrease in tactile sensitivity may place the client at risk for burns and other types of tissue injury.

- When the client demonstrates factors that increases the risk for injury (regardless of age), a home hazard evaluation should be conducted by the nurse, a physical therapist, and/or occupational therapist. The client is made aware of the environmental factors that may pose a risk to safety and suggestion modifications to be made.

- Modifications that can be made to improve home safety include:

  □ Removing items that could cause the client to trip, such as throw rugs and loose carpets.

  □ Placing electrical cords and extension cords that against a wall behind furniture.

  □ Monitoring gait and balance, and providing aids as needed.

  □ Making sure that steps and sidewalks are in good repair.

  □ Placing grab bars near the toilet and in the tub or shower, and installing a stool riser.

  □ Using a nonskid mat in the tub or shower.

  □ Placing a shower chair in the shower and bedside commode if needed.

  □ Ensuring that lighting is adequate both inside and outside of the home.

Fire Safety in the Home

- Home fires continue to be a major cause of death and injury for people of all ages.

- Nurses should educate clients about the importance of a home safety plan.

- A home safety plan should include:

  ○ Keeping emergency numbers near the phone for prompt use in the event of an emergency of any type.

  ○ Ensuring that the number and placement of fire extinguishers and smoke alarms are adequate, that they are operable, and that family members understand how to operate. Set a specific time to routinely change the batteries in the smoke alarms (for example: in the fall when the clocks are set back to standard time and spring when reset at Daylight Saving Time).

  ○ Having a family exit plan for fires that is reviewed and practiced regularly. Be sure to include closing windows and doors if able and to exit a smoke-filled area by covering the mouth and nose with a damp cloth and getting down as close to the floor as possible.

  ○ Reviewing with clients of all ages that in the event that the client's clothing or skin is on fire, the mnemonic "stop, drop, and roll" should be used to extinguish the fire.

  ○ Reviewing oxygen safety measures. Because oxygen can cause materials to combust more easily and burn more rapidly, the client and family must be provided with information on use of the oxygen delivery equipment and the dangers of combustion. The following information should be included in the teaching plan:

    - Using and storing oxygen equipment according to the manufacturer's recommendations.

    - Placing a "No Smoking" sign in a conspicuous place near the front door of the home. A sign may also be placed on the door to the client's bedroom.

    - Informing the client and family of the danger of smoking in the presence of oxygen. Family members and visitors who smoke should do so outside the home.

    - Ensuring that electrical equipment is in good repair and well grounded.

- Replacing bedding that can generate static electricity (wool, nylon, synthetics) with items made from cotton.

- Keeping flammable materials, such as heating oil and nail polish remover, away from the client when oxygen is in use.

- Following general measures for fire safety in the home, such as having a fire extinguisher readily available and an established exit route if a fire occurs.

Additional Risks in the Home and Community

- Additional risks in the home and community include passive smoking, carbon monoxide poisoning, and food poisoning. Bioterrorism also has become a concern, making disaster plans a mandatory part of community safety.

- Nurses should teach clients about the dangers of these additional risks.

- Passive smoking

  - Passive smoking is the unintentional inhalation of tobacco smoke.

  - Exposure to nicotine and other toxins places people at risk for numerous diseases including cancer, heart disease, and lung infections.

  - Low-birth-weight infants, prematurity, stillbirths, and sudden infant death syndrome (SIDS) have been associated with maternal smoking.

  - Smoking in the presence of children is associated with the development of bronchitis, pneumonia, and middle ear infections.

  - For children with asthma, exposure to passive smoke can result in an increase in the frequency and the severity of asthma attacks.

  - The nurse should inform the client who smokes and his family about:

    - The hazards of smoking

    - Available resources to stop smoking (smoking cessation programs, medication support, self-help groups)

    - The effect that visiting individuals who smoke or riding in the automobile of a smoker has on a nonsmoker

- Carbon monoxide

  - Carbon monoxide is a very dangerous gas because it binds with hemoglobin and ultimately reduces the oxygen supplied to the tissues in the body.

  - Carbon monoxide cannot be seen, smelled, or tasted.

  - Symptoms of carbon monoxide poisoning include nausea, vomiting, headache, weakness, and unconsciousness.

  - Death may occur with prolonged exposure.

  - Measures to prevent carbon monoxide poisoning include ensuring proper ventilation when using fuel-burning devices (lawn mowers, wood-burning and gas fireplaces, charcoal grills).

  - Gas-burning furnaces, water heaters, and appliances should be inspected annually.

  - Flues and chimneys should be unobstructed.

  - Carbon monoxide detectors should be installed and inspected regularly.

- Food poisoning
  - Food poisoning is a major cause of illness in the United States.
  - Most food poisoning is caused by bacteria such as *Escherichia coli, Listeria monocytogenes,* and *Salmonella.*
  - Healthy individuals usually recover from the illness in a few days.
  - Very young, very old, and immunocompromised individuals, as well as pregnant women, are at risk for complications.
  - Clients who are especially at risk are instructed to follow a low-microbial diet.
  - Most food poisoning occurs because of unsanitary food practice.
  - Performing proper hand hygiene, ensuring that meat and fish are cooked to the correct temperature, handling raw and fresh food separately to avoid cross contamination, and refrigerating perishable items are measures that may prevent food poisoning.
  - Check expiration dates, and clean fresh fruit and vegetables.
- Bioterrorism
  - Bioterrorism is the dissemination of harmful toxins, bacteria, viruses, and pathogens for the purpose of causing illness or death.
  - Anthrax, variola, *Clostridium botulism*, and *Yersinia pestis* are examples of agents used by terrorists.
  - Nurses and other health professionals must be prepared to respond to an attack by being proficient in early detection, recognizing the causative agent, identifying the affected community, and providing early treatment to affected persons.

Primary Survey

- A primary survey is a rapid assessment of life-threatening conditions. It should take no longer than 60 seconds to perform.
- The primary survey should be completed systematically so conditions are not missed.
- Standard precautions (gloves, gowns, eye protection, face masks, and shoe covers) must be worn to prevent contamination with bodily fluids.
- The ABCDE principle guides the primary survey. Emergency care is guided by the principle of ABCDE.
  - Airway/Cervical Spine – This is the most important step in performing the primary survey. If a patent airway is not established, subsequent steps of the primary survey are futile.
  - Breathing – Once a patent airway is achieved, the presence and effectiveness of breathing should be assessed.
  - Circulation – Once adequate ventilation is accomplished, circulation is assessed.
  - Disability – A quick assessment should be performed to determine the client's level of consciousness.
  - Exposure – A quick physical assessment should be performed to determine the client's exposure to adverse elements such as heat or cold.
- See the chapter on *Emergency Nursing Principles and Management* in the *Adult Medical Surgical Nursing Review Module* for further detail on the primary survey.

Basic First-Aid

- Complete the primary survey before performing first aid.
- Bleeding – Identify any sources of external bleeding and apply direct pressure to the wound site.
  - DO NOT remove impaled objects.
    - Internal bleeding may require intravascular volume replacement with fluids and/or blood products or surgical intervention.
- Fractures and splinting
  - Assess the site for swelling, deformity, and skin integrity.
  - Assess temperature, distal pulses, and mobility.
  - Apply a splint to immobilize the fracture. Cover any open areas with a sterile cloth if available.
  - Reassess neurovascular status after splinting.
- Sprains
  - Refrain from weight-bearing.
  - Apply ice to decrease inflammation.
  - Apply a compression dressing to minimize swelling.
  - Elevate the affected limb.
- Heat stroke
  - Heat stroke must be identified quickly and treated aggressively.
  - Manifestations of a heat stroke include hot, dry skin, hypotension, tachypnea, tachycardia, anxiety, confusion, unusual behavior, seizures, and coma.
    - Rapid cooling must be achieved.
      - Remove the client's clothing.
      - Place ice packs over the major arteries (axillae, chest, groin, neck).
      - Immerse the client in a cold-water bath.
      - Wet the client's body, then fan with rapid movement of air.
- Frostnip and frostbite
  - Frostnip does not lead to tissue injury and may be treated by warming.
  - Frostbite presents as white, waxy areas on exposed skin, and tissue injury occurs.
  - Frostbite may be full- or partial-thickness.
  - Warm the affected area in a 38° to 41° C (100.4° to 105.8° F) water bath.
  - Provide pain medication.
  - Administer a tetanus vaccination.
- Burns
  - Burns may result from an electrical current, chemicals, radiation, and/or flames.
    - Remove the agent (electrical current, radiation source, chemical).
    - Smother any flames that are present. Perform a primary survey.
    - Cover the client and maintain NPO status.
    - Elevate the client's extremities if not contraindicated (presence of a fracture).
    - Perform a head-to-toe assessment and estimate the surface area and thickness of burns.
    - Administer fluids and a tetanus toxoid.

- Altitude-related illnesses
  - Clients may become hypoxic in high altitudes.
  - Clinical findings
    - Throbbing headache
    - Nausea
    - Vomiting
    - Dyspnea
    - Anorexia
  - Nursing interventions
    - Administer oxygen.
    - Descend to a lower altitude.
    - Provide pharmacological therapy, such as steroids and diuretics, if indicated.
  - Altitude sickness can progress to cerebral and pulmonary edema and should be treated immediately.

CPR

- CPR is a combination of basic interventions designed to sustain oxygen and circulation to vital organs until more advanced interventions can be initiated to correct the root cause of the cardiac arrest.
- Basic interventions can be delivered by trained individuals, but advanced interventions require more sophisticated training and certification and the use of emergency equipment.
- CPR is directed at artificially providing a client with circulation (chest compressions) and oxygenation (ventilations) in the absence of cardiac output.
- CPR is a component of basic life support (BLS).
- The goal of BLS is to provide oxygen to the vital organs until appropriate advanced resuscitation measures can be initiated or until resuscitative efforts are ordered to be stopped.
- BLS involves the CABs (Chest Compression, Airway, and Breathing) of CPR.
  - Assess victim for a response and look for breathing. Do not take time to perform a "look, listen, and feel" assessment of breathing. If there is no breathing or no normal breathing (only gasping), call for help.
  - If alone, activate emergency response system and get an AED or defibrillator, if available, and return to the victim. If a second person is available, send him or her to activate the emergency response system and get an AED or defibrillator.
  - Check pulse. If a pulse can't be felt, begin CPR compressions and breaths.
- For further detail on CPR, visit the American Heart Association website, www.heart.org.
- The role of the nurse in client education
  - Encourage family members to take basic first aid and CPR courses. Refer client and/or family members to a community agency where basic first aid and CPR are taught.
  - Ensure client and family members keep emergency numbers (poison control, fire/rescue, providers, and nearest hospitals and urgent care facilities) available in the home.

APPLICATION EXERCISES

1. A nurse is providing discharge instructions to a client who has a prescription for the use of oxygen in his home. Which of the following should the nurse teach the client about using oxygen safely in his home? (Select all that apply.)

_____ A. Family members who smoke must be at least 10 ft from the client when oxygen is in use.

_____ B. Nail polish should not be used near a client who is receiving oxygen.

_____ C. A "No Smoking" sign should be placed on the front door.

_____ D. Cotton bedding and clothing should be replaced with items made from wool.

_____ E. A fire extinguisher should be readily available in the home.

2. A nurse educator is conducting a parenting class for new parents. Which of the following statements made by a participant indicates a need for further clarification and instruction?

A. "I will begin swimming lessons as soon as my baby can close her mouth under water."

B. "Once my baby can sit up, he should be safe in the bathtub."

C. "I will test the temperature of the water before placing my baby in the bath."

D. "Once my infant starts to push up, I will remove the mobile from over the bed."

3. A home health nurse is discussing the dangers of carbon monoxide poisoning with a client. Which of the following information should the nurse include in her counseling?

A. Carbon monoxide has a distinct odor.

B. Water heaters should be inspected every 5 years.

C. The lungs are damaged from carbon monoxide inhalation.

D. Carbon monoxide binds with hemoglobin in the body.

4. A nurse educator is presenting a module on basic first aid for newly licensed home health nurses. The nurse educator evaluates the teaching as effective when the newly licensed nurse states the client who has heat stroke will have which of the following?

A. Hypotension

B. Bradycardia

C. Clammy skin

D. Bradypnea

5. A home health nurse is discussing the dangers of food poisoning with a client. Which of the following information should the nurse including in her counseling? (Select all that apply.)

_____ A. Most food poisoning is caused by a virus.

_____ B. Immunocompromised individuals are at risk for complications from food poisoning

_____ C. Clients who are especially at risk are instructed to eat or drink only pasteurized milk, yogurt, cheese, or other dairy products.

_____ D. Healthy individuals usually recover from the illness in a few weeks.

_____ E. Handling raw and fresh food separately to avoid cross contamination may prevent food poisoning.

6. A nurse educator is teaching a module on the basic principles of creating a home safety plan during nursing orientation to a group of newly appointed home health nurses. Use the ATI Active Learning Template: Basic Concept to complete this item. Under Nursing Interventions, list four key elements that a home safety plan should include.

APPLICATION EXERCISES KEY

1. A. INCORRECT: Family members who smoke should do so outside.

    B. **CORRECT:** Nail polish and other flammable materials may cause a fire and should not be used.

    C. **CORRECT:** A "No Smoking" sign should be placed near the front door. A sign also may be placed on the client's bedroom door.

    D. INCORRECT: Woolen and synthetic materials create static electricity; cotton materials do not and should be used instead.

    E. **CORRECT:** A readily available fire extinguisher should be placed in all homes, including the home of a client who is receiving oxygen.

    (N) NCLEX® Connection: Safety and Infection Control, Safe Use of Equipment

2. A. INCORRECT: It is recommended to begin swimming lessons when the infant's developmental status allows for protective responses such as closing her mouth under water.

    B. **CORRECT:** Although the baby can hold his head above the water by sitting up, this does not make the child safe in the bathtub. Parents should never leave an infant or toddler alone in the bathtub.

    C. INCORRECT: It is recommended to test the temperature of bath water prior to placing an infant in the bath.

    D. INCORRECT: It is recommended to remove crib toys, such as mobiles, from over the bed as soon as the infant begins to push up.

    (N) NCLEX® Connection: Safety and Infection Control, Home Safety

3. A. INCORRECT: Carbon monoxide cannot be seen, smelled, or tasted.

    B. INCORRECT: Gas-burning furnaces, water heaters, and appliances should be inspected annually.

    C. INCORRECT: Although carbon monoxide reduces the amount of oxygen supplied to the body, the lungs are not damaged.

    D. **CORRECT:** Carbon monoxide is a very dangerous gas because it binds with hemoglobin and ultimately reduces the oxygen supplied to the tissues in the body.

    (N) NCLEX® Connection: Safety and Infection Control, Home Safety

FUNDAMENTALS FOR NURSING

4. A. **CORRECT:** A clinical manifestation of heat stroke is hypotension.

    B. INCORRECT: A clinical manifestation of heat stroke is tachycardia, not bradycardia.

    C. INCORRECT: A clinical manifestation of heat stroke is hot, dry skin, not clammy skin.

    D. INCORRECT: A clinical manifestation of heat stroke is tachypnea, not bradypnea.

    Ⓝ NCLEX® Connection: Physiological Adaptations, Pathophysiology

5. A. INCORRECT: Most food poisoning is caused by bacteria such as *Escherichia coli*, *Listeria monocytogenes*, and *Salmonella*.

    B. **CORRECT:** Very young, very old, and immunocompromised individuals, as well as pregnant women, are at risk for complications from food poisoning.

    C. **CORRECT:** Clients who are especially at risk are instructed to follow a low-microbial diet, which includes eating or drinking only pasteurized milk, yogurt, cheese, or other dairy products.

    D. INCORRECT: Healthy individuals usually recover from the illness in a few days.

    E. **CORRECT:** Performing proper hand hygiene, ensuring that meat and fish are cooked to the correct temperature, handling raw and fresh food separately to avoid cross contamination, and refrigerating perishable items may prevent food poisoning.

    Ⓝ NCLEX® Connection: Physiological Adaptations, Pathophysiology

6. *Using the ATI Active Learning Template: Basic Concept*
    - Nursing Interventions
      - A home safety plan should include:
        - Keeping emergency numbers near the phone for prompt use in the event of an emergency of any type.
        - Ensuring that the number and placement of fire extinguishers and smoke alarms are adequate, that they are operable, and that family members know how to operate. Set a specific time to routinely change the batteries in the smoke alarms (for example, in the fall when the clocks are set back to standard time and spring when reset at Daylight Saving Time).
        - Having a family exit plan for fires that the family reviews and practices regularly. Be sure to include closing windows and doors if able and to exit a smoke filled area by covering the mouth and nose with a damp cloth and getting down as close to the floor as possible.
        - Reviewing with clients of all ages that in the event that the client's clothing or skin is on fire, the client should use the mnemonic "stop, drop, and roll" to extinguish the fire.
        - Reviewing oxygen safety measures. Because oxygen can cause materials to combust more easily and burn more rapidly, the client and family must be provided with information on use of the oxygen delivery equipment and the dangers of combustion.

    Ⓝ NCLEX® Connection: Safety and Infection Control, Home Safety

chapter **14**

Overview

- Ergonomics are the factors or qualities in an object's design and/or use that contribute to comfort, safety, efficiency, and ease of use.

- Using good body mechanics when positioning and moving clients promotes safety for the client as well as for health care providers.

- Before attempting to position or move a client, the nurse should perform a mobility assessment. Begin this assessment with the easiest movements (range of motion) and progress as long as the client tolerates it (balance, gait, and exercise).

Ergonomic Principles and Body Mechanics

- Body mechanics is the proper use of muscles to maintain balance, posture, and body alignment when performing a physical task. Nurses use body mechanics when providing care to clients by lifting, bending, and carrying out the activities of daily living.

- The risk of injury to the client and the nurse is reduced with the use of good body mechanics. Whenever possible, mechanical lift devices should be used to lift and transfer clients. Many health care agencies have "no manual lift" and "no solo lift" policies.

- Center of gravity

 View Video: Ergonomic Principles

- The center of gravity is the center of a mass.

- Weight is a quantity of matter acted on by the force of gravity.

- To lift an object, the nurse must overcome the weight of the object and know the center of gravity of the object.

- When the human body is in the upright position, the center of gravity is the pelvis.

- When an individual moves, the center of gravity shifts.

- The closer the line of gravity is to the center of the base of support, the more stable the individual is.

- To lower the center of gravity, bend the hips and knees.

- Greater stability and balance occurs by lowering the center of gravity and broadening the base of support.

- To broaden the base of support, spread the feet apart.

- Lifting
  - Use the major muscle groups to prevent back strain, and tighten the abdominal muscles to increase support to the back muscles.
  - Distribute the weight between the large muscles of the arms and legs to decrease the strain on any one muscle group and avoid strain on smaller muscles.
  - When lifting an object from the floor, flex the hips, knees, and back. Get the object to thigh level, keeping the knees bent and the back straightened. Stand up while holding the object as close as possible to the body, bringing the load to the center of gravity to increase stability and decrease back strain.
  - Use assistive devices whenever possible, and seek assistance whenever it is needed.
- When pushing or pulling a load:
  - Widen the base of support.
  - When opportunity allows, pull objects toward the center of gravity rather than pushing away.
  - If pushing, move the front foot forward, and if pulling, move the rear leg back to promote stability.
  - Face the direction of movement when moving a client.
  - Use own body as a counterweight when pushing or pulling to make the movement easier.
  - Sliding, rolling, and pushing require less energy than lifting and offer less risk for injury.
  - Avoid twisting the thoracic spine and bending the back while the hips and knees are straight.
- Guidelines to Prevent Injury
  - Know your agency's policies regarding lifting and safe patient handling.
  - It is preferred that two or more personnel assist with any positioning.
  - Plan ahead for activities that require lifting, transfer, or ambulation of a client, and ask others to be ready to assist at the planned time.
  - Prepare environment to remove obstacles prior to procedure.
  - Explain process to client and assistants to clarify roles.
  - Be aware that the safest way to lift a client may be with the use of assistive equipment.
  - Rest between heavy activities to decrease muscle fatigue.
  - Maintain good posture and exercise regularly to increase the strength of arm, leg, back, and abdominal muscles, so these activities will require less energy.
  - Use smooth movements when lifting and moving clients to prevent injury through sudden or jerky muscle movements.
  - When standing for long periods of time, flex the hip and knee through use of a foot rest. When sitting for long periods of time, keep the knees slightly higher than the hips.
  - Avoid repetitive movements of the hands, wrists, and shoulders. Take a break every 15 to 20 min to flex and stretch joints and muscles.
  - Maintain good posture (head and neck in straight line with pelvis) to avoid neck flexion and hunched shoulders, which can cause impingement of nerves in the neck.
  - Avoid twisting the spine or bending at the waist (flexion) to minimize the risk for injury.

Client Positioning

- The nurse is responsible for positioning clients so that good body alignment is maintained. Many clients are able to reposition themselves when they are uncomfortable. It is especially important for the nurse to ensure proper positioning of clients who are unable to move themselves due to disability or injury. Frequent position changes prevent discomfort, contractures, pressure on tissue, nerve and circulatory damage, and stimulate postural reflexes and muscle tone.

- Pillows, bath blankets, hand rolls, boots, splints, trochanter rolls, ankle support devices, and other aids are used to maintain proper body alignment for the client.

- Transfers and Use of Assistive Devices

  ○ Assess each situation and use an algorithm to determine the safest method of transfer or client movement. Questions included in the algorithm should include: Can the client bear weight? Can the client assist? Is the client cooperative?

  ○ Assess the client's ability to help with transfers (balance, muscle strength, endurance).

  ○ Determine the need for additional personnel or assistive devices (transfer belt, hydraulic lift, sliding board).

  ○ Assess and monitor the client's proper use of mobility aids (canes, walkers, crutches).

  ○ Include assistance or mobility aids needed for safe transfers and ambulation in the plan of care.

Bed and Client Positions

POSITION	DESCRIPTION
Semi-Fowler's position	› The client lies supine with the head of the bed elevated approximately 30°, and his knees may be slightly elevated (about 15°). › This position is frequently used to prevent regurgitation of enteral feedings and aspiration in clients who have difficulty swallowing.
Fowler's position	› The client lies supine with the head of the bed slightly elevated approximately 45°, and his knees may be slightly elevated (about 15°). › This position is frequently used during procedures such as nasogastric tube insertion and suctioning. It allows for better chest expansion and ventilation, as well as better dependent drainage, after abdominal surgeries.
High-Fowler's position	› The client lies supine with the head of the bed elevated approximately 90°, and his knees may or may not be elevated. › This position promotes lung expansion by lowering the diaphragm and is used for clients experiencing severe dyspnea.
Supine or dorsal recumbent position	› The client lies on his back with his head and shoulders elevated on a pillow. The client's forearms may be placed on pillows or placed at the side. A foot support prevents footdrop and maintains proper alignment.
Prone position	› The client lies flat on his abdomen with his head to one side. › This position promotes drainage from the mouth for clients following throat or oral surgery, but inhibits chest expansion.

POSITION	DESCRIPTION
Lateral or side-lying position	› The client lies on his side with most of his weight on the dependent hip and shoulder. His arms should be flexed in front of the body. A pillow is placed under his head and neck, the upper arm, and under the leg and thigh to maintain body alignment.
	› This is a good sleeping position, but the client must be turned regularly to prevent development of pressure ulcers on the dependent areas. A 30° lateral position is recommended for clients at risk for pressure ulcers.
Sims' or semi-prone position	› The client is on his side halfway between lateral and prone positions. (Weight is on the anterior ileum, humerus, and clavicle.) The lower arm is behind the client while the upper arm is in front. Both legs are flexed, but the upper leg is flexed at a greater angle than the lower leg at the hip as well as at the knee.
	› This is a comfortable sleeping position for many clients, and it promotes oral drainage.
Orthopneic position	› The client sits in the bed or at the bedside. A pillow is placed on the over-bed table, which is placed across the client's lap. The client rests his arms on the over-bed table.
	› This position allows for chest expansion and is especially beneficial to clients who have COPD.
Trendelenburg position	› The entire bed is tilted with the head of the bed lower than the foot of the bed.
	› This position is used during postural drainage, and it facilitates venous return.
Reverse Trendelenburg	› The entire bed is tilted with the foot of the bed lower than the head of the bed.
	› This position promotes gastric emptying and prevents esophageal reflux.
Modified Trendelenburg	› Client remains flat with legs elevated above the level of the heart.
	› This position is used to prevent and treat hypovolemia and facilitates venous return.

APPLICATION EXERCISES

1. A nurse is caring for a client receiving enteral tube feedings due to dysphagia. Which of the following bed positions is appropriate for safe care of this client?

    A. Supine

    B. Semi-Fowler's

    C. Semi-prone

    D. Trendelenburg

2. A nurse is caring for a client who is sitting in a chair and asks to return to bed. Which of the following is the priority action for the nurse to take at this time?

    A. Obtain a walker for the client to use to transfer back to bed.

    B. Call for additional personnel to assist with the transfer.

    C. Use a transfer belt and assist the client to bed.

    D. Assess the client's ability to help with the transfer.

3. A nurse is completing discharge teaching to a client who has COPD. The client verbalizes understanding of the orthopneic position when he states, "When I have difficulty breathing at night, I will

    A. lie on my back with my head and shoulders elevated on a pillow."

    B. lie flat on my stomach with my head to one side."

    C. sit on the side of my bed and rest my arms over pillows on top of my raised bedside table."

    D. lie on my side with my weight on my hips and shoulder with my arms flexed in front of me."

4. A nurse manager is reviewing guidelines to prevent injury with staff nurses. Which of the following should the nurse manager include in the teaching? (Select all that apply.)

    _____ A. Request assistance when repositioning a client.

    _____ B. Avoid twisting the spine or bending at the waist.

    _____ C. Keep the knees slightly lower than the hips when sitting for long periods of time.

    _____ D. Use smooth movements when lifting and moving clients.

    _____ E. Take a break from repetitive movements every 2 to 3 hr to flex and stretch joints and muscles.

5. A nurse educator is teaching a module on proper body mechanics during employee orientation. Which of the following statements by a newly hired nurse indicates the need for further teaching?

    A. "My line of gravity should fall outside my base of support."

    B. "The lower my center of gravity, the more stability I have."

    C. "To broaden my base of support, I should spread my feet apart."

    D. "When I lift an object, I should hold it as close to my body as possible."

6. A nurse educator is teaching basic principles of proper lifting techniques to a group of newly hired nurses. Use the ATI Active Learning Template: Basic Concept to complete this item. Under the section Underlying Principles, list four key elements of proper lifting techniques.

APPLICATION EXERCISES KEY

1.   A. INCORRECT: In the supine position, the client lies on his back with his head and shoulders elevated on a pillow. This angle is not adequate to prevent regurgitation.

   B. **CORRECT:** In the semi-Fowler's position, the client lies supine with the head of the bed elevated approximately 30°. This position is frequently used to prevent regurgitation and aspiration in clients who have difficulty swallowing. This is the safest position for the client receiving a tube feeding.

   C. INCORRECT: In the semi-prone or Sims' position, the client is on his side halfway between lateral and prone positions. This position is not safe because it may promote regurgitation.

   D. INCORRECT: In the Trendelenburg position, the entire bed is tilted with the head of the bed lower than the foot of the bed. This position is not safe because it may promote regurgitation.

   Ⓝ NCLEX® Connection: Reduction of Risk Potential, Potential for Complications of Diagnostic Tests/ Treatments/Procedures

2.   A. INCORRECT: Although this might be a necessary assistive device for this client, it is not the priority action the nurse should take.

   B. INCORRECT: Although this might be necessary for a safe transfer, it is the not the priority action the nurse should take.

   C. INCORRECT: Although this might be a necessary assistive device for the transfer of this client, it is not the priority action the nurse should take.

   D. **CORRECT:** The first action the nurse should take using the nursing process is to assess/collect data from the client. The nurse should assess the client's ability to help with transfers (balance, muscle strength, endurance). Then the nurse can proceed with a safe transfer of the client.

   Ⓝ NCLEX® Connection: Safety and Infection Control, Ergonomic Principles

3.   A. INCORRECT: The client is describing the supine position, not the orthopneic position.

   B. INCORRECT: The client is describing the prone position, not the orthopneic position.

   C. **CORRECT:** The client is describing the orthopneic position. This position allows for chest expansion and is especially beneficial to clients who have COPD.

   D. INCORRECT: The client is describing the lateral or side-lying position, not the orthopneic position.

   Ⓝ NCLEX® Connection: Safety and Infection Control, Ergonomic Principles

4.   A. **CORRECT:** It is preferred that two or more personnel assist with any positioning in order to reduce the risk of injury.

    B. **CORRECT:** Twisting the spine or bending at the waist (flexion) increases the nurse's risk for injury.

    C. INCORRECT: When sitting for long periods of time, the nurse should keep knees slightly higher than, not lower than, the hips in order to decrease strain on the lower back

    D. **CORRECT:** Using smooth movements instead of sudden or jerky muscle movements is recommended to prevent injury

    E. INCORRECT: The nurse should take a break every 15 to 20 min, not every 2 to 3 hr, from repetitive movements to flex and stretch joints and muscles.

 NCLEX® Connection: Safety and Infection Control, Ergonomic Principles

5.   A. **CORRECT:** The line of gravity should fall within the base of support, not outside, which increases the risk of falling.

    B. INCORRECT: Being closer to the ground causes a lower center of gravity, which leads to greater stability and balance.

    C. INCORRECT: Spreading the feet apart increases and widens the base of support.

    D. INCORRECT: Holding an object as close to the body as possible helps avoid displacement of the center of gravity, which can prevent injury and instability.

 NCLEX® Connection: Safety and Infection Control, Ergonomic Principles

6.   *Using the ATI Active Learning Template: Basic Concept*

- Underlying Principles
  - Use the major muscle groups to prevent back strain, and tighten the abdominal muscles to increase support to the back muscles.
  - Distribute the weight between the large muscles of the arms and legs to decrease the strain on any one muscle group and avoid strain on smaller muscles.
  - When lifting an object from the floor, flex the hips, knees, and back. Get the object to thigh level, keeping the knees bent and the back straightened. Stand up while holding the object as close as possible to the body, bringing the load to the center of gravity to increase stability and decrease back strain.
  - Use assistive devices whenever possible, and seek assistance whenever it is needed.

 NCLEX® Connection: Safety and Infection Control, Ergonomic Principles

chapter 15

Overview

- A disaster is a mass casualty or intra-facility event that overwhelms or interrupts, at least temporarily, the normal flow of services of a hospital.
- Disasters that health care facilities face include internal and external emergencies.
  - Internal emergencies include loss of electric power or potable water and severe damage or casualties within the facility related to fire, weather (tornado, hurricane), an explosion, or a terrorist act. Internal emergency readiness includes safety and hazardous materials protocols, and infection control policies and practices.
  - External emergencies include hurricanes, floods, volcano eruptions, earthquakes, pandemic flu, industrial accidents, chemical plant explosions, major transportation accidents, building collapse, and terrorist acts (including biological and chemical warfare). External emergency readiness includes a plan for participation in community-wide emergencies and disasters.

The Joint Commission and Emergency Preparedness

- The Joint Commission established emergency preparedness management standards for various types of health care facilities. These standards mandate that an institutional emergency preparedness plan is developed by all health care institutions and that these plans include institution-specific procedures for:
  - Notifying and assigning personnel.
  - Notifying external authorities of emergencies.
  - Managing space and supplies and providing security.
  - Isolating and decontaminating radioactive or chemical agents (measures to contain contamination, decontamination at the scene of exposure).
  - Evacuating and setting up an alternative care site when the environment cannot support adequate client care and treatment. Critical processes when an alternative care site is necessary include:
    - Client information/care packaging (medications, supplies, admissions, medical records, and tracking).
    - Interfacility communication.
    - Transportation of clients, staff, and equipment.
    - Cross-privileging of medical staff.
  - Performing triage of incoming clients.
  - Managing clients during emergencies, including scheduling, modification or discontinuation of services, control of client information, and client discharge and transportation.
  - Interacting with family members and the media and responding to public reaction.
  - Identifying backup resources (electricity, water, fire protection, fuel sources, medical gas and vacuum) for utilities and communication.

○ Orienting and educating personnel participating in implementation of the emergency preparedness plan.

○ Providing crisis support for health care workers (access to vaccines, infection control recommendations, mental health counseling).

○ Providing performance monitoring and evaluation related to emergency preparedness.

○ Conducting two emergency preparedness drills each year.

  ▪ Drills should include an influx of clients beyond those being treated by the facility.

  ▪ Drills should include either an internal or an external disaster (a situation beyond the normal capacity of the facility).

○ Participating in one community-wide practice drill per year.

Nursing Role in Disaster Planning and Emergency Response Plans

- Emergency Response Plans

  ○ Each health care institution must have an emergency preparedness plan that has been developed by a planning committee. This committee reviews information regarding the potential for various types of natural and man-made emergencies depending on the characteristics of the community. Resources necessary to meet the potential emergency are determined and a plan developed that takes into consideration all of the above factors.

  ○ Nurses, as well as a cross-section of other members of the health care team, are involved in the development of a disaster plan for such emergencies. Criteria under which the disaster plan is activated must be clear. Roles for each employee are outlined and administrative control determined. A designated area for the area command center is identified as well as a person to serve as the incident control manager.

  ○ Communication, using common terminology, is important within any emergency management plan.

  ○ Nurses are expected to set up an emergency action plan for personal family needs.

- Triage

  ○ Principles of triage are followed in health care facilities involved in a mass casualty event.

  ○ These differ from the principles of triage that are typically followed during provision of day-to-day services in an emergency or urgent care setting. During mass casualty events, casualties are separated in relation to their potential for survival, and treatment is allocated accordingly.

  ○ Categories of Triage During Mass Casualty Events

    ▪ Emergent Category (Class I) – Highest priority is given to clients who have life-threatening injuries but also have a high possibility of survival once they are stabilized.

    ▪ Urgent Category (Class II) – Second-highest priority is given to clients who have major injuries that are not yet life-threatening and can usually wait 45 to 60 min for treatment.

    ▪ Nonurgent Category (Class III) – The next highest priority is given to clients who have minor injuries that are not life-threatening and do not need immediate attention.

    ▪ Expectant Category (Class IV) – The lowest priority is given to clients who are not expected to live and are allowed to die naturally. Comfort measures may be provided, but restorative care is not.

- Discharge/Relocation of Clients
  - During an emergency such as a fire or a mass casualty event, decisions are made regarding discharging clients or relocating them so their beds can be given to clients who have higher-priority needs.
  - Criteria are followed when identifying clients who can be safely discharged.
    - Ambulatory clients requiring minimal care are discharged or relocated first.
    - Clients requiring assistance are next and arrangements are made for continuation of their care.
    - Clients who are unstable and/or require nursing care are not discharged or relocated unless they are in imminent danger.
- Fire
  - If evacuation of the unit is necessary, horizontal evacuation is done first. Lateral evacuation is done if client safety cannot be maintained.
  - If a nurse discovers a fire that threatens the safety of a client, the nurse uses the RACE (Rescue, Alarm, Contain, and Extinguish) mnemonic to guide the order of actions.

RACE MNEMONIC	
R – Rescue	› **Rescue** the client and other individuals from the area.
A – Alarm	› Sound the fire **alarm**, which activates the EMS response system. › Systems that could increase fire spread are automatically shut down with activation of the alarm.
C – Contain	› Once the room or area has been cleared, the door leading to the area in which the fire is located as well as the fire doors are kept closed in order to **contain** the fire. › Fire doors are kept closed as much as possible when moving from area to area within the facility to avoid the spread of smoke and fire.
E – Extinguish	› Make an attempt to **extinguish** small fires using a single fire extinguisher, smothering them with a blanket, or dousing with water (except with an electrical or grease fire). › Complete evacuation of the area occurs if the nurse cannot put the fire out with these methods. › Attempts at extinguishing the fire are only made when the employee is properly trained in the safe use of a fire extinguisher and when only one extinguisher is needed.

- Severe Thunderstorm/Tornado
  - Draw shades and close drapes to protect against shattering glass.
  - Lower beds to the lowest position and move away from the windows.
  - Place blankets over all clients who are confined to beds.
  - Close all doors.
  - Relocate as many ambulatory clients as possible into the hallways (away from windows).
  - Do not use elevators.
  - Monitor for severe weather warnings using television, radio, or Internet.

- Biological Pathogens
  - Be alert to indications of a possible bioterrorism attack, as early detection and management is key.
  - Use appropriate isolation measures, as indicated.
  - In most instances, infection from biological agents is not spread from one client to another. However, vigilance is of the utmost importance. Management of the incident includes recognition of the occurrence (often the clinical manifestations are similar to other illnesses), directing personnel in the proper use of personal protective equipment, and, in some situations, decontamination and isolation.
  - Transport or move clients only if needed for treatment and care.
  - Take measures to protect self and others.
  - Recognize indications of infection/poisoning and appropriate treatment.

BIOLOGICAL PATHOGENS

INHALATIONAL ANTHRAX

Clinical Manifestations	› Small lesion that becomes a blister, then an ulcer with a black area in the center	› Sore throat › Fever › Cough › Shortness of breath	› Muscle aches › Severe dyspnea › Meningitis › Shock
Treatment/ Prevention	› Oral ciprofloxacin (Cipro) › IV ciprofloxacin › In addition to IV ciprofloxacin, one or two additional antibiotics such as vancomycin, penicillin		

CUTANEOUS ANTHRAX

Clinical Manifestations	› Starts as a lesion that may be itchy › Develops into a vesicular lesion that later becomes necrotic with the formation of black eschar › Fever, chills
Treatment/ Prevention	› Oral ciprofloxacin (Cipro) › Doxycycline (Doryx)

BOTULISM

Clinical Manifestations	› Difficulty swallowing › Double vision	› Slurred speech › Descending progressive weakness	› Nausea, vomiting, abdominal cramps › Difficulty breathing
Treatment/ Prevention	› Airway management	› Antitoxin	› Elimination of toxin

VIRAL HEMORRHAGIC FEVERS (E.G., EBOLA, YELLOW FEVER)

Clinical Manifestations	› Sore throat › Headache	› Elevated temperature › Nausea, vomiting, diarrhea	› Internal and external bleeding › Shock
Treatment/ Prevention	› Treatment: no cure › Supportive care: minimize invasive procedures › Prevention: vaccine		

BIOLOGICAL PATHOGENS	
PLAGUE	
Clinical Manifestations	› These forms may occur separately or in combination: » Pneumonic plague infects the lungs. The first signs of illness are fever, headache, weakness, and rapidly developing pneumonia with shortness of breath, chest pain, cough, and sometimes bloody or watery sputum. The pneumonia progresses for 2 to 4 days and can cause respiratory failure and shock. » Bubonic plague – swollen, tender lymph glands, fever, headache, chills, and weakness. » Septicemic plague occurs when plague bacteria multiply in the blood. Manifestations include fever, chills, prostration, abdominal pain, shock, and bleeding into skin and other organs.
Treatment/ Prevention	› Treatment: Early treatment of pneumonic plague is essential. To reduce the chance of death, antibiotics must be given within 24 hr of first manifestations. Streptomycin, gentamicin, the tetracyclines, and chloramphenicol are all effective against pneumonic plague.
SMALLPOX	
Clinical Manifestations	› High fever › Rash › Vomiting › Fatigue › Chills › Delirium › Severe headache
Treatment/ Prevention	› Treatment: no cure › Supportive care: prevent dehydration, provide skin care, medications for pain and fever › Prevention: vaccine
TULAREMIA	
Clinical Manifestations	› Sudden fever › Muscle aches › Progressive weakness › Chills › Joint pain › If airborne, life-threatening pneumonia and systemic infection › Headache › Dry cough › Diarrhea
Treatment/ Prevention	› Treatment: streptomycin IV or gentamicin IV or IM are the medications of choice; in mass causality, use doxycycline or ciprofloxacin › Prevention: vaccine under review by the Food and Drug Administration

- Chemical Incidents
  - Chemical incidents may occur as result of an accident or due to a purposeful action such as terrorism.
  - Take measures to protect self and to avoid contact.
  - Assess and intervene to maintain the client's airway, breathing, and circulation. Administer first aid as needed.
  - Remove the offending chemical by undressing the client, removing all identifiable particulate matter. Provide immediate and prolonged irrigations of contaminated areas. The client's skin is irrigated with running water with the exception of dry chemicals, such as lye or white phosphorus. In the case of exposure to a dry chemical, brush the agent off of the client's clothing and skin.

- Gather a specific history of the injury, if possible (name and concentration of the chemical, duration of exposure).

- In the event of chemical attack, have knowledge of which facilities are open to exposed clients and which are only open to unexposed clients.

- Follow the facility's emergency response plans (personal protection measures, the handling and disposal of wastes, use of space and equipment, reporting procedures).

- Hazardous Material Incidents

  - Take measures to protect self and to avoid contact.

  - Approach the scene with caution.

  - Identify the hazardous material with available resources (emergency response guidebook, poison control centers). Know the location of the material safety data sheets (MSDS) manual.

  - Try to contain the material in one place prior to the arrival of the hazardous materials team.

  - If individuals are contaminated, decontaminate them as much as possible at the scene or as close as possible to the scene.

    - With few exceptions, water is the universal antidote. For biological hazardous materials, wash skin with copious amounts of water and antibacterial soap.

    - Don gloves, gown, mask, and shoe covers to protect self from contamination.

    - Carefully and slowly remove contaminated clothing so that deposited material does not become airborne

    - Place all contaminated material into large plastic bags and seal them.

- Radiological Incidents

  - The amount of exposure is related to the duration of the exposure, distance from source, and amount of shielding.

  - The facility where victims are treated activates interventions to prevent contamination of treatment areas (floors and furniture are covered, air vents and ducts are covered, radiation-contaminated waste is disposed of according to procedural guidelines).

  - Staff wear water-resistant gowns, double glove, and fully cover their bodies with caps, shoe covers, masks, and goggles.

  - Staff wear radiation or dosimetry badges to monitor the amount of their radiation exposure.

  - Clients initially are surveyed with a radiation meter to determine the amount of contamination.

  - Decontamination with soap, water, and disposable towels occurs prior to entering the facility. Water runoff is contaminated and contained.

  - After decontamination, clients are resurveyed for residual contamination and irrigation of the skin is continued until the client is clean of all contamination.

- Bomb Threat

  - When a phone call is received

    - Extend the conversation as long as possible.

    - Listen for distinguishing background noises (music, voices, traffic, airplanes).

    - Note distinguishing voice characteristics of the caller.

    - Ask where and when the bomb is set to explode.

- Note whether the caller is familiar with the physical arrangement of the facility.

- If a bomblike device is located, do not touch it. Clear the area, and isolate the device as much as possible by closing doors, for example.

- Notify the appropriate authorities and personnel (police, administrator, director of nursing).

- Cooperate with police and others – Assist to conduct a search as needed, provide copies of floor plans, have master keys available, and watch for and isolate suspicious objects such as packages and boxes.

- Keep elevators available for authorities.

- Remain calm and alert and try not to alarm clients.

SECURITY PLAN

Overview

- All health care facilities have security plans in place that include preventive, protective, and response measures designed for identified security needs.

- Security issues faced by health care facilities include: admission of potentially dangerous individuals, vandalism, infant abduction, and information theft.

- The International Association for Healthcare Security & Safety (IAHSS) provides recommendations for the development of security plans.

Nursing Role in Security Plan

- Nurses should be aware that security measures include:
  - An identification system that identifies employees, volunteers, physicians, students, and regularly scheduled contract services staff as authorized personnel of the health care facility.
  - Electronic security systems in high-risk areas (maternal newborn to prevent infant abductions, the emergency department to prevent unauthorized entrance). Examples include:
    - Key code access into and out of areas such as the maternal newborn unit.
    - Wristbands that electronically link parents and their infants.
    - Alarms integrated with closed-circuit television cameras.
- Nurses should prepare to take immediate action when breaches in security occur. Time is of the essence in preventing or stopping a breach in security.

APPLICATION EXERCISES

1. A nurse is caring for multiple clients during a mass casualty event. Which of the following clients is the highest priority?

    A. A client who received crush injuries to the chest and abdomen and is expected to die

    B. A client who has a 4-inch laceration to the head

    C. A client who has partial-thickness and full-thickness burns to his face, neck, and chest

    D. A client who has a fractured fibula and tibia

2. A nurse on a medical-surgical unit is informed that a mass casualty event occurred in the community and that it is necessary to discharge clients to make beds available for injury victims. Which of the following clients can be safely discharged? (Select all that apply.)

    _____ A. A client who is dehydrated and receiving IV fluid and electrolytes

    _____ B. A client who has a nasogastric tube to treat a small bowel obstruction

    _____ C. A client who is scheduled for a transurethral resection of the prostate (TURP)

    _____ D. A client who is 24 hr postoperative following a mastectomy

    _____ E. A client who is scheduled for an appendectomy

3. A nurse educator is discussing the facility protocol in the event of a tornado with the staff. Which of the following should the nurse include in the instructions? (Select all that apply.)

    _____ A. Open doors to client rooms.

    _____ B. Place blankets over clients who are confined to beds.

    _____ C. Move beds away from the windows.

    _____ D. Draw shades and close drapes.

    _____ E. Relocate ambulatory clients in the hallways back into their rooms.

4. An occupational health nurse is caring for an employee who was exposed to an unknown dry chemical, resulting in a chemical burn. Which of the following interventions should the nurse include in the plan of care?

    A. Irrigate the affected area with running water.

    B. Wash the affected area with antibacterial soap.

    C. Brush the chemical off the skin and clothing.

    D. Apply a neutralizing agent.

5. A security officer is reviewing actions to take in the event of a bomb threat by phone to a group of nurses. Which of the following statements by a nurse indicates understanding of proper procedure?

    A. "I will get the caller off the phone as soon as possible so I can alert the staff."

    B. "I will use overhead paging to alert the entire facility."

    C. "I will not ask any questions and just let the caller talk."

    D. "I will listen for background noises."

6. A nurse educator is teaching a module on biological pathogens during orientation to a group of newly hired nurses. What information should the nurse educator include? Use the ATI Active Learning Template: Basic Concept to complete this item to include Related Content: List four clinical manifestations and the recommended treatment for anthrax, botulism, pneumonic plague, and tularemia.

APPLICATION EXERCISES KEY

1. A. INCORRECT: The nurse should give the lowest priority to a client who is not expected to live. The nurse should provide comfort measures for this client (Expectant Category – Class IV).

   B. INCORRECT: The nurse should give third priority to the client who has minor injury that is not life-threatening, such as a laceration to the head (Nonurgent Category – Class III).

   C. **CORRECT:** The nurse should give first priority to the client who has the greatest chance of survival with prompt intervention. If not treated immediately, a client who has burns to his face, neck, and chest is at risk for airway obstruction, but is still expected to live. Therefore, this client is the highest priority (Emergent Category – Class I).

   D. INCORRECT: The nurse should give second priority to the client who has major fractures (Urgent Category – Class II).

   Ⓝ NCLEX® Connection: Management of Care, Establishing Priorities

2. A. INCORRECT: A client who is dehydrated and receiving IV fluid and electrolytes is unstable for discharge.

   B. INCORRECT: A small bowel obstruction that is not treated could result in the death of the client.

   C. **CORRECT:** A client who is scheduled for a TURP could be safely discharged because a TURP is not an emergent surgery.

   D. **CORRECT:** A client who 24 hr postoperative following a mastectomy is stable and could be safely discharged.

   E. INCORRECT: A client who has appendicitis needs immediate surgery to prevent rupture of the appendix and subsequent peritonitis.

   Ⓝ NCLEX® Connection: Management of Care, Establishing Priorities

3.   A. INCORRECT: In the event of a tornado, the nurse should close all client doors to minimize the threat of flying glass and debris, not open them.

     B. **CORRECT:** In the event of a tornado, placing blankets over clients protects them from shattering glass or flying debris.

     C. **CORRECT:** In the event of a tornado, the nurse should move all beds away from windows to protect clients from shattering glass or flying debris.

     D. **CORRECT:** In the event of a tornado, the nurse should draw shades and close drapes to protect clients against shattering glass.

     E. INCORRECT: In the event of a tornado, the nurse should relocate ambulatory clients to the hallways, away from windows.

      NCLEX® Connection: Safety and Infection Control, Accident/Error/Injury Prevention

4.   A. INCORRECT: In a dry chemical exposure, it is not recommended to wet the skin.

     B. INCORRECT: Washing the skin with antibacterial soap is not recommended in the event of a dry chemical exposure.

     C. **CORRECT:** In the event of a dry chemical exposure, the recommendation is to brush the chemical off the skin and clothing.

     D. INCORRECT: The nurse should not apply a neutralizing agent until after the chemical is identified.

      NCLEX® Connection: Safety and Infection Control, Handing Hazardous and Infectious Materials

5.   A. INCORRECT: In the event of a bomb threat, the nurse should keep the caller on the line in order to trace the call and to collect as much information as possible.

     B. INCORRECT: The nurse should avoid announcing that a bomb threat has occurred using the paging system because it could cause mass panic.

     C. INCORRECT: It is recommended to ask to caller about the location of the bomb and the time it is set to explode in order to gather as much information as possible.

     D. **CORRECT:** In order to identify the location of the caller, the nurse should listen for background noises such as church bells, train whistles, or other distinguishing noises.

      NCLEX® Connection: Safety and Infection Control, Handing Hazardous and Infectious Materials

6. *Using the ATI Active Learning Template: Basic Concept*
    - Related Content
        - Anthrax
            - Clinical Manifestations
                - Sore throat
                - Fever
                - Cough
                - Shortness of breath
                - Muscle aches
                - Severe dyspnea
                - Meningitis
                - Shock
            - Nursing Interventions
                - Oral ciprofloxacin (Cipro)
                - IV ciprofloxacin
                - One or two additional antibiotics, such as vancomycin or penicillin
        - Botulism
            - Clinical Manifestations
                - Difficulty swallowing
                - Double vision
                - Slurred speech
                - Descending progressive weakness
                - Nausea, vomiting, abdominal cramps
                - Difficulty breathing
            - Nursing Interventions
                - Airway management
                - Antitoxin
                - Elimination of toxin
        - Pneumonic plague
            - Clinical Manifestations
                - Fever
                - Headache
                - Weakness
                - Rapidly developing pneumonia
                - Shortness of breath
                - Chest pain
                - Cough
                - Bloody or watery sputum.
                - Progresses for 2 to 4 days
                - May cause respiratory failure and shock.
            - Nursing Interventions
                - Early treatment is essential.
                - Administer antibiotics within 24 hr of first symptoms. Streptomycin, gentamicin, the tetracyclines, and chloramphenicol are all effective against pneumonic plague.
        - Tularemia
            - Clinical Manifestations
                - Sudden fever
                - Chills
                - Headache
                - Diarrhea
                - Muscle aches
                - Joint pain
                - Dry cough
                - Progressive weakness
                - If airborne, life-threatening pneumonia and systemic infection
            - Nursing Interventions
                - Streptomycin IV or gentamicin IV or IM are the drugs of choice.
                - In mass casualty, use doxycycline or ciprofloxacin.

(N) NCLEX® Connection: Safety and Infection Control, Handing Hazardous and Infectious Materials

UNIT 2   Health Promotion

SECTION: NURSING THROUGHOUT THE LIFESPAN

› Health Promotion and Disease Prevention
› Client Education
› Infants (1 Month to 1 Year)
› Toddlers (1 to 3 Years)
› Preschoolers (3 to 6 Years)
› School-Age Children (6 to 12 Years)
› Adolescents (12 to 20 Years)
› Young Adults (20 to 35 Years)
› Middle Adults (35 to 65 Years)
› Older Adults (65 Years and Older)

NCLEX® CONNECTIONS

When reviewing the chapters in this unit, keep in mind the relevant sections of the NCLEX® outline, in particular:

Client Needs: Safety and Infection Control	Client Needs: Health Promotion and Maintenance	Client Needs: Basic Care and Comfort

› Relevant topics/tasks include:
» Accident/Injury Prevention
  › Identify factors that influence accident/injury prevention.
» Home Safety
  › Educate the client on home safety issues.
	› Relevant topics/tasks include:
	» Developmental Stages and Transitions
	  › Identify expected physical, cognitive, and psychosocial stages of development.
	» Health and Wellness
	  › Identify the client's health-oriented behaviors.
	» Health Promotion/Disease Prevention
	  › Educate the client on actions to promote/maintain health and prevent disease.
		› Relevant topics/tasks include:
		» Mobility/Immobility
		  › Assess the client for mobility, gait, strength, and motor skills.

chapter 16

Overview

- Nurses use traditional nursing measures and complementary therapies, such as guided imagery, massage, relaxation, and music, to help promote health and prevent disease.

- Levels of prevention address health-related activities that are primary, secondary, and tertiary. Levels of prevention are not the same as levels of care.

Risk Factor Assessment

- Genetics – Heredity creates a predisposition for various disorders (heart disease, cancers, mental illnesses).

- Gender – Some diseases are more common in one gender than in the other. For example, women have a higher incidence of autoimmune disorders, while men have a higher suicide rate.

- Physiologic factors – Various physiologic states place clients at an increased risk for health problems (body mass index [BMI] above 25, pregnancy).

- Environmental factors – Toxic substances and chemicals can affect health where clients live and work (water quality, pesticide exposure, air pollution).

- Lifestyle-risk behaviors – Clients have control over how they choose to live, and making positive choices can reduce risk factors. Risk behaviors to screen for include stress, substance use disorders, diet deficiencies, lack of exercise, and sun exposure.

- Age – Screening guidelines from the American Diabetes Association, the American Heart Association, and the American Cancer Society promote early detection and intervention. Ages vary with individual practices (for example, a woman who is sexually active before the age of 20 should start screenings when sexual activity begins).

- Frequency of some major examinations and screenings for clients who are asymptomatic and do not have risk factors:

TEST	FREQUENCY
› Routine physical examination	› Variable, generally every 3 to 5 years from age 20 to 40, more often after 40
› Dental assessments	› Every 6 months
› Blood pressure	› At least every 2 years, annually if previously elevated
› Body mass index (BMI)	› At each routine health care visit
› Blood cholesterol	› Starting at age 20, a minimum of every 5 years

TEST	FREQUENCY
› Blood glucose	› Starting at age 45, a minimum of every 3 years
› Colorectal screening	› Starting at age 50, high-sensitivity fecal occult blood testing every year, or flexible sigmoidoscopy every 5 years, or colonoscopy every 10 years
Tests Specific for Females	
› Cervical cancer screening	› Ages 21 to 29, Papanicolaou test (Pap smear) every 3 years; ages 30 to 65, Pap and human papilloma virus test every 5 years
› Breast cancer screening	› Ages 20 to 40, clinical breast examination every 3 years, then annually; ages 50 to 74, mammogram every 2 years
Tests Specific for Males	
› Clinical testicular examination	› At each routine health care visit starting at age 20
› Prostate-specific antigen test, digital rectal examination	› Starting at age 50 if indicated

Prevention

- The terms primary prevention, secondary prevention, and tertiary prevention describe the focus of activities and the level of prevention.

 View Video: Health Screening

LEVEL OF PREVENTION	EXAMPLES OF PREVENTION ACTIVITIES
› Primary prevention addresses the needs of healthy clients to promote health and prevent disease with specific protections.	› Immunization programs › Child car seat education › Nutrition, fitness activities › Health education in schools
› Secondary prevention focuses on identifying illness, providing treatment, and conducting activities that help prevent a worsening health status.	› Communicable disease screening, case finding › Early detection, treatment of diabetes mellitus › Exercise programs for older adults who are frail
› Tertiary prevention aims to prevent the long-term consequences of a chronic illness or disability and to support optimal functioning.	› Prevention of pressure ulcers after spinal cord injury › Promoting independence after traumatic brain injury

Nursing Interventions

- Examine risk factors to identify modifications, adopt mutually agreeable goals, and identify support systems.

  - Refer clients to educational/community/support resources.

  - Help clients recognize benefits (not smoking reduces the risk of lung cancer) and overcome barriers (not smoking covers expenses for healthful pursuits).

- Use behavior-change strategies.

  - Identify clients' readiness to receive and apply health information.

  - Identify acceptable interventions.

  - Help motivate change by setting realistic timelines.

  - Reinforce steps toward change.

  - Encourage clients to maintain the change.

- Promote healthy lifestyle behaviors by instructing clients to:

  - Use stress management strategies.

  - Get adequate sleep and rest.

  - Eat a nutritious diet to achieve and maintain a healthy weight.

  - Avoid saturated fats.

  - Participate in regular physical activity most days.

  - While outdoors, wear protective clothing, use sunscreen, and avoid sun exposure between 10 a.m. and 4 p.m.

  - Wear safety gear (bike helmets, knee and elbow pads) when participating in physical activity.

  - Avoid tobacco products, alcohol, and illegal drugs.

  - Practice safer sex.

  - Seek medical care when necessary, get routine screenings, and perform recommended self-examinations (breast, testicular).

APPLICATION EXERCISES

1. A nurse is caring for a 19-year-old client who is sexually active and has come to the college health clinic for the first time for a checkup. Which of the following interventions should the nurse perform first to determine the client's need for health promotion and disease prevention?

    A. Measure the client's vital signs.

    B. Encourage HIV screening.

    C. Determine the client's risk factors.

    D. Instruct the client to use condoms.

2. A nurse in a health clinic is caring for a 21-year-old client who reports a sore throat. The client tells the nurse that he has not seen a doctor since high school. Which of the following health screenings should the nurse expect the provider to perform for this client?

    A. Testicular examination

    B. Blood glucose

    C. Fecal occult blood

    D. Prostate-specific antigen

3. A nurse at a provider's office is talking with a 45-year-old client who has no specific family history of cancer or diabetes mellitus about planning her routine screeings. Which of the following client statements indicates that the client understands how to proceed?

    A. "So I don't need the colon cancer procedure for another 2 or 3 years."

    B. "For now, I should continue to have a mammogram each year."

    C. "Because the doctor just did a Pap smear, I'll come back next year for another one."

    D. "I had my blood glucose test last year, so I won't need it again till next year."

4. A nurse is talking with a client who recently attended a cholesterol screening event and a heart-healthy nutrition presentation at a neighborhood center. His total cholesterol result from the screening was 248 mg/dL, so he saw his provider and received a medication prescription to improve his cholesterol level. The client was later hospitalized for severe chest pain, and subsequently enrolled in a cardiac rehabilitation program. Which of the following activities of this client is an example of primary prevention?

    A. Cholesterol screening

    B. Nutrition presentation

    C. Medication therapy

    D. Cardiac rehabilitation

5. A nurse in a clinic is caring for a client who has multiple risk factors for cardiovascular disease. When planning health promotion and disease prevention strategies for this client, which of the following interventions should the nurse include? (Select all that apply.)

_____ A. Help the client see the benefits of her actions.

_____ B. Identify the client's support systems.

_____ C. Suggest and recommend community resources.

_____ D. Devise and set goals for the client.

_____ E. Teach stress management strategies.

6. A nurse is caring for a client in a spinal cord injury rehabilitation center following head and neck injuries he sustained while riding his bicycle. The client had surgery during the acute phase of treatment to relieve intracranial pressure and to stabilize his cervical spine. Now, he and his spouse are learning essential self-management strategies. Use the ATI Active Learning Template: Basic Concept to complete this item. Under Related Content, list each of the three levels of prevention with an example of each level from this client's history or from what this client might have done to prevent this injury and its life-altering consequences.

APPLICATION EXERCISES KEY

1. A. INCORRECT: Vital signs are a part of any health care visit, but they are not the priority for a 19-year-old client.

    B. INCORRECT: It might be appropriate to suggest HIV screening, but there is a higher priority action the nurse must take before doing this.

    C. **CORRECT:** The first action the nurse should take using the nursing process is assessment. The nurse should talk with the client first to determine what risk factors the client might have before initiating the appropriate health promotion and disease prevention measures.

    D. INCORRECT: It might be appropriate to suggest condom use, but there is a higher priority action the nurse must take before doing this.

    Ⓝ NCLEX® Connection: Health Promotion and Maintenance, Health Screening

2. A. **CORRECT:** Starting at age 20, examinations for testicular cancer are appropriate, along with blood pressure and body mass index measurements and cholesterol determinations.

    B. INCORRECT: Blood glucose testing begins at age 45.

    C. INCORRECT: Testing for fecal occult blood usually begins at age 50.

    D. INCORRECT: Testing for prostate-specific antigen usually begins at age 50.

    Ⓝ NCLEX® Connection: Health Promotion and Maintenance, Health Screening

3. A. INCORRECT: Clients who have no specific family or personal history of colorectal cancer should begin screening procedures at age 50.

    B. **CORRECT:** Between the ages of 40 and 50, women should have a mammogram annually.

    C. INCORRECT: Between the ages of 30 and 65, women with no family or personal history of cervical cancer should have a Pap smear and a human papilloma virus test every 5 years.

    D. INCORRECT: Starting at age 45, clients should have a blood glucose test at least every 3 years. Unless there is a specific family or personal history of diabetes mellitus, annual blood glucose determinations are not necessary.

    Ⓝ NCLEX® Connection: Health Promotion and Maintenance, Health Promotion/Disease Prevention

4. A. INCORRECT: The cholesterol screening is an example of secondary prevention.

    B. **CORRECT:** Primary prevention encompasses strategies that actually help prevent illness or injury. This level of prevention includes health information about nutrition, exercise, stress management, and protection from injuries and illness.

    C. INCORRECT: The medication therapy is an example of secondary prevention.

    D. INCORRECT: Cardiac rehabilitation is an example of tertiary prevention.

    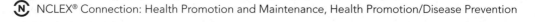 NCLEX® Connection: Health Promotion and Maintenance, Health Promotion/Disease Prevention

5. A. **CORRECT:** The nurse should help the client recognize the benefits of her health-promoting actions while also overcoming barriers to taking implementing actions.

    B. **CORRECT:** Once the nurse has collected information about who can help the client change her unhealthful behaviors, she can suggest ways the client's supportive friends and family can get involved.

    C. **CORRECT:** The nurse should promote the client's use of any available community or online resources that can help her progress toward meeting her goals.

    D. INCORRECT: The nurse and the client should work together to devise and set mutually agreeable goals that are also realistic and achievable.

    E. **CORRECT:** Stress is a contributing factor to cardiovascular disease, as well as many other specific and systemic disorders.

    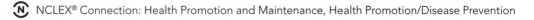 NCLEX® Connection: Health Promotion and Maintenance, Health Promotion/Disease Prevention

6. *Using the ATI Active Learning Template: Basic Concept*
    - Related Content
        ○ Primary: take various courses, read about bicycle safety (wear a helmet, use reflective accessories and lights for visibility to drivers, follow the rules of the road for cyclists)
        ○ Secondary: emergency care, surgery
        ○ Tertiary: rehabilitative care, learning self-management procedures, strategies

    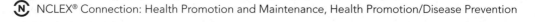 NCLEX® Connection: Health Promotion and Maintenance, Health Promotion/Disease Prevention

chapter 17

Overview

- Nurses provide health education to individual clients, families, and communities. Factors influencing client education needs include health status, educational level, socioeconomic status, cultural and family influences, emotional status, spiritual factors, perception of functioning, willingness to participate, and developmental stage.

    View Video: Client Education

- Teaching is a goal-driven interactive process.

- Learning is an intentional gain of new information and promotes behavioral change.

- Motivation influences how much and how quickly a person learns.

- Information technology can enhance access to and delivery of knowledge.

- Client education provides clients with information and skills to:
  - Maintain and promote health and prevent illness (immunizations, lifestyle changes, prenatal care).
  - Restore health (self-administering insulin).
  - Adapt to permanent illness or injury (ostomy care, swallowing techniques, speech therapy).

- Domains of learning:
  - Cognitive learning is obtaining new information, applying the information, and evaluating the information. For example, cognitive learning takes place when clients learn the signs and symptoms of hypoglycemia and then can verbalize when to notify the provider.
  - Affective learning involves feelings, beliefs, and ideals. For example, affective learning takes place when clients learn about the life changes necessary to manage diabetes mellitus and then discuss their feelings about having diabetes.
  - Psychomotor learning is gaining skills that require mental and physical activity. For example, psychomotor learning takes place when clients practice preparing insulin injections.

Assessment/Data Collection

- Assess/monitor learning needs.
- Evaluate the learning environment.
- Assess/monitor learning style (auditory, visual, kinesthetic).
- Identify areas of concern (low literacy levels, pain, distractions).
- Assess/monitor available resources (financial, social, community).
- Identify developmental stage.
- Determine physical and cognitive ability.
- Identify special needs (visual impairment, decreased manual dexterity, learning challenges).
- Determine motivation and readiness to learn.

Planning

- Identify mutually agreeable outcomes.
- Prioritize the learning objectives with clients' needs in mind.
- Use methods that emphasize the learning style.
- Select age-appropriate teaching methods/material.
- Provide electronic educational resources (CDs, DVDs, software programs, mobile applications).
- Use reliable Internet sources to access information and support services.
- Organize learning activities to move from simple to more complex tasks, and known to unknown concepts.
- Incorporate active participation in the learning process.
- Schedule teaching sessions at optimal times for learning (teaching ostomy care when replacing the bag).

Implementation

- Create an environment conducive to learning (minimize distractions and interruptions, provide privacy).
- Use therapeutic communication (active listening, empathy) to develop trust and promote sharing of concerns.

- Review previous knowledge and experiences.
- Explain the therapeutic regimen or procedure.
- Present steps that build toward more complex tasks.
- Demonstrate psychomotor skills.
- Allow time for return demonstrations.
- Provide positive reinforcement.

Evaluation

- Ask clients to explain the information in their own words.
- Observe return demonstrations (psychomotor learning).
- Use written tools to measure the accuracy of information.
- Ask clients to evaluate their own progress.
- Observe nonverbal communication.
- Reevaluate learning during follow-up telephone calls or contacts, such as home health visits or appointments with the provider.
- Revise the care plan accordingly.

Factors Affecting Learning

FACTORS THAT ENHANCE LEARNING	BARRIERS TO LEARNING
› Perceived benefit	› Fear, anxiety, depression
› Cognitive and physical ability	› Physical discomfort, pain, fatigue
› Health and cultural beliefs	› Environmental distractions
› Active participation	› Health and cultural beliefs
› Age/educational level-appropriate methods	› Sensory and perceptual deficits
	› Psychomotor deficits

APPLICATION EXERCISES

1. When a nurse is observing a client drawing up and mixing insulin injections, which of the following best demonstrates that psychomotor learning has taken place?

    A. The client is able to discuss the appropriate technique.

    B. The client is able to demonstrate the appropriate technique.

    C. The client states that he understands.

    D. The client is able to write the steps on a piece of paper.

2. A nurse in a provider's office is collecting data from the mother of a 1-year-old child. The client states that her child is old enough for toilet training. Following an educational session by the nurse, the client now states that her earlier ideas have changed. She is now willing to postpone toilet training until the child is older. Learning has occurred in which of the following domains?

    A. Cognitive

    B. Affective

    C. Psychomotor

    D. Kinesthetic

3. A nurse is providing preoperative teaching for a client who is scheduled for a mastectomy the next day. Which of the following client statements indicates that the client is ready to learn?

    A. "I don't want my spouse to see my incision."

    B. "Will you be able to give me pain medicine after the surgery?"

    C. "Can you tell me about how long the surgery will take?"

    D. "My roommate listens to everything I say."

4. A nurse is preparing an instructional session about managing stress incontinence for an older adult. Which of the following actions should the nurse take first when meeting with the client?

    A. Encourage the client to participate actively in learning.

    B. Select instructional materials appropriate for the older adult.

    C. Identify goals the nurse and the client agree are reasonable.

    D. Determine what the client knows about stress incontinence.

5. A nurse is evaluating how well a client learned the information presented in an instructional session about following a heart-healthy diet. The client states that she understands what to do now. Which of the following actions by the nurse should assist the nurse in evaluating the client's learning?

    A. Encourage the client to ask questions.

    B. Ask the client to explain how to select or prepare meals.

    C. Encourage the client to fill out an evaluation form.

    D. Ask the client if she has resources for further instruction on this topic.

6. A nurse is preparing a presentation at a community center for a group of parents who are interested in learning how to prevent childhood obesity. Use the ATI Active Learning Template: Basic Concept to complete this item. Include the following Related Content:

    A. List at least three factors the nurse should consider when incorporating ways to enhance learning.

    B. List at least three barriers the nurse might encounter among the attendees.

APPLICATION EXERCISES ANSWER KEY

1. A. INCORRECT: Discussing the appropriate technique demonstrates learning, but it does not involve the use of motor skills.

    B. **CORRECT:** Demonstrating the appropriate technique indicates that psychomotor learning has taken place.

    C. INCORRECT: Verbalizing understanding demonstrates learning, but it does not involve the use of motor skills.

    D. INCORRECT: Writing steps on paper demonstrates learning, but it does not involve the motor skills essential for performing the procedure.

    Ⓝ NCLEX® Connection: Health Promotion and Maintenance, Health Promotion/Disease Prevention

2. A. INCORRECT: An example of cognitive learning is stating the behavior the child will demonstrate when ready to toilet train.

    B. **CORRECT:** Affective learning has taken place, as evidenced by the client's changed ideas about toilet training.

    C. INCORRECT: An example of psychomotor learning is performing the proper techniques for introducing the child to toilet training.

    D. INCORRECT: Kinesthetic learning is a learning style, not a domain of learning.

    Ⓝ NCLEX® Connection: Health Promotion and Maintenance, Health Promotion/Disease Prevention

3. A. INCORRECT: The client's concern about her spouse seeing the incision may indicate anxiety or depression.

    B. INCORRECT: The client's request for pain medicine may indicate fear and anxiety.

    C. **CORRECT:** Asking a concrete question about the surgery indicates that the client is ready to discuss the surgery. The client's new diagnosis of cancer may cause anxiety, fear, or depression, all of which can interfere with the learning process.

    D. INCORRECT: The lack of privacy due to the presence of a roommate may be a barrier to learning.

    Ⓝ NCLEX® Connection: Reduction of Risk Potential, Therapeutic Procedures

4. A. INCORRECT: Active participation in the learning process is essential for the success of the session. However, this is not the priority action.

   B. INCORRECT: It is essential for the nurse to prepare and select instructional materials appropriate for the client's age, developmental level, and other parameters. However, this is not the priority action.

   C. INCORRECT: Establishing mutually agreeable goals is essential for the success of the session. However, this is not the priority action.

   D. **CORRECT:** The first action the nurse should take using the nursing process is to assess or collect data from the client. The nurse should determine how much the client knows about stress incontinence, the accuracy of this knowledge, and what the client needs to learn to manage this condition before proceeding to instructing the client.

   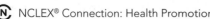 NCLEX® Connection: Health Promotion and Maintenance, Health Promotion/Disease Prevention

5. A. INCORRECT: The client stated that she understood the content, so she might not ask any questions that would help the nurse evaluate learning.

   B. **CORRECT:** A useful strategy for evaluating learning is to ask the client to explain in her own words how she will implement what she learned.

   C. INCORRECT: An evaluation form usually gives the client a means of evaluating the teaching. It might not offer clues about what the client has learned.

   D. INCORRECT: The nurse should identify the client's resources early in the instructional process. At this point, the exploration of resources does not help the nurse evaluate the client's learning.

   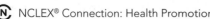 NCLEX® Connection: Health Promotion and Maintenance, Health Promotion/Disease Prevention

6. *Using the ATI Active Learning Template: Basic Concept*

   A. Factors that enhance learning
      - Perceived benefit
      - Cognitive and physical ability
      - Health and cultural beliefs
      - Active participation
      - Age
      - Educational level-appropriate methods

   B. Barriers to learning
      - Fear
      - Anxiety
      - Depression
      - Physical discomfort
      - Pain
      - Fatigue
      - Environmental distractions
      - Health and cultural beliefs
      - Sensory and perceptual deficits
      - Psychomotor deficits

   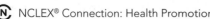 NCLEX® Connection: Health Promotion and Maintenance, Health Promotion/Disease Prevention

UNIT 2   **HEALTH PROMOTION**
SECTION: NURSING THROUGHOUT THE LIFESPAN

CHAPTER 18   Infants (1 Month to 1 Year)

Expected Growth and Development

- Physical Development
  - ○ The infant's posterior fontanel closes by 2 to 3 months of age.
  - ○ The infant's anterior fontanel closes by 12 to 18 months of age.
  - ○ Tracking parameters for infants:
    - ▪ Weight: Infants gain about 150 to 210 g (about 5 to 7 oz) per week in the first 6 months. Birth weight should double by 4 to 6 months and triple by the end of the first year.
    - ▪ Height: Infants grow about 2.5 cm (1 in) per month in the first 6 months, and then about 1.25 cm (0.5 in) per month until the end of the first year.
    - ▪ Head circumference: Head circumference increases about 1.25 cm (0.5 in) per month in the first 6 months and then about 0.5 cm (0.2 in) between 6 and 12 months.
  - ○ Dentition – Six to eight teeth erupt in the infant's mouth by the end of the first year.

    - ▪ Use cold teething rings, over-the-counter teething gels, and acetaminophen (Tylenol) or ibuprofen (Advil).
    - ▪ Use a cool, wet washcloth to clean the teeth.
    - ▪ Do not give infants a bottle when they are falling asleep. Prolonged exposure to milk or juice can cause dental caries (bottle-mouth caries).
  - ○ Fine and Gross Motor Development

AGE	GROSS MOTOR SKILLS	FINE MOTOR SKILLS
1 month	› Demonstrates head lag	› Has a grasp reflex
2 months	› Lifts head off mattress	› Holds hands in an open position
3 months	› Raises head and shoulders off mattress	› No longer has a grasp reflex › Keeps hands loosely open
4 months	› Rolls from back to side	› Places objects in mouth
5 months	› Rolls from front to back	› Uses palmar grasp dominantly
6 months	› Rolls from back to front	› Holds bottle
7 months	› Bears full weight on feet	› Moves objects from hand to hand
8 months	› Sits unsupported	› Begins using pincer grasp
9 months	› Pulls to a standing position	› Has a crude pincer grasp
10 months	› Changes from prone to sitting position	› Grasps rattle by its handle
11 months	› Walks while holding on to something	› Can place objects into a container
12 months	› Sits down from a standing position without assistance	› Tries to build a two-block tower without success

- Cognitive Development
  - Piaget – Sensorimotor stage (birth to 24 months)
    - Separation is the sense of being distinct from other objects in the environment.
    - Object permanence develops at about 9 months. This is the process of knowing that an object still exists when it is hidden from view.
    - Mental representation is the recognition of symbols.
  - Language Development
    - Responds to noises
    - Vocalizes with "ooos" and "aahs"
    - Laughs and squeals
    - Turns head to the sound of a rattle
    - Pronounces single-syllable words
    - Begins speaking two- and then three-word phrases
- Psychosocial Development
  - An infant's stage of psychosocial development, according to Erikson, is trust vs. mistrust.
    - Infants trust that others will meet their feeding, comfort, stimulation, and caring needs.
    - Infants' reflexive behavior (attachment, separation recognition/anxiety, and stranger fear) influences their social development.
    - Attachment, when infants begin to bond with their parents, develops within the first month, but actually begins before birth. The process is optimal when the infant and parents are in good health, have positive feeding experiences, and receive adequate rest.
    - Separation recognition occurs during the first year as infants recognize the boundaries between themselves and others. Learning how to respond to people in their environment is the next phase of development. Positive interactions with parents, siblings, and other caregivers help establish trust.
    - Separation anxiety develops between 4 and 8 months of age. Infants protest loudly when separated from parents, which can cause considerable anxiety for the parents.
    - Stranger fear becomes evident between ages 6 to 8 months, when infants are less likely to accept strangers.
  - Self-Concept Development
    - By the end of the first year, infants distinguish themselves as separate from their parents.
  - Body-Image Changes
    - Infants discover that the mouth is a pleasure producer.
    - Hands and feet are objects of play.
    - Smiling makes others react.
- Age-Appropriate Activities
  - Infants have a short attention span and do not interact with other children during play (solitary play). Appropriate toys and activities that stimulate the senses and encourage development include rattles, mobiles, teething toys, nesting toys, playing pat-a-cake, playing with balls, and reading books.

Health Promotion

- Immunizations
  - Follow the latest Centers for Disease Control and Prevention (CDC) immunization recommendations (see www.cdc.gov) for healthy infants. During the first year, these generally include immunizations against hepatitis B, diphtheria, tetanus, pertussis, rotavirus, polio, influenza, and pneumococcal pneumonia. The recommendations change periodically, so check them often.

- Nutrition
  - Feeding alternatives:
    - Breastfeeding provides a complete diet for infants during the first 6 months.
    - Iron-fortified formula is an acceptable alternative to breast milk. Cow's milk is inadequate.
  - Solid food is appropriate around 4 to 6 months.
    - Indicators for readiness include voluntary control of the head and trunk and disappearance of the extrusion reflex (pushing food out of the mouth).
    - Introduce iron-fortified rice cereal first.
    - Start new foods one at a time over a 5- to 7-day period to observe for signs of allergy or intolerance (fussiness, rash, vomiting, diarrhea, constipation). Vegetables, fruits, and meats follow, generally in that order.
    - Delay milk, eggs, wheat, citrus fruits, peanuts, peanut butter, and honey until the second half of first year of life, as they can trigger allergies, and honey can also cause infant botulism.
    - Appropriate finger foods to introduce around 9 months include ripe bananas, toast strips, graham crackers, cheese cubes, noodles, and peeled chunks of apples, pears, and peaches.
    - Remind parents that solid food is not a substitute for breast milk or formula until after 12 months.
  - Weaning is appropriate when infants can drink from a cup (after 6 months).
    - Replace feeding with breast milk or formula in a cup.
    - Replace the bedtime feeding last.

- Injury Prevention
  - Aspiration
    - Avoid small objects, such as grapes, coins, and candy, that can become lodged in the throat.
    - Provide age-appropriate toys.
    - Check clothing for safety hazards (loose buttons).
  - Bodily harm
    - Keep sharp objects out of reach.
    - Keep infants away from heavy objects they can pull down.
    - Do not leave infants alone with animals.
    - Monitor for shaken baby syndrome.
  - Burns
    - Check the temperature of bath water.
    - Turn down the thermostat on the hot water heater.

- Have smoke detectors in the home and change their batteries regularly.
- Turn handles of pots and pans toward the back of the stove.
- Apply sunscreen when outdoors during daylight hours.
- Cover electrical outlets.
  - Drowning
    - Do not leave infants unattended in the bathtub.
  - Falls
    - Keep the crib mattress in the lowest position with the rails all the way up.
    - Use restraints in infant seats.
    - Place the infant seat on the ground or floor when outside of a vehicle, and do not leave it unattended or on elevated surfaces.
    - Use safety gates across stairs.
  - Poisoning
    - Avoid lead paint exposure.
    - Keep toxins and plants out of reach.
    - Keep safety locks on cabinets that contain cleaners and other household chemicals.
    - Keep a poison control number handy or program it into the phone.
    - Keep medications in childproof containers and out of reach.
    - Have a carbon monoxide detector in the home.
  - Motor-Vehicle Injuries
    - Use an approved rear-facing car seat in the back seat, preferably in the middle, (away from air bags and side impact). Infants should be in rear-facing car seats until age 2 or until they reach the maximum height and weight for the seat (as long as the top of the head is below the top of the seat back). Convertible restraints should have a five-point harness or a T-shield.
  - Suffocation
    - Avoid plastic bags.
    - Keep balloons away from infants.
    - Be sure the crib mattress fits tightly.
    - Ensure crib slats are no farther apart than 6 cm (2.4 in).
    - Remove crib mobiles or crib gyms by 4 to 5 months of age.
    - Do not use pillows in the crib.
    - Place infants on the back for sleep.
    - Keep toys that have small parts out of reach.
    - Remove drawstrings from jackets and other clothing.

APPLICATION EXERCISES

1. A nurse is talking with the parents of a 6-month-old infant about gross motor development. Which of the following gross motor skills are expected findings in the next 3 months? (Select all that apply.)

_____ A. Rolls from back to front

_____ B. Bears weight on legs

_____ C. Walks holding onto furniture

_____ D. Sits unsupported

_____ E. Sits down from a standing position

2. A nurse is cautioning the mother of an 8-month-old infant about safety. Which of the following statements by the mother indicates an understanding of safety for the infant?

A. "My baby loved to play with his crib gym, but I took it away from him."

B. "I just bought a soft mattress so my baby will sleep better."

C. "My baby really likes sleeping on the fluffy pillow we just got for him."

D. "I just bought a child-safety gate that folds like an accordion."

3. A nurse is reviewing car-seat safety with parents of a 1-month-old infant. When reviewing car-seat use, which of the following instructions should the nurse include?

A. Use a car seat that has a three-point harness system.

B. Position the car seat so that the infant is rear-facing.

C. Secure the car seat in the front passenger seat of the vehicle.

D. Put soft padding in the car seat behind the infant's back and neck.

4. The mother of a 7-month-old infant tells the nurse at the pediatric clinic that her baby has been fussy with occasional loose stools since she started feeding him fruits and vegetables. Which of the following responses by the nurse are appropriate? (Select all that apply.)

_____ A. "It might be good to add bananas, as they can help with loose stools."

_____ B. "Let's make a list of the foods he is eating so we can spot any problems."

_____ C. "Did the changes begin after you started one particular food?"

_____ D. "Has he been vomiting since he started these new foods?"

_____ E. "Most babies react with a little indigestion when you start new foods."

5. A parent brings a 5-month-old infant to the clinic for a well-infant check. The infant weighed 3.2 kg (7 lb) at birth. If the infant has followed the usual pattern of growth for 5 months, how much should the infant weigh? (Round the answer to the nearest tenth.)

_____ lb

6. A nurse is explaining to the parents of a 4-month-old infant what milestones they can expect their infant to achieve during this first year of her life and what they can do to encourage her development. Use the ATI Active Learning Template: Growth and Development to complete this item. Include the following:

A. Cognitive Development:

  • Name the developmental stage Piaget has identified for the first two years of life.

  • Identify three essential components that comprise this stage.

B. Age-Appropriate Activities

  • Identify at least two toys and two activities the nurse should suggest that the parents provide for their infant.

APPLICATION EXERCISES KEY

1. A. **CORRECT:** The infant should be able to roll from back to front by 6 months.

    B. **CORRECT:** The infant should be able to bear weight on legs by 7 months.

    C. INCORRECT: The infant should be able to do this by 11 months.

    D. **CORRECT:** The infant should be able to do this by 8 months.

    E. INCORRECT: The infant should be able to do this by 12 months.

     NCLEX® Connection: Health Promotion and Maintenance, Developmental Stages and Transitions

2. A. **CORRECT:** Parents should remove gyms and mobiles by 4 months because injury can occur from choking or strangulation.

    B. INCORRECT: The infant's crib mattress should be firm and fit tightly to prevent suffocation.

    C. INCORRECT: Parents should not place any pillows in the crib, as they pose a risk for strangulation.

    D. INCORRECT: Child-safety gates should expand by a horizontal mechanism and not like an accordion to prevent injury to hands and arms.

     NCLEX® Connection: Health Promotion and Maintenance, Developmental Stages and Transitions

3. A. INCORRECT: A three-point harness system protects the upper body only. Infants should have car seats with five-point harness systems.

    B. **CORRECT:** Infants in a car seat should face the rear of the vehicle until age 2 or until they reach the maximum height and weight for the seat.

    C. INCORRECT: Infants in a car seat in the front passenger seat are at risk for injury from the airbag in the event of a crash.

    D. INCORRECT: Padding creates some slack in the harnessing, which could allow the infant to slip out of the harness in a crash.

     NCLEX® Connection: Safety and Infection Control, Accident/Error/Injury Prevention

4.   A. INCORRECT: This response is an attempt to eliminate a symptom without attempting to determine if there is a problem that requires intervention.

   B. **CORRECT:** Before the nurse can determine that there is a problem, such as a food allergy or intolerance, she should determine the components of the child diet.

   C. **CORRECT:** Fussiness and diarrhea, as well as a rash and vomiting or constipation, can all be signs of a food allergy or intolerance. Before the nurse can intervene, she has to collect data that can help her plan the appropriate interventions.

   D. **CORRECT:** Vomiting and constipation can also be signs of a food allergy or intolerance. Before the nurse can intervene, she has to collect data that can help her plan the appropriate interventions.

   E. INCORRECT: This response is nontherapeutic because it offers false reassurance without any attempt to determine if there is a problem that requires intervention.

   (N) NCLEX® Connection: Basic Care and Comfort, Nutrition and Oral Hydration

5.   **14.5** lb: The infant should gain 0.7 kg (1.5 lb) per month in the first 6 months.
   1.5 lb x Age 5 months + Birthweight 7 lb = 14.5 lb

   (N) NCLEX® Connection: Health Promotion and Maintenance, Developmental Stages and Transitions

6.   *Using the ATI Active Learning Template: Growth and Development*

   A. Cognitive Development
   - Piaget's sensorimotor stage (first 2 years)
     - Separation
     - Object permanence
     - Mental representation

   B. Age-Appropriate Activities
   - Toys and activities
     - Rattles
     - Mobiles
     - Teething toys
     - Nesting toys
     - Playing pat-a-cake
     - Playing with balls
     - Reading books

   (N) NCLEX® Connection: Health Promotion and Maintenance, Developmental Stages and Transitions

Expected Growth and Development

- Physical Development
  - The anterior fontanel closes by 18 months.
  - Weight: At 24 months, toddlers should weigh four times their birth weight.
  - Height: Toddlers grow by 7.5 cm (3 in) per year.

AGE	GROSS MOTOR SKILLS	FINE MOTOR SKILLS
15 months	› Walks without help. Creeps up stairs.	› Uses cup well. Builds tower of two blocks.
18 months	› Assumes standing position. Jumps in place with both feet.	› Manages spoon without rotation. Turns pages in book two or three at a time.
2 years	› Walks up and down stairs.	› Builds a tower with six or seven blocks.
2.5 years	› Jumps with both feet. Stands on one foot momentarily.	› Draws circles. Has good hand-finger coordination.

- Cognitive Development
  - Piaget – Sensorimotor transitions to preoperational.
    - The concept of object permanence is fully developed.
    - Toddlers have and demonstrate memories of events that relate to them.
    - Domestic mimicry is evident (playing house).
    - Preoperational thought does not allow toddlers to understand other viewpoints, but it does allow them to symbolize objects and people in order to imitate activities they have seen.
  - Language Development
    - Language increases to about 400 words, with toddlers speaking in two- to three-word phrases.
- Psychosocial Development
  - Toddlers' stage of psychosocial development, according to Erikson, is autonomy vs. shame and doubt.
    - Independence is paramount as toddlers attempt to do everything for themselves.
    - Separation anxiety continues when parents leave.
  - Moral Development
    - Moral development parallels cognitive development.
    - Egocentric – Toddlers are unable to see another's perspective; they can only view things from their point of view.
    - Punishment and obedience orientation begins with a sense that others reward good behavior and punish bad behavior.

- Self-Concept Development
  - Toddlers progressively see themselves as separate from their parents and increase their explorations away from them.
- Body-Image Changes
  - Toddlers appreciate the usefulness of various body parts.
  - Toddlers develop gender identity by age 3.

- Age-Appropriate Activities
  - Solitary play evolves into parallel play where toddlers observe other children and then engage in activities nearby.
  - Appropriate activities include:
    - Filling and emptying containers
    - Playing with blocks
    - Looking at books
    - Playing with push and pull toys
    - Tossing a ball
  - Temper tantrums result when toddlers are frustrated with restrictions on independence. Providing consistent, age-appropriate expectations helps them work through their frustration.
  - Toilet training can begin with awareness of the sensation of needing to urinate or defecate. Parents should demonstrate patience and consistency with toilet training. Nighttime control may develop last.
  - Discipline should be consistent with well-defined boundaries that help develop appropriate social behavior.

Health Promotion

- Immunizations
  - Follow the latest Centers for Disease Control and Prevention (CDC) immunization recommendations (see www.cdc.gov) for healthy toddlers 12 months to 3 years of age. These generally include immunizations against hepatitis A, diphtheria, tetanus, pertussis, measles, mumps, rubella, varicella, polio, influenza, and pneumococcal pneumonia. The recommendations change periodically, so check them often.
- Nutrition
  - Toddlers are picky eaters with repeated requests for favorite foods.
  - Toddlers should consume 24 to 30 oz of milk per day and may switch from drinking whole milk to drinking low-fat or fat-free milk at 2 years of age.
  - Limit juice to 4 to 6 oz a day.
  - Food serving size is 1 tbsp for each year of age.
  - Toddlers may be reluctant to try or accept foods new to them.
  - If there is a family history of allergy, introduce cow's milk, chocolate, citrus fruits, egg white, seafood, and nut butters gradually while monitoring for reactions.
  - As toddlers become more autonomous, they tend to prefer finger foods.

- Regular meal times and nutritious snacks best meet nutrient needs.

- Avoid snacks and desserts that are high in sugar, fat, or sodium.

- Avoid foods that pose choking hazards (nuts, grapes, hot dogs, peanut butter, raw carrots, tough meats, popcorn).

- Supervise toddlers during snack and mealtimes.

- Cut food into small, bite-sized pieces to make it easier to swallow and to prevent choking.

- Do not allow toddlers to eat or drink during play activities or while lying down.

- Suggest that parents follow U.S. Department of Agriculture nutrition recommendations (www.myplate.gov).

- Injury Prevention

  - Aspiration

    - Avoid small objects (grapes, coins, candy) that can lodge in the throat.

    - Keep toys with small parts out of reach.

    - Provide age-appropriate toys.

    - Check clothing for safety hazards, such as loose buttons.

    - Keep balloons away from toddlers.

  - Bodily Harm

    - Keep sharp objects out of reach.

    - Keep firearms in a locked box or cabinet.

    - Do not leave toddlers unattended with animals present.

    - Teach stranger safety.

  - Burns

    - Check the temperature of bath water.

    - Turn down the thermostat on the hot water heater.

    - Have smoke detectors in the home and replace their batteries regularly.

    - Turn pot handles toward the back of the stove.

    - Cover electrical outlets.

    - Use sunscreen when outside.

  - Drowning

    - Do not leave toddlers unattended in the bathtub.

    - Keep toilet lids closed.

    - Closely supervise toddlers at the pool or any other body of water.

    - Teach toddlers to swim.

  - Falls

    - Keep doors and windows locked.

    - Keep the crib mattress in the lowest position with the rails all the way up.

    - Use safety gates across stairs.

- Motor-vehicle injuries
  - Use an approved car seat in the back seat, away from air bags.
  - Toddlers should be in a rear-facing car seat until age 2 or until they exceed the height and weight limit of the car seat. They can then sit in an approved forward-facing car seat in the back seat, using a five-point harness or T-shield until they exceed the manufacturer's recommended height and weight for the car seat.
- Poisoning
  - Avoid exposure to lead paint.
  - Place safety locks on cabinets that contain cleaners and other chemicals.
  - Keep plants out of reach.
  - Keep a poison control number handy or program it into the phone.
  - Keep medications in childproof containers out of the child's reach.
  - Have a carbon monoxide detector in the home.
- Suffocation
  - Avoid plastic bags.
  - Be sure the crib mattress fits tightly.
  - Ensure crib slats are no further apart than 6 cm (2.4 in).
  - Keep pillows out of the crib.
  - Remove drawstrings from jackets and other clothing.

APPLICATION EXERCISES

1. A nurse is giving a presentation about accident prevention to a group of parents of toddlers. Which of the following accident-prevention strategies should the nurse include? (Select all that apply.)

_____ A. Keep toxic agents in locked cabinets.

_____ B. Keep toilet seats up.

_____ C. Turn pot handles toward the back of the stove.

_____ D. Place safety gates across stairways.

_____ E. Make sure balloons are fully inflated.

2. A nurse is planning diversionary activities for children on an inpatient unit. Which of the following should the nurse incorporate as appropriate play activities for a toddler? (Select all that apply.)

_____ A. Building simple models

_____ B. Working with clay

_____ C. Filling and emptying containers

_____ D. Playing with blocks

_____ E. Looking at books

3. A nurse is talking with the parents of toddler. Which of the following should the nurse suggest regarding discipline?

A. Establish consistent boundaries.

B. Place him in a room with the door closed.

C. Have him learn by trial and error.

D. Use favorite snacks as rewards.

4. A mother tells the nurse that her 2-year-old child has temper tantrums. The child says "no" every time the mother tries to help her get dressed. The nurse explains that, developmentally, the toddler is

A. trying to increase her independence.

B. developing a sense of trust.

C. manifesting an anger management problem.

D. attempting to finish a project she started.

5. A nurse is reviewing nutritional guidelines with the parents of a 2-year-old toddler. Which of the following parents' statements should indicate to the nurse that they understand the feeding guidelines for this age group?

    A. "I should keep feeding my son whole milk until he is 3 years old."

    B. "It's okay for me to give my son a cup of apple juice with each meal."

    C. "I'll give my son about 2 tablespoons of each food at mealtimes."

    D. "My son loves popcorn, and I know it is better for him than sweets."

6. A nurse is explaining to the parents of a 14-month-old toddler what physical and cognitive development they can expect from now until their son is 3 years old. Use the ATI Active Learning Template: Growth and Development to complete this item. Include the following:

    A. Physical Development: Identify at least four gross or fine motor skills the parents can expect at specific ages.

    B. Cognitive Development: Describe at least three parameters the parents can expect to observe during the toddler stage.

APPLICATION EXERCISES KEY

1.   A. **CORRECT:** Parents must prevent toddlers from accessing dangerous substances.

    B. INCORRECT: Easy access to the water in the toilet bowl could result in aspiration or drowning.

    C. **CORRECT:** If toddlers can reach a pot handle, they can pull the pot and its contents down on themselves and incur serious injuries.

    D. **CORRECT:** At the bottom of a staircase, they prevent toddlers from climbing stairs and falling backward. At the top of a staircase, they prevent toddlers from falling down the stairs.

    E. INCORRECT: Toddlers should not have access to balloons at all, as balloons can easily burst and toddlers can put fragments of the balloon or the entire deflated balloon in the mouth and asphyxiate.

    Ⓝ NCLEX® Connection: Safety and Infection Control, Accident/Error/Injury Prevention

2.   A. INCORRECT: This play activity is more appropriate for school-age children.

    B. INCORRECT: Toddlers can easily swallow bits of clay.

    C. **CORRECT:** This activity is toddler-appropriate and helps develop fine motor skills and coordination.

    D. **CORRECT:** This activity is toddler-appropriate and helps develop fine motor skills.

    E. **CORRECT:** This activity is toddler-appropriate and helps with preparation for learning to read.

    Ⓝ NCLEX® Connection: Health Promotion and Maintenance, Developmental Stages and Transitions

3.   A. **CORRECT:** Toddlers need to have consistent boundaries for discipline to be effective.

    B. INCORRECT: Placing toddlers in a room with the door closed may cause anxiety and fear.

    C. INCORRECT: Trial and error lacks consistent boundaries and increases the risk for harmful consequences.

    D. INCORRECT: Using favorite foods as rewards may promote unhealthy eating habits.

    Ⓝ NCLEX® Connection: Health Promotion and Maintenance, Developmental Stages and Transitions

4. A. **CORRECT:** Toddlers express a drive for independence by opposing the desires of those in authority and attempting to do everything themselves.

    B. INCORRECT: Developing trust is a developmental task for infants.

    C. INCORRECT: This behavior is expected for a 2-year-old child and does not indicate an anger management problem.

    D. INCORRECT: Finishing a project is a developmental task of school-age children.

    Ⓝ NCLEX® Connection: Health Promotion and Maintenance, Developmental Stages and Transitions

5. A. INCORRECT: When toddlers turn 2 years old, the parents should give them low-fat or fat-free milk, not whole milk. This reduces fat and cholesterol intake and helps prevent childhood obesity.

    B. INCORRECT: Toddlers should have 4 to 6 oz of juice per day. Juices do not have the whole fiber that fruit has, plus they contain sugar, so parents should limit their use.

    C. **CORRECT:** Serving sizes for toddlers should be about 1 tbsp of solid food per year of age, so 2-year-olds should have about 2 tbsp per serving.

    D. INCORRECT: Popcorn poses a choking hazard, so it is an inappropriate snack food for toddlers.

    Ⓝ NCLEX® Connection: Health Promotion and Maintenance, Developmental Stages and Transitions

6. *Using the ATI Active Learning Template: Growth and Development*

    A. Physical Development
    - At 15 months, gross motor skills: walks without help, creeps up stairs
    - At 15 months, fine motor skills: uses cup well, builds tower of two blocks
    - At 18 months, gross motor skills: assumes standing position, jumps in place with both feet
    - At 18 months, fine motor skills: manages spoon without rotation, turns pages in book two or three at a time
    - At 2 years, gross motor skills: walks up and down stairs
    - At 2 years, fine motor skills: builds a tower with six or seven blocks
    - At 2.5 years, gross motor skills: jumps with both feet, stands on one foot momentarily
    - At 2.5 years, fine motor skills: draws circles, has good hand-finger coordination

    B. Cognitive Development
    - During toddler stage: object permanence, memories of events that relate to them, domestic mimicry (playing house), symbolization of objects and people, use of 400 words, use of two- to three-word phrases

    Ⓝ NCLEX® Connection: Health Promotion and Maintenance, Developmental Stages and Transitions

Expected Growth and Development

- Physical Development
  - Weight: Preschoolers gain about 2.3 kg (5 lb) per year.
  - Height: Preschoolers grow about 6.2 to 7.5 cm (2.5 to 3 in) per year.
    - Preschoolers evolve from the characteristically unsteady wide stance and protruding abdomen of toddlers to the more graceful, posturally erect, and sturdy physicality of this age group.
  - Fine and gross motor skills
    - Preschoolers show an improvement in fine motor skills, such as copying figures on paper and dressing themselves.

GROSS MOTOR SKILLS BY AGE		
3-year-old	4-year-old	5-year-old
› Ride a tricycle	› Skip and hop on one foot	› Jump rope
› Jump off bottom step	› Throw ball overhead	› Walk backward with heel to toe
› Stand on one foot for a few seconds		› Move up and down stairs easily

- Cognitive Development
  - Piaget – Preschoolers are still in the preoperational phase of cognitive development. They participate in preconceptual thought (from 2 to 4 years of age) and intuitive thought (from 4 to 7 years of age).
    - Preconceptual thought – Preschoolers make judgments based on visual appearances. Misconceptions in thinking during this stage include:
      - Artificialism – Everything is made by humans.
      - Animism – Inanimate objects are alive.
      - Imminent justice – A universal code exists that determines law and order.
    - Intuitive thought – Preschoolers can classify information and become aware of cause-and-effect relationships.
  - Time – Preschoolers begin to understand the concepts of the past, present, and future. By the end of the preschool years, they might may comprehend days of the week.
  - Language – Vocabulary continues to increase. Preschoolers speak in sentences, identify colors, and enjoy talking.

- Psychosocial Development
  - Erikson – Initiative vs. Guilt.
    - Preschoolers take on many new experiences, despite not having all of the physical abilities necessary to be successful at everything. When children are unable to accomplish a task, they might feel guilty and believe they have misbehaved. Guiding preschoolers to attempt activities within their capabilities while setting limits is appropriate.
  - Moral Development
    - Preschoolers continue in the good-bad orientation of the toddler years but begin to understand behavior in terms of what is socially acceptable.
  - Self-Concept Development
    - Preschoolers feel good about themselves for mastering skills, such as dressing and feeding, that allow independence. During stress, insecurity, or illness, they tend to regress to previous immature behavior or develop habits such as nose picking, bed wetting, or thumb sucking.
  - Body-Image Changes
    - Mistaken perceptions of reality coupled with misconceptions in thinking lead to active fantasies and fears. Preschoolers fear bodily harm, the dark, ghosts, and animals.
    - Sex-role identification is typical.
  - Social Development
    - During the preschool time period, children generally do not exhibit stranger anxiety and have less separation anxiety. However, prolonged separation, such as during hospitalization, can provoke anxiety. Favorite toys and play help ease fears.
    - Pretend play is healthy and allows children to determine the difference between reality and fantasy.
    - Sleep disturbances are common during early childhood, and problems range from difficulties going to bed to night terrors. Advise parents to:
      - Assess whether the bedtime is too early for children who still take naps. Preschoolers average about 12 hr of sleep a day. Some still require a daytime nap.
      - Keep a consistent bedtime routine, and help children slow down in preparation for bedtime.
      - Use a night light.
      - Reassure children who are frightened, but do not allow them to sleep in the parents' bed.
- Age-Appropriate Activities
  - Parallel play shifts to associative play during the preschool years. Play is not highly organized, and preschoolers do not cooperate during play. Appropriate activities include:
    - Playing ball.
    - Putting puzzles together.
    - Riding tricycles.
    - Pretend and dress-up activities.
    - Musical toys.
    - Painting, drawing, and coloring.
    - Sewing cards.
    - Cooking and housekeeping toys.
    - Looking at illustrated books.

Health Promotion

Q
EBP

- Immunizations

  - Follow the latest Centers for Disease Control and Prevention (CDC) immunization recommendations (www.cdc.gov) for healthy preschoolers.

    - These generally include immunizations against diphtheria, tetanus, pertussis, measles, mumps, rubella, varicella, seasonal influenza, and polio.

    - Recommendations change periodically, so check them often.

- Health Screenings

  - Vision screening is routine in the preschool population as part of the prekindergarten physical examination. It is essential to detect and treat myopia and amblyopia before poor visual acuity impairs the learning environment.

- Nutrition

  - Preschoolers consume about half the amount of energy that adults do (1,800 kcal).

  - Picky eating remains a problem for some preschoolers, but often by age 5 they become a bit more willing to sample different foods.

  - Preschoolers need 13 to 19 g/day of complete protein in addition to adequate calcium, iron, folate, and vitamins A and C.

  - Parents should provide a balance of nutrients. See www.choosemyplate.gov for nutritional guidelines for preschoolers.

Q
S

- Injury Prevention

  - Bodily harm

    - Keep firearms in a locked cabinet or container.

    - Teach stranger safety.

    - Wear helmets when riding a bicycle or tricycle and during any other activities that increase head-injury risk.

      □ Wear protective equipment (helmet and pads) during physical activity.

  - Burns

    - Reduce the temperature setting on the hot water heater.

    - Have smoke detectors in the home and replace the batteries regularly.

    - Use sunscreen while outdoors.

  - Drowning

    - Do not leave children unattended in the bathtub.

    - Closely supervise children at a pool or any other body of water.

    - Teach children to swim.

- ○ Motor-vehicle injuries
  - Preschoolers must sit in a forward-facing car seat with a harness in the back seat away from airbags for as long as possible, at least to 4 years of age. Children who outgrow the seat before age 4 should use a seat with a harness approved for higher weights and heights. Preschoolers whose weight or height exceed the forward-facing limit for their car seat should use a belt-positioning booster seat until the vehicle's seat belt fits properly, typically beyond the preschooler stage.
- ○ Poisoning
  - Avoid exposure to lead paint.
  - Keep plants out of reach.
  - Place safety locks on cabinets with cleaners and other chemicals.
  - Keep a poison control number handy or program it into the phone.
  - Keep medications in childproof containers out of reach.
  - Have a carbon monoxide detector in the home.

APPLICATION EXERCISES

1. A nurse is talking with the father of a 4-year-old child who states that his daughter goes to bed at 8:30 p.m. and wakes up at about 7:30 a.m., but she often lies in bed talking to herself or gets up a few times before falling asleep 40 min later. At her preschool, the children take a 2-hr afternoon nap. Which of the following recommendations should the nurse make to help improve the child's sleep behavior?

    A. Offer the child a snack of her favorite treat right before bedtime.

    B. Allow the child to watch an extra 30 min of TV in the evening.

    C. Change the child's bedtime to 9 p.m. on days she napped.

    D. Request that the preschool staff limit her nap time to 1 hr.

2. A nurse is planning diversionary activities for children on an inpatient pediatric unit. Which of the following should the nurse incorporate as appropriate play activities for preschoolers? (Select all that apply.)

    _____ A. Assembling puzzles

    _____ B. Pulling wheeled toys

    _____ C. Using musical toys

    _____ D. Using finger paints

    _____ E. Coloring with crayons

3. A nurse is caring for a 5-year-old client whose parents report that she fears painful procedures, such as injections. Which of the following strategies should the nurse use to try to help ease the child's fear? (Select all that apply.)

    _____ A. Invite the child to assist with mealtime activities.

    _____ B. Cluster invasive procedures whenever possible.

    _____ C. Assign caregivers with whom the child is familiar.

    _____ D. Have the parents bring in a favorite toy from home.

    _____ E. Engage the child in pretend play with a toy medical kit.

4. A nurse is reviewing the Centers for Disease Control and Prevention's (CDC's) immunization recommendations with the parents of two preschoolers. Which of the following recommendations should the nurse include in this discussion? (Select all that apply.)

_____ A. *Haemophilus influenzae* type b

_____ B. Varicella

_____ C. Polio

_____ D. Hepatitis A

_____ E. Seasonal influenza

5. A nurse is talking with parents of a preschooler who describe several issues that concern them. Which of the following problems the parents verbalized should the nurse identify as the priority for further assessment and intervention?

A. "Our son will only eat a few things, like burgers and bananas, and pretty much refuses everything else."

B. "Our son has these temper tantrums every time we tell him to do something he doesn't want to do."

C. "We think our son truly believes that his toys have personalities and talk to him, especially at night."

D. "We feel bad when we see our son trying so hard to button his shirt. We just tell him this is something he'll just have to learn to do."

6. A nurse is making safety recommendations to the parents of a two preschoolers. Use the ATI Active Learning Template: Growth and Development to complete this item. Under Injury Prevention, list at least four key areas of safety and age-appropriate instructions for addressing each area.

APPLICATION EXERCISES KEY

1. A. INCORRECT: Eating a snack, especially one with a high sugar content, is likely to provide stimulation that will make it more difficult for the child to fall asleep.

    B. INCORRECT: Watching TV is likely to provide stimulation that will make it more difficult for the child to fall asleep.

    C. **CORRECT:** Preschoolers start to need less sleep than they did in previous stages. Putting the child to bed 30 min later, when she might be more tired, could help her fall asleep more readily.

    D. INCORRECT: It is impractical and inappropriate to ask preschool staff to limit nap time because one child has difficulty falling asleep at night. Also, if the child is napping for that amount of time, she probably needs that rest during the day.

     NCLEX® Connection: Basic Care and Comfort, Rest and Sleep

2. A. **CORRECT:** Putting puzzles together is appropriate for preschoolers and helps develop fine motor and cognitive skills.

    B. INCORRECT: Pulling or pushing toys with wheels is more appropriate for toddlers.

    C. **CORRECT:** Playing with musical toys is appropriate for preschoolers and helps develop fine motor skills and coordination.

    D. INCORRECT: Using finger paints is more appropriate for toddlers.

    E. **CORRECT:** Using crayons to color on paper or in coloring books is appropriate for preschoolers and helps develop fine motor skills and coordination.

     NCLEX® Connection: Health Promotion and Maintenance, Developmental Stages and Transitions

3. A. **CORRECT:** Preschoolers enjoy mastering tasks they can perform independently. Assisting with routine, nonthreatening tasks can help improve their self-esteem during hospitalization.

    B. INCORRECT: This creates an unnecessarily lengthy painful period for the child, which is likely to increase her fear.

    C. INCORRECT: Preschoolers have less stranger anxiety than toddlers, so this is not necessary and not always possible on hospital units.

    D. **CORRECT:** Having familiar and cherished objects nearby is therapeutic for children during their hospitalization.

    E. **CORRECT:** Pretend play helps children determine the difference between reality and fantasy (imagined fears), especially with the assistance of the nurse during hospitalization.

     NCLEX® Connection: Health Promotion and Maintenance, Developmental Stages and Transitions

4. A. INCORRECT: The CDC recommends *Haemophilus influenzae* type b immunizations during infancy, but not generally beyond 18 months of age.

   B. **CORRECT:** The CDC recommends a varicella (chickenpox) immunization during the preschool years.

   C. **CORRECT:** The CDC recommends a polio immunization during the preschool years.

   D. INCORRECT: The CDC recommends hepatitis A immunizations during infancy, but not generally beyond 24 months of age.

   E. **CORRECT:** The CDC recommends seasonal influenza immunizations during the preschool years.

   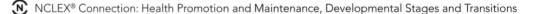 NCLEX® Connection: Health Promotion and Maintenance, Health Promotion/Disease Prevention

5. A. INCORRECT: It is common for preschoolers to continue to be picky eaters, as in the toddler stage. This usually resolves by the end of the preschool stage and is not the priority for assessment and intervention.

   B. **CORRECT:** When using the urgent vs. nonurgent approach to client care, the nurse determines that the priority issue is the problem that reflects a lack of completion of the previous stage of development and progression to the current stage of development. According to Erikson, it is a task of the toddler stage to develop autonomy vs. shame and doubt. This preschooler is still acting out with negativism, which is a persistent negative response to requests, often manifested in tantrums. He is still struggling with this task and needs assistance in working through that stage.

   C. INCORRECT: It is common for preschoolers to manifest misperceptions in thinking, such as animism – the belief that inanimate objects are alive. This problem is not the priority for assessment and intervention.

   D. INCORRECT: It is common for preschoolers, who are in the stage Erikson describes as initiative vs. guilt, to face the challenge of mastering activities they can perform independently, such as dressing themselves. This problem is not the priority for assessment and intervention.

   NCLEX® Connection: Health Promotion and Maintenance, Developmental Stages and Transitions

6. *Using the ATI Active Learning Template: Growth and Development*

- Injury Prevention
  - Bodily harm
    - Keep firearms in a locked cabinet or container.
    - Teach stranger safety.
    - Wear helmets when riding a bicycle or tricycle and during any other activities that increase head-injury risk.
    - Wear protective equipment (helmet and pads) during physical activity.
  - Burns
    - Reduce the temperature setting on the hot water heater.
    - Have smoke detectors in the home and replace the batteries regularly.
    - Use sunscreen while outdoors.
  - Drowning
    - Do not leave children unattended in the bathtub.
    - Closely supervise children at a pool or any other body of water.
    - Teach children to swim.
  - Motor-vehicle injuries
    - Use a forward-facing car seat with a harness in the back seat.
    - If weight or height exceeds the forward-facing limit, use a belt-positioning booster seat.
  - Poisoning
    - Avoid exposure to lead paint.
    - Keep plants out of reach.
    - Place safety locks on cabinets with cleaners and other chemicals.
    - Keep a poison control number handy or program it into the phone.
    - Keep medications in childproof containers out of reach.
    - Have a carbon monoxide detector in the home.

Ⓝ NCLEX® Connection: Health Promotion and Maintenance, Developmental Stages and Transitions

chapter 21

Expected Growth and Development

- Physical Development
  - Weight: School-age children gain about 1.8 to 3.2 kg (4 to 7 lb) per year.
  - Height: School-age children grow by about 5 cm (2 in) per year.
  - Changes related to puberty begin to appear in girls. These changes include:
    - Budding of breasts.
    - Appearance of pubic hair.
    - Menarche.
  - Changes related to puberty begin to appear in boys. These changes include:
    - Enlargement of testicles with changes in the scrotum, such as increased looseness.
    - Appearance of pubic hair.
  - Permanent teeth erupt.
  - Visual acuity improves to 20/20.
  - Auditory acuity and sense of touch fully develop.
  - Fine and gross motor development – coordination continues to improve.
- Cognitive Development
  - Piaget – Concrete Operations
    - See weight and volume as unchanging
    - Understand simple analogies
    - Understand time (days, seasons)
    - Classify more complex information
    - Understand various emotions
    - Become self-motivated
    - Solve problems
  - Language – Define many words and understands rules of grammar.
    - Understand that a word may have multiple meanings
- Psychosocial Development
  - School-age children's stage of psychosocial development, according to Erikson, is industry vs. inferiority.
    - School-age children develop a sense of industry through advances in learning.
    - Tasks that increase self-worth motivate them.
    - Fears of ridicule by peers and teachers over school-related issues are common. Some children manifest nervous behavior to deal with the stress, such as nail biting.

- Moral Development
  - Early on, school-age children might not understand the reasoning behind many rules and will try to find ways around them. Instrumental exchange is in place ("I'll help you if you help me."). They want to make the best deal and do not consider elements of loyalty, gratitude, or justice when making decisions.
  - In the latter part of the school years, they move into a law-and-order orientation, placing more emphasis on justice.
- Self-Concept Development
  - School-age children strive to develop healthy self-respect by finding out in what areas they excel.
  - School-age children need parents to encourage them in educational or extracurricular successes.
- Body-Image Changes
  - This is the age at which body image solidifies.
  - Education should address curiosity about sexuality, sexual development, and the reproductive process.
  - School-age children are more modest than preschoolers and place more emphasis on privacy.
- Social Development
  - Peer groups play an important part in social development. However, peer pressure begins to take effect.
  - Friendships begin to form among same-gender peers. Clubs and best friends are popular.
  - Children at this age prefer the company of same-gender companions.
  - Most relationships come from school associations.
  - Children at this age may rival the same-gender parent.
  - Conformity becomes evident.

- Age-Appropriate Activities
  - Competitive and cooperative play predominates.
  - 6- to 9-year-olds:
    - Play board, video, and number games.
    - Play hopscotch.
    - Jump rope.
    - Collect rocks, stamps, cards, coins, or stuffed animals.
    - Ride bicycles.
    - Build simple models.
    - Play team sports – skill building.
  - 9- to 12-year-olds:
    - Make crafts.
    - Read books.
    - Build models.
    - Develop in hobbies.
    - Assemble jigsaw puzzles.
    - Play video games.
    - Play team sports.

Health Promotion

- Immunizations

  - Follow the latest Centers for Disease Control and Prevention (CDC) immunization recommendations (see www.cdc.gov) for healthy school-age children. These generally include immunizations against diphtheria, tetanus, pertussis, human papillomavirus, hepatitis A and B, measles, mumps, rubella, varicella, seasonal influenza, polio, meningococcal infections, and for some high-risk individuals, pneumococcal infections. The recommendations change periodically, so check them often.

- Health Screenings

  - Scoliosis – Screening for idiopathic scoliosis, a lateral curvature of the spine with no apparent cause, is essential, especially for girls, during the school-age stage.

- Nutrition

  - By the end of the school-age stage, children eat adult servings of food and also need nutritious snacks.

  - Obesity predisposes school-age children to low self-esteem, diabetes mellitus, heart disease, and high blood pressure. Advise parents to:

    - Not use food as a reward.

    - Emphasize physical activity.

    - Provide a balanced diet. See www.choosemyplate.gov for nutritional guidelines for school-age children.

    - Teach children to make healthy food selections for meals and snacks.

    - Avoid eating meals at fast-food restaurants.

    - Avoid skipping meals.

- Dental health

  - Brush daily.

  - Floss daily.

  - Get regular check-ups.

- Injury Prevention

  - Bodily Harm

    - Keep firearms in a locked cabinet or box.

    - Assist with identifying "safe" play areas.

    - Teach stranger safety.

    - Teach children to wear helmets and/or pads when rollerskating, skateboarding, bicycling, riding scooters, skiing, and during any other activities that increase injury risk.

  - Burns

    - Teach fire safety and elimination of potential burn hazards.

    - Have working smoke and carbon monoxide detectors in the home.

    - Promote sunscreen use.

- ○ Drowning
  - ▪ Supervise children when swimming or near a body of water.
    - ▢ Teach swimming skills and safety.
- ○ Motor-Vehicle Injuries
  - ▪ Have children use a car or booster seat until adult seat belts fit correctly.
  - ▪ Children younger than 13 years of age are safest in the back seat.
- ○ Substance Abuse/Poisoning
  - ▪ Keep cleaners and chemicals in locked cabinets or out of reach.
  - ▪ Teach children to say "no" to illegal drugs and alcohol.

APPLICATION EXERCISES

1. A nurse is talking with parents of a school-age child who describe several issues that concern them. Which of the following problems the parents verbalized should the nurse identify as the priority for further assessment and intervention?

    A. "We just don't understand why our son can't keep up with the other kids in simple activities like running and jumping."

    B. "Our son keeps trying to find ways around our household rules. He always wants to make deals with us."

    C. "We think our son is trying too hard to excel in math just to get the top grades in his class."

    D. "Our son is always afraid the kids in school will laugh at him because he likes to sing and write little poems."

2. A nurse is planning diversionary activities for children on an inpatient pediatric unit. Which of the following should the nurse incorporate as appropriate play activities for school-age children? (Select all that apply.)

    _____ A. Building models

    _____ B. Playing video games

    _____ C. Reading books

    _____ D. Using toy carpentry tools

    _____ E. Shaping modeling clay

3. A nurse is reviewing nutritional guidelines with the parents of an 11-year-old child. Which of the following parents' statements should indicate to the nurse that they understand the guidelines for school-age children?

    A. "She wants to eat as much as we do, but we're afraid she'll soon be overweight."

    B. "She skips lunch sometimes, but we figure it's okay as long as she has a healthy breakfast and dinner."

    C. "We limit fast-food restaurant meals to three times a week now."

    D. "We reward her school achievements with a point system instead of a pizza or ice cream."

4. A nurse is talking with the parents of a 10-year-old child who express concern that their son is suddenly becoming secretive, for example, closing the door when he showers, dresses, and does his homework in his room. Which of the following responses by the nurse is appropriate?

    A. "Perhaps you should try to find out what he is doing behind those closed doors."

    B. "Suggest that he leave the door ajar for his own safety."

    C. "At this age, children tend to become more modest and value their privacy."

    D. "Tell him it's okay to close the door when he is undressed, but he has to do his homework where you can see him."

5. A nurse at an elementary school is planning a health promotion and primary prevention class. Which of the following topics are appropriate to include for the parents of school-age children? (Select all that apply.)

_____ A. Childhood obesity

_____ B. Substance use disorders

_____ C. Scoliosis screening

_____ D. Front-seat seatbelt use

_____ E. Stranger awareness

6. A nurse is explaining to a group of parents in a community center what cognitive development characteristics they should expect of their school-age children. Use the ATI Active Learning Template: Growth and Development to complete this item. Under Cognitive Development, list at least eight cognitive and language development expectations during young adulthood.

APPLICATION EXERCISES KEY

1. A. **CORRECT:** When using the urgent vs. nonurgent approach to client care, the priority issue is the problem that reflects a lack of completion of the previous stage of development and progression to the current stage of development. According to Erikson, it is a task of the preschool stage to develop initiative vs. guilt. This school-age child is still trying to develop the physical abilities he needs to feel a sense of accomplishment. He is still struggling with this task and needs assistance with motor skills and agility.

   B. INCORRECT: It is common for school-age children to fail to understand the reasoning behind many rules and to try to find ways around them and make the best deal. This problem is not the priority for assessment and intervention.

   C. INCORRECT: It is common for school-age children, who are in the stage Erikson describes as industry vs. inferiority, to strive to develop a sense of industry through advances in learning. This problem is not the priority for assessment and intervention.

   D. INCORRECT: It is common for school-age children, who are in the stage Erikson describes as industry vs. inferiority, to face the challenge of acquiring new skills and achieving success socially. This problem is not the priority for assessment and intervention.

   Ⓝ NCLEX® Connection: Health Promotion and Maintenance, Developmental Stages and Transitions

2. A. **CORRECT:** Building simple models is appropriate for school-age children and helps develop fine motor and cognitive skills.

   B. **CORRECT:** Playing video games, especially educational and nonviolent ones, is appropriate for school-age children and helps develop fine motor and cognitive skills.

   C. **CORRECT:** Reading books is appropriate for school-age children and helps develop cognitive and communication skills.

   D. INCORRECT: Using toy carpentry tools is more appropriate for preschoolers.

   E. INCORRECT: Shaping modeling clay is more appropriate for preschoolers.

   Ⓝ NCLEX® Connection: Health Promotion and Maintenance, Developmental Stages and Transitions

3. A. INCORRECT: By the end of the school-age stage, parents should expect children to eat adult-size portions of food.

   B. INCORRECT: Skipping meals can lead to unhealthful snacking and overeating later in the day.

   C. INCORRECT: Parents should avoid fast-food restaurants completely to keep children from eating food high in sugar, fat, and starches.

   D. **CORRECT:** Parents should avoid rewarding children with food for good behavior or achievements. Associations children form between food and feeling good can lead to weight problems.

   Ⓝ NCLEX® Connection: Basic Care and Comfort, Nutrition and Oral Hydration

4. A. INCORRECT: This response unnecessarily casts suspicion and implies that the child is doing something wrong.

    B. INCORRECT: This response unnecessarily suggests that the child has something to fear in his own home.

    C. **CORRECT:** From a developmental perspective, it is an expectation that school-age children develop privacy. They have their own way of doing things and spend more time alone.

    D. INCORRECT: This suggestion sounds like a punishment, and the parents have not presented any evidence that the child is doing anything wrong.

     NCLEX® Connection: Health Promotion and Maintenance, Developmental Stages and Transitions

5. A. **CORRECT:** Parents of school-age children need to be aware of nutritional strategies for preventing childhood obesity.

    B. **CORRECT:** Parents of school-age children need to know how to teach children to say no to illegal drugs, alcohol, and all other harmful or addictive substances.

    C. **CORRECT:** School-age children and adolescents require screening for scoliosis.

    D. INCORRECT: Children younger than 13 years are safest in the back seat.

    E. **CORRECT:** Parents need to reinforce stranger safety as soon as their children are old enough to understand it, and throughout all stages of childhood.

     NCLEX® Connection: Health Promotion and Maintenance, Health Promotion/Disease Prevention

6. *Using the ATI Active Learning Template: Growth and Development*
    - Cognitive Development
        - See weight and volume as unchanging
        - Understand simple analogies
        - Understand time (days, seasons)
        - Classify more complex information
        - Understand various emotions people experience
        - Become self-motivated
        - Solve problems
        - Define many words and understands rules of grammar
        - Understand that a word may have multiple meanings
        - Have a carbon monoxide detector in the home

     NCLEX® Connection: Health Promotion and Maintenance, Developmental Stages and Transitions

chapter 22

Expected Growth and Development

- Physical Development
  - Adolescents gain the final 20% to 25% of height during puberty.
  - Girls grow 5 to 20 cm (2 to 8 in), and 7 to 25 kg (15.5 to 55 lb) during the prepuberty growth spurt.
  - Girls stop growing around 16 to 17 years of age; boys stop growing at around 18 to 20 years of age. Boys grow 10 to 30 cm (4 to 12 in) and 7 to 29 kg (15 to 65 lb) during the prepuberty growth spurt.
  - Girls mature sexually in the following order:
    - Appearance of breast buds.
    - Growth of pubic hair (although some girls may have hair growth prior to breast bud development).
    - Onset of menstruation.
  - Boys mature in the following order:
    - Increase in the size of the testes and scrotum.
    - Appearance of pubic hair.
    - Rapid growth of genitalia.
    - Growth of axillary hair.
    - Appearance of downy hair on the upper lip.
    - Change in voice.
  - Sleep habits change with puberty due to increased metabolism and rapid growth during the adolescent years. Adolescents stay up late, sleep later in the morning, and perhaps sleep longer than they did during the school-age years.
- Cognitive Development
  - Piaget – Formal operations
    - Think at an adult level
    - Think abstractly and deal with principles
    - Evaluate the quality of their own thinking
    - Have a longer attention span
    - Are highly imaginative and idealistic
    - Make decisions through logical operations
    - Are future-oriented
    - Are capable of deductive reasoning
    - Understand how actions of an individual influence others
  - Language – Adolescents develop jargon within the peer group. They communicate one way with the peer group and another way with adults.

- Psychosocial Development
  - Adolescents' stage of psychosocial development, according to Erikson, is identity vs. role confusion.
    - They develop a sense of personal identity that family expectations influence.
      - Group identity – They become part of a peer group that greatly affects behavior.
  - Vocationally – Work habits and plans for college and career begin to solidify.
  - Sexually – Sexual identity develops during adolescence, with increasing interest in the opposite gender, the same gender, or both genders, according to self-identification with heterosexuality, homosexuality, or bisexuality. Self-identification may shift as sexual maturity progresses.
  - Health perceptions – Adolescents often feel invincible to bad outcomes of risky behaviors.
  - Moral Development
    - Conventional law and order – Adolescents do not see rules as absolutes, instead looking at each situation and adjusting the rules. They thrive on flexibility. Not all adolescents attain this level of moral development during these years.
  - Self-Concept Development
    - Adolescents develop a healthy self-concept by having healthy relationships with peers, family, and teachers. Identifying a skill or talent helps them maintain a healthy self-concept. Participation in sports, hobbies, or the community can have a positive outcome.
  - Body-Image Changes
    - Adolescents seem particularly concerned with the body images the media portray. Changes during puberty result in comparisons between adolescents and peers. Parents also give their input for hair styles, dress, and activity. Adolescents require help if depression or eating disorders result due to poor body image.
  - Social Development
    - Peer relationships develop as a support system.
    - Best-friend relationships are more stable and long-lasting than in previous years.
    - Parent-child relationships change to allow more independence.
- Age-Appropriate Activities
  - Nonviolent video games, music, movies
  - Sports, social events
  - Caring for a pet
  - Career-training programs
  - Reading

Health Promotion

- Immunizations
  - Follow the latest Centers for Disease Control and Prevention (CDC) immunization recommendations (see www.cdc.gov) for healthy adolescents. These generally include immunizations against diphtheria, tetanus, pertussis, human papillomavirus, hepatitis A and B, measles, mumps, rubella, varicella, seasonal influenza, and polio, and for some high-risk individuals, meningococcal and pneumococcal infections. The recommendations change periodically, so check them often.

- Health Screenings
  - Scoliosis – Screening for idiopathic scoliosis, a lateral curvature of the spine with no apparent cause, is essential, especially for girls, during the adolescent growth spurt because it is most evident at that time.
- Nutrition
  - Rapid growth and high metabolism require increases in high-quality nutrients. Nutrients that tend to be deficient during this stage of life are iron, calcium, and vitamins A and C.
  - Eating disorders commonly develop during adolescence (more in girls than in boys) due to a fear of being overweight, fad diets, or as a mechanism of maintaining control over some aspect of life. These include:
    - Anorexia nervosa
    - Bulimia nervosa
    - Overeating
  - Advise parents to:
    - Not use food as a reward.
    - Emphasize physical activity.
    - Provide a balanced diet. See www.choosemyplate.gov for nutritional guidelines for adolescents.
    - Teach adolescents to make healthy food selections for meals and snacks.
- Dental health
  - Brush daily.
  - Floss daily.
  - Get regular check-ups.

- Injury Prevention
  - Bodily harm
    - Keep firearms in a locked cabinet or box.
    - Teach proper use of sporting equipment prior to use.
    - Insist on helmet use and/or pads when rollerskating, skateboarding, bicycling, riding scooters, skiing, and during any other activities that increase injury risk.
    - Avoid trampolines.
    - Be aware of changes in mood and monitor for self-harm in at-risk adolescents. Watch for:
      - Poor school performance
      - Lack of interest in things of previous interest.
      - Social isolation
      - Disturbances in sleep or appetite
      - Expression of suicidal thoughts
  - Burns
    - Teach fire safety.
    - Promote sunscreen use.

- ○ Drowning
    - ▪ Teach swimming skills and safety.
- ○ Motor-vehicle injury
    - ▪ Encourage attendance at drivers' education courses.
    - ▪ Emphasize seat belt use.
    - ▪ Discourage use of cell phones, including texting, while driving.
    - ▪ Teach the dangers of combining substance use with driving.
- ○ Substance use disorders
    - ▪ Monitor at-risk adolescents.
    - ▪ Teach adolescents to say "no" to drugs and alcohol.
    - ▪ Present a no-tolerance attitude.
- ○ Sexually transmitted infections (STIs)
    - ▪ Provide education and resources for treatment.
- ○ Pregnancy prevention
    - ▪ Provide education.

APPLICATION EXERCISES

1. A nurse is talking with the father of a 12-year-old boy who is concerned that he hasn't observed any indications that his son is approaching puberty. The nurse should explain that the first sign of sexual maturation in boys is

    A. the appearance of downy hair on the upper lip.

    B. hair growth in the axillae.

    C. enlargement of the testes and the scrotum.

    D. deepening of the voice.

2. A nurse on a pediatric unit is caring for an adolescent who has multiple fractures. Which of the following interventions are appropriate for this client? (Select all that apply.)

    _____ A. Suggest that his parents room in with him.

    _____ B. Provide a television and DVDs for him to watch.

    _____ C. Limit visitors to immediate family.

    _____ D. Devise a regular schedule for inpatient routines.

    _____ E. Allow him to perform his own morning care.

3. A nurse is talking with an adolescent who describes having difficulty dealing with several issues. Which of the following problems the client verbalized should the nurse identify as the priority for further assessment and intervention?

    A. "I kind of like this girl in my class. She doesn't like me back, though, not that way."

    B. "I like hanging out with the guys in the science club, but the jocks pick on them."

    C. "I just don't seem to be any good at anything. I can't play any sports at all."

    D. "My dad wants me to be a lawyer like him, but I don't want to learn all that stuff."

4. A nurse is reviewing the Centers for Disease Control and Prevention's (CDC's) immunization recommendations with the parents of an adolescent. Which of the following recommendations should the nurse include in this discussion? (Select all that apply.)

    _____ A. Rotavirus

    _____ B. Varicella

    _____ C. Herpes zoster

    _____ D. Human papilloma virus

    _____ E. Seasonal influenza

5. A nurse is preparing a wellness presentation for families at a community center. When discussing health screenings for adolescents, which of the following information about scoliosis should the nurse include? (Select all that apply.)

_____ A. Scoliosis is more common among girls than it is among boys.

_____ B. Loss of height is often the first sign of scoliosis.

_____ C. Scoliosis screening is essential during the adolescent growth spurt.

_____ D. Slouching is a common cause of scoliosis, especially in adolescents.

_____ E. Scoliosis is a forward curvature of the spine.

6. A nurse on a pediatric unit is reviewing with a group of nursing students the cognitive developmental milestones to expect from adolescent clients. Use the ATI Active Learning Template: Growth and Development to complete this item. Under Cognitive Development, list at least five cognitive development expectations during adolescence.

APPLICATION EXERCISES KEY

1. A. INCORRECT: Emerging facial hair is a later pubescent change.

    B. INCORRECT: Hair growth in nongenital areas is a later pubescent change.

    C. **CORRECT:** The first prepubescent change in boys is an increase in the size of the testicles along with a thinning and expanding of the scrotum.

    D. INCORRECT: Changing vocal quality is a later pubescent change.

    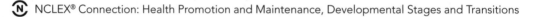 NCLEX® Connection: Health Promotion and Maintenance, Developmental Stages and Transitions

2. A. INCORRECT: Rooming in is more appropriate for younger children.

    B. **CORRECT:** Nonviolent DVDs are appropriate diversional activities for an adolescent.

    C. INCORRECT: There is no reason to restrict visitors. Allowing his friends to visit helps prevent feelings of isolation.

    D. INCORRECT: Flexible routines and activities, such as wearing his own clothes and having his favorite snacks on hand, help adolescents feel more comfortable in inpatient settings.

    E. **CORRECT:** Allowing him to perform his own morning care helps promote a sense of independence.

    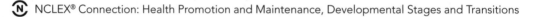 NCLEX® Connection: Health Promotion and Maintenance, Developmental Stages and Transitions

3. A. INCORRECT: It is common for adolescents, who are in the stage Erikson describes as identity vs. role confusion, to face the challenge of forming peer relationships and dating relationships. This problem is not the priority for assessment and intervention.

    B. INCORRECT: It is common for adolescents, who are in the stage Erikson describes as identity vs. role confusion, to face the challenge of becoming part of a peer group and establishing a group identity. This problem is not the priority for assessment and intervention.

    C. **CORRECT:** When using the urgent vs. nonurgent approach to client care, the nurse determines that the counseling priority is the problem that reflects a lack of completion of the previous stage and progression to the current stage of development. According to Erikson, it is a task of the school-age years to develop industry (such as by learning new skills and experiencing achievements in them) vs. inferiority. This adolescent is still struggling with this task and needs assistance in working through that dilemma.

    D. INCORRECT: It is common for adolescents, who are in the stage Erikson describes as identity vs. role confusion, to face the challenge of forming an identity that will lead to higher education and a career. This problem is not the priority for assessment and intervention.

    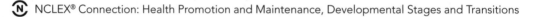 NCLEX® Connection: Health Promotion and Maintenance, Developmental Stages and Transitions

4. A. INCORRECT: The CDC recommends rotavirus immunizations during infancy and not generally beyond 8 months of age.

    B. **CORRECT:** The CDC recommends varicella (chickenpox) immunizations during adolescence.

    C. INCORRECT: The CDC recommends herpes zoster (shingles) immunizations during middle adulthood, typically one dose at age 60 or beyond.

    D. **CORRECT:** The CDC recommends human papilloma virus (genital warts) immunizations during adolescence.

    E. **CORRECT:** The CDC recommends seasonal influenza immunizations during adolescence.

    Ⓝ NCLEX® Connection: Health Promotion and Maintenance, Health Promotion/Disease Prevention

5. A. **CORRECT:** Girls are more likely than boys to have adolescent idiopathic scoliosis.

    B. INCORRECT: Loss of height is often the first sign of osteoporosis. Asymmetry in shoulder or hip height is a sign of scoliosis.

    C. **CORRECT:** Idiopathic scoliosis is most noticeable during the adolescent growth spurt.

    D. INCORRECT: In most cases, scoliosis has no apparent cause.

    E. INCORRECT: Scoliosis is a lateral curvature of the spine.

    Ⓝ NCLEX® Connection: Health Promotion and Maintenance, Health Screening

6. *Using the ATI Active Learning Template: Growth and Development*
    - Cognitive Development
        ○ Think at an adult level
        ○ Think abstractly and deal with principles
        ○ Evaluate the quality of their own thinking
        ○ Have a longer attention span
        ○ Are highly imaginative and idealistic
        ○ Make decisions through logical operations
        ○ Are future-oriented
        ○ Are capable of deductive reasoning
        ○ Understand how actions of an individual influence others

    Ⓝ NCLEX® Connection: Health Promotion and Maintenance, Developmental Stages and Transitions

chapter 23

Expected Growth and Development

- Physical Development
  - Growth has concluded around age 20.
  - Physical senses peak.
  - Cardiac output and efficiency peak.
  - Muscles function optimally at ages 25 to 30.

  - Metabolic rate decreases 2% to 4% every decade after age 20.
  - Libido is high for men.
  - Libido for women peaks during the later part of this stage.
  - Time for childbearing is optimal.
  - Pregnancy-related changes occur.
- Cognitive Development
  - Piaget – Formal operations
    - The young adult years are an optimal time for education – both formal and informal. In young adults:
      - Critical thinking skills improve.
      - Memory peaks in the 20s.
      - There is an increased ability for creative thought.
      - The values/norms of friends (social groups) are relevant.
- Psychosocial Development
  - According to Erikson, young adults must achieve intimacy vs. isolation.
  - Young adults may take on more adult commitments and responsibilities.
  - Young adults' occupational choices relate to:
    - High goals/dreams
    - Exploration/experimentation
  - Moral Development
    - Young adults may personalize values and beliefs.
    - They may base reasoning on ethical fairness principles, such as justice.

- ○ Self-Concept Development
  - ▪ Influences on the formation of a healthy self-concept during the young adult years include:
    - ▫ Avoidance of substance use disorders
    - ▫ Late formation of a family
    - ▫ Frequent interactions with family and friends
    - ▫ Choosing to behave in an ethical manner
- ○ Body-Image Changes
  - ▪ What young adults eat and how much exercise they get affect body image.
  - ▪ Pregnancy-related body image changes may also occur.
- ○ Social Development
  - ▪ Young adults may:
    - ▫ Leave home and establish independent living situation.
    - ▫ Establish close friendships (intimacy).
    - ▫ Transition from being single to being a member of a new family.
    - ▫ Question their ability to parent.
    - ▫ Experience increased anxiety and/or depression, especially after the birth of a child.

Health Promotion

- Young adults are especially at risk for alterations in health from:
  - ○ Substance use disorders
  - ○ Periodontal disease due to poor oral hygiene
  - ○ Unplanned pregnancies – a source of high stress
  - ○ Sexually transmitted infections (STIs)
  - ○ Infertility
  - ○ Work-related injuries or exposures
  - ○ Violent death and injury
- Immunizations
  - ○ Follow the latest Centers for Disease Control and Prevention (CDC) immunization recommendations (see www.cdc.gov). These generally include immunizations against hepatitis A and B, diphtheria, tetanus, pertussis, measles, mumps, rubella, varicella, influenza, human papillomavirus, and pneumococcal and meningococcal infections. The recommendations change periodically, so check them often.
- Health Screenings
  - ○ Young adults should follow age-related guidelines for screening.
- Nutrition
  - ○ Monitor for adequate nutrition and proper physical activity.
  - ○ Women – Monitor calcium intake.
  - ○ See myplate.gov for nutritional recommendations.

- Routine health care visits should include obtaining height, weight, vital signs, and family history; screening for stress; education related to STIs, substance use disorders, and contraception; and encouragement of good nutrition and regular physical activity.

- Injury prevention for young adults includes:

  ○ Avoiding drugs, including alcohol, that can lead to substance use disorders.

  ○ Avoiding driving a vehicle during or after drinking alcohol or taking drugs that impair sensory and motor functions.

  ○ Wearing a seat belt when operating a vehicle.

  ○ Wearing a helmet while bike riding, skiing, and other recreational activities that increase head-injury risk.

  ○ Installing smoke and carbon monoxide detectors in the home.

  ○ Securing firearms in a safe location.

APPLICATION EXERCISES

1. A nurse is teaching a young adult client about health promotion and illness prevention. Which of the following statements by the client indicates an understanding of the teaching?

    A. "I already had my immunizations as a child, so I'm protected in that area."

    B. "It is important to schedule routine health care visits even if I am feeling well."

    C. "If I am having any discomfort, I'll just go to an urgent care center."

    D. "If I am feeling stressed, I will remind myself that this is something I should expect."

2. A nursing instructor is explaining the various stages of the lifespan to a group of nursing students. The nurse should offer which of the following behaviors by a young adult as an example of appropriate psychosocial development?

    A. Becoming actively involved in providing guidance to the next generation

    B. Adjusting to major changes in roles and relationships due to losses

    C. Devoting a great deal of time to establishing an occupation

    D. Finding oneself "sandwiched" in between and being responsible for two generations

3. A nurse is counseling a young adult who describes having difficulty dealing with several issues. Which of the following problems the client verbalized should the nurse identify as the priority for further assessment and intervention?

    A. "I have my own apartment now, but it's not easy living away from my parents."

    B. "It's been so stressful for me to even think about having my own family."

    C. "I don't even know who I am yet, and now I'm supposed to know what to do."

    D. "My girlfriend is pregnant, and I don't think I have what it takes to be a good father."

4. A nurse is reviewing safety precautions with a group of young adults at a community health fair. Which of the following recommendations should the nurse include specifically for this age group? (Select all that apply.)

    _____ A. Install bath rails and grab bars in bathrooms.

    _____ B. Wear a helmet while skiing.

    _____ C. Install a carbon monoxide detector.

    _____ D. Secure firearms in a safe location.

    _____ E. Remove throw rugs from the home.

5. A nurse is reviewing the Centers for Disease Control and Prevention's (CDC's) immunization recommendations with a young adult client. Which of the following recommendations should the nurse include in this discussion? (Select all that apply.)

_____ A. Human papillomavirus

_____ B. Measles, mumps, rubella

_____ C. Varicella

_____ D. *Haemophilus influenzae* type b

_____ E. Polio

6. A nurse is explaining to a group of young adults in a community center what physical and cognitive development characteristics they should expect at this stage of life. Use the Growth and Development ATI Active Learning Template to complete this item. Under Physical Development, list at least five physical development expectations. Under Cognitive Development, list at least three cognitive development expectations during young adulthood.

APPLICATION EXERCISES KEY

1. A. INCORRECT: For protection against a wide variety of communicable illnesses, adults should obtain the immunizations the CDC recommends throughout the lifespan, not just during childhood.

    B. **CORRECT:** Young adulthood is a time of relative health, but routine screenings and health care visits are still important.

    C. INCORRECT: Urgent care centers offer limited services, typically for acute injuries or problems that cannot wait until a primary care provider is available. Young adults should establish a relationship with a primary care provider to consult for nonurgent health problems.

    D. INCORRECT: Although it is true that stress is inevitable, chronic stress can lead to severe health alterations. Young adults who have stress that is recurrent or escalating should seek medical care.

    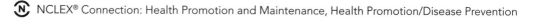 NCLEX® Connection: Health Promotion and Maintenance, Health Promotion/Disease Prevention

2. A. INCORRECT: Active involvement in the next generation is a developmental task for middle adults.

    B. INCORRECT: Adjusting to major role changes is a developmental task for older adults.

    C. **CORRECT:** Exploring career options and then establishing oneself in a specific occupation is a major developmental task for a young adult.

    D. INCORRECT: Assuming responsibility for the previous as well as the next generation is a developmental task for middle adults.

    NCLEX® Connection: Health Promotion and Maintenance, Developmental Stages and Transitions

3. A. INCORRECT: It is common for young adults to face the challenge of leaving home and establishing independent living. This problem is not the priority for assessment and intervention.

    B. INCORRECT: It is common for young adults to face the challenge of transitioning from being single to being a member of a new family. This problem is not the priority for assessment and intervention.

    C. **CORRECT:** When using the urgent vs nonurgent approach to client care, the nurse determines that the counseling priority is the problem that reflects a lack of completion of the previous stage and progression to the current stage of development. According to Erikson, it is a task of adolescence to develop identity vs role confusion. This young adult is still struggling with this task and needs assistance in working through that dilemma.

    D. INCORRECT: It is common for young adults to face the challenge involved in questioning their ability to parent. This problem is not the priority for assessment and intervention.

    NCLEX® Connection: Health Promotion and Maintenance, Developmental Stages and Transitions

4. A. INCORRECT: Although bath rails and grab bars add a measure of safety to bathing activities, this recommendation is specific for the older adult population due to their risk for falls.

    B. **CORRECT:** Wearing a helmet while skiing helps reduce the risk of head injury. Although it applies to other age groups, many young adults engage in winter sports, so this is an age-appropriate recommendation for this developmental group.

    C. **CORRECT:** Having a carbon monoxide detector in the home is an essential safety precaution for young adults as well as for all other developmental stages.

    D. **CORRECT:** Securing firearms in a safe location helps reduce the risk of accidental gunshot injuries. Although it applies to all age groups, many young adults own firearms, so this is an age-appropriate recommendation for this developmental group.

    E. INCORRECT: Although throw rugs can pose a safety hazard, this recommendation is specific for the older adult population due to their risk for falls.

    Ⓝ NCLEX® Connection: Health Promotion and Maintenance, Developmental Stages and Transitions

5. A. **CORRECT:** The CDC recommends human papillomavirus immunizations during adulthood. This virus, which causes genital warts, is most prevalent during adolescence and young adulthood.

    B. **CORRECT:** The CDC recommends measles, mumps, rubella immunizations during adulthood.

    C. **CORRECT:** The CDC recommends varicella (chickenpox) immunizations during adulthood.

    D. INCORRECT: The CDC recommends *Haemophilus influenzae* type b immunizations during infancy and not generally beyond 18 months of age.

    E. INCORRECT: The CDC recommends polio immunizations during childhood, but not generally beyond 18 years.

    Ⓝ NCLEX® Connection: Health Promotion and Maintenance, Health Promotion/Disease Prevention

6. *Use the Growth and Development ATI Active Learning Template*
    - Physical Development
      - Completion of growth
      - Peak in physical senses
      - Peak in cardiac output, efficiency
      - Optimal muscle function
      - Gradual decline in metabolic rate
      - High libido (men)
      - Eventual peak in libido (women)
      - Optimal childbearing
      - Pregnancy-related changes
    - Cognitive Development
      - Improvement in critical thinking
      - Peak in memory
      - Increased ability for creative thought
      - Relevance of values/norms of friends

    Ⓝ NCLEX® Connection: Health Promotion and Maintenance, Developmental Stages and Transitions

Expected Growth and Development

- Physical Development
  - Decreases in:
    - Skin turgor and moisture
    - Subcutaneous fat
    - Melanin in hair (graying)
    - Hair
    - Visual acuity, especially for near vision
    - Auditory acuity, especially for high-pitched sounds
    - Sense of taste
    - Skeletal muscle mass
    - Height
    - Calcium/bone density
    - Blood vessel elasticity
    - Respiratory vital capacity
    - Large intestine muscle tone
    - Gastric secretions
    - Estrogen/testosterone
    - Glucose tolerance
- Cognitive Development
  - Piaget – Formal operations
    - Reaction time and speed of performance slow slightly.
    - Memory is intact.
    - Crystallized intelligence remains (stored knowledge).
    - Fluid intelligence (how to learn and process new information) declines slightly.

- Psychosocial Development
  - According to Erikson, middle adults must achieve generativity vs. stagnation.
    - Middle adults strive for generativity.
      - Use life as an opportunity for creativity and productivity.
      - Have concern for others.
      - Consider parenting an important task.
      - Contribute to the well-being of the next generation.
      - Strive to do well in one's own environment.
      - Adjust to changes in physical appearance and abilities.
  - Moral Development
    - Religious maturity
      - Spiritual beliefs and religion may take on added importance.
      - Middle adults may become more secure in their convictions.
      - Middle adults often have advanced moral development.
  - Self-Concept Development
    - Some middle adults have issues related to:
      - Menopause
      - Sexuality
      - Depression
      - Irritability
      - Difficulty with sexual identity
      - Job performance and ability to provide support
      - Marital changes with the death of a spouse or divorce
  - Body Image Changes
    - Women – Symptoms of menopause can represent a:
      - Loss of the reproductive role or femininity
      - New interest in intimacy
    - Men – Decreasing strength can be frustrating or frightening.
    - Sex drive can decrease as a result of declining hormones, chronic disorders, or medications.
    - Changes in physical appearance can raise concerns about desirability.
  - Social Development
    - Need to maintain and strengthen intimacy.
    - Provide assistance to aging parents, adult children, and grandchildren.

Health Promotion

- Middle adults are especially at risk for alterations in health from:
  - Obesity, type 2 diabetes mellitus
  - Cardiovascular disease
  - Cancer
  - Substance use disorders (alcoholism)
  - Psychosocial stressors
- Immunizations
  - Follow the latest Centers for Disease Control and Prevention (CDC) immunization recommendations (see www.cdc.gov). These generally include immunizations against diphtheria, tetanus, pertussis, varicella, seasonal influenza, and herpes zoster, and for some high-risk individuals, measles, mumps, rubella, hepatitis A and B, and pneumococcal and meningococcal infections. The recommendations change periodically, so check them often.
- Health Screenings
  - Middle adults should follow age-related guidelines for screening.
  - Other screenings include:
    - Dual-energy x-ray absorptiometry (DEXA) screening for osteoporosis
    - Eye examination for glaucoma and other disorders every 2 to 3 years or annually depending on provider.
    - Mental health screening for depression
- Nutrition
  - See www.choosemyplate.gov for nutritional recommendations.
  - Nutrition counseling for middle adults generally includes:
    - Obtaining adequate protein.
    - Increasing the consumption of whole grains and fresh fruits and vegetables.
    - Limiting fat and cholesterol.
    - Increasing vitamin D and calcium supplementation (especially for women).
- Injury Prevention
  - Avoid drugs, including alcohol, that can lead to substance use disorders.
  - Avoid driving a vehicle during or after drinking alcohol or taking drugs that impair sensory and motor functions.
  - Wear a seat belt when operating a vehicle.
  - Wear a helmet while bike riding, skiing, and other recreational activities that increase head-injury risk.
  - Install smoke and carbon monoxide detectors in the home.
  - Secure firearms in a safe location.

APPLICATION EXERCISES

1. A nursing instructor is explaining the various stages of the lifespan to a group of nursing students. The nurse should offer which of the following behaviors by a young adult as an example of accomplishing Erikson's tasks for psychosocial development during middle adulthood?

    A. The client evaluates his behavior after a social interaction.

    B. The client states he is learning to trust others.

    C. The client wishes to find meaningful friendships.

    D. The client expresses concerns about the next generation.

2. A nurse is collecting data to evaluate a middle adult's psychosocial development. The nurse should expect middle adults to demonstrate which of the following capabilities? (Select all that apply.)

_____ A. Develop an acceptance of diminished strength and increased dependence on others.

_____ B. Feel frustrated that time is too short for attempting to start another life.

_____ C. Welcome opportunities to be creative and productive.

_____ D. Commit to finding friendship and companionship.

_____ E. Become involved with community issues and activities.

3. A nurse is collecting history and physical examination data from a middle adult. The nurse should expect to find decreases in which of the following physiologic functions? (Select all that apply.)

_____ A. Metabolism

_____ B. Ability to hear low-pitched sounds

_____ C. Gastric secretion

_____ D. Far vision

_____ E. Glomerular filtration

4. A nurse is reviewing the Centers for Disease Control and Prevention's (CDC's) immunization recommendations with a middle adult client. Which of the following recommendations should the nurse include in this discussion? (Select all that apply.)

_____ A. *Haemophilus influenzae* type b

_____ B. Varicella

_____ C. Herpes zoster

_____ D. Human papilloma virus

_____ E. Seasonal influenza

5. A nurse is counseling a middle adult who describes having difficulty dealing with several issues. Which of the following problems the client verbalized should the nurse identify as the priority for further assessment and intervention?

A. "I am struggling to accept that my parents are aging and need so much help."

B. "It's been so stressful for me to think about having intimate relationships."

C. "I know I should volunteer my time for a good cause, but maybe I'm just selfish."

D. "I love my grandchildren, but my son expects me to relive my parenting days."

6. A nurse is explaining to a group of middle adults in a community center what moral and cognitive development characteristics they should expect at this stage of life. Use the ATI Active Learning Template: Growth and Development to complete this item to include the following:

A. Cognitive Development:
  • List at least two moral development expectations during middle adulthood.
  • List at least five cognitive development expectations during middle adulthood.

APPLICATION EXERCISES KEY

1. A. INCORRECT: This is a task middle adults should have accomplished to master an earlier developmental stage.

    B. INCORRECT: This is a task middle adults should have accomplished to master an earlier developmental stage.

    C. INCORRECT: This is a task middle adults should have accomplished to master an earlier developmental stage.

    D. **CORRECT:** The task for a middle adult is generativity vs. stagnation. Concern for the next generation is a positive sign that the middle adult is meeting the task.

    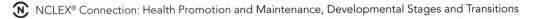 NCLEX® Connection: Health Promotion and Maintenance, Developmental Stages and Transitions

2. A. INCORRECT: Acceptance of diminished strength and increased dependence is a developmental task crucial for older adults.

    B. INCORRECT: Feeling frustrated that time is too short affects adults who are having difficulties with the developmental tasks of middle age.

    C. **CORRECT:** Psychosocially healthy middle adults accept life's opportunities for creativity and productivity and use these opportunities for achieving Erikson's stage of generativity vs. stagnation.

    D. INCORRECT: Seeking and forming friendships is a developmental task crucial for young adults.

    E. **CORRECT:** Psychosocially healthy middle adults achieve Erikson's stage of generativity vs. stagnation by contributing to future generations through community involvement as well as teaching and parenting.

    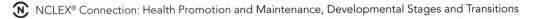 NCLEX® Connection: Health Promotion and Maintenance, Health Screening

3. A. **CORRECT:** In middle adulthood, metabolism declines and weight gain is likely.

    B. INCORRECT: In middle adulthood, the ability to hear high-pitched sounds declines.

    C. **CORRECT:** In middle adulthood, decreases in secretions of bicarbonate and gastric mucus begin and persist into older age. This increases the risk of peptic ulcer disease.

    D. INCORRECT: In middle adulthood, near vision declines (presbyopia).

    E. **CORRECT:** Middle adults begin to lose nephron units, which results in a decline in glomerular filtration rates.

    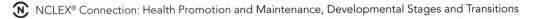 NCLEX® Connection: Health Promotion and Maintenance, Health Promotion/Disease Prevention

4. A. INCORRECT: The CDC recommends *Haemophilus influenzae* type b immunizations during infancy and not generally beyond 18 months of age

    B. **CORRECT:** The CDC recommends varicella (chickenpox) immunizations during middle adulthood.

    C. **CORRECT:** The CDC recommends herpes zoster (shingles) immunizations during middle adulthood, typically one dose at age 60 or beyond.

    D. INCORRECT: The CDC recommends human papilloma virus (genital warts) immunizations during adolescence and young adulthood.

    E. **CORRECT:** The CDC recommends seasonal influenza immunizations during middle adulthood.

    (N) NCLEX® Connection: Basic Care and Comfort, Nutrition and Oral Hydration

5. A. INCORRECT: It is common for middle adults to face the challenge involved in adjusting to and caring for aging parents. This problem is not the priority for assessment and intervention.

    B. **CORRECT:** When using the urgent vs. nonurgent approach to client care, the nurse determines that the counseling priority is the problem that reflects a lack of completion of the previous stage and progression to the current stage of development. According to Erikson, it is a task of young adulthood to develop intimacy vs. isolation. This middle adult is still struggling with this task and needs assistance in working through searching for and developing intimate relationships with others.

    C. INCORRECT: It is common for middle adults to face the challenge involved in contributing to their community. This problem is not the priority for assessment and intervention.

    D. INCORRECT: It is common for middle adults to face the challenge involved in questioning their ability to contribute to future generations in a grandparenting role. This problem is not the priority for assessment and intervention.

    (N) NCLEX® Connection: Health Promotion and Maintenance, Developmental Stages and Transitions

6. *Using the ATI Active Learning Template: Growth and Development*
    A. Cognitive Development
       - Moral Development
         - Spiritual beliefs and religion may take on added importance.
         - Middle adults may become more secure in their convictions.
         - Middle adults often have advanced moral development.
       - Cognitive Development
         - Reaction time and speed of performance slow slightly.
         - Memory is intact.
         - Crystallized intelligence remains (stored knowledge).
         - Fluid intelligence (how to learn and process new information) declines slightly.

    (N) NCLEX® Connection: Safety and Infection Control, Accident/Error/Injury Prevention

chapter 25

Expected Growth and Development

- Physical Development
  - Physical changes related to older adults
    - A decrease in skin turgor, subcutaneous fat, and connective tissue (dermis), which leads to wrinkles and dry, transparent skin
    - A loss of subcutaneous fat, which makes it more difficult for older adults to adjust to cold temperatures
    - Thinning and graying of the hair, as well as a more sparse distribution
    - Thickening of the fingernails and toenails
    - A decrease in chest wall movement, vital capacity, and cilia, which increases the risk for respiratory infections
    - A slower reaction time
    - A decrease in touch, smell, and taste sensations
    - A decrease in the production of saliva
    - A decline in visual acuity
    - A decrease in the ability for the eyes to adjust from light to dark leading to night blindness, which is especially dangerous when driving
    - An inability to hear high-pitched sounds (presbycusis)
    - A decrease in height due to intervertebral disk changes
    - A decrease in muscle strength and tone
    - A decrease in digestive enzymes
    - A decrease in intestinal motility, which can lead to an increase in the risk of constipation
    - An increase in dental problems
    - Decalcification of bones
    - Degeneration of joints
    - A decrease in bladder capacity
    - Prostate hypertrophy in men
    - A decline in estrogen or testosterone production
    - A decline in triiodothyronine (T3) production, yet overall function remains effective
    - Decrease in sensitivity of tissue cells to insulin
    - Atrophy of breast tissue in women

- Cognitive Development
  - Piaget – formal operations
  - Many older adults maintain their cognitive function. There is some decline in speed of the cognitive function versus cognitive ability.
  - A number of factors influence older adults' abilities to function, such as overall health, the number of stressors, and lifelong mental well-being.
  - Slowed neurotransmission, vascular circulation impairment, disease states, poor nutrition, and structural brain changes can result in the following cognitive disorders:
    - Delirium – Acute, temporary, and usually relates to other physiologic problems. Delirium is often the first symptom of infection (urinary tract infection) in older adults.
    - Dementia – Chronic, progressive, and possibly with an unknown cause (Alzheimer's disease, vascular dementia).
    - Depression – Chronic, acute, or gradual onset (present for at least 6 weeks).
- Psychosocial Development
  - Older adults' stage of psychosocial development, according to Erikson, is integrity vs. despair.
  - Older adults need to:
    - Adjust to lifestyle changes related to retirement (decrease in income, living situation, loss of work role).
    - Adapt to changes in family structure (may be role reversal in later years).
    - Deal with multiple losses (death of a spouse, friends, siblings).
    - Face death.
  - Self-Concept Development
    - Older adults face difficulties in the area of self-concept, which include:
      - Seeing oneself as an aging person.
      - Finding ways to maintain a good quality of life.
      - Becoming more dependent on others for activities of daily living.
  - Body Image Changes
    - Adjustments to decreases in physical strength and endurance may be difficult, especially for older adults who are cognitively active and engaged. Many older adults feel frustrated that their bodies are limiting what they desire to do.
  - Social Development
    - Find ways to remain socially active and to overcome isolation.
    - Maintain sexual health.

Health Promotion

- Health Risks
  - Cardiovascular diseases that can affect older adults
    - Coronary artery disease
    - Hypertension
    - Cerebrovascular accident

- ○ Factors affecting mobility of older adults
  - ▪ Arthritis
  - ▪ Osteoporosis
  - ▪ Falls
- ○ Mental health disorders that can affect older adults
  - ▪ Depression
  - ▪ Dementia
  - ▪ Suicide
- ○ Other disorders that can affect older adults
  - ▪ Diabetes mellitus
  - ▪ Cancer
  - ▪ Incontinence
  - ▪ Abuse and neglect
  - ▪ Cataracts
  - ▪ Alcoholism
  - ▪ Pain

Q EBP

- Immunizations
  - ○ Follow the latest Centers for Disease Control and Prevention (CDC) immunization recommendations (www.cdc.gov) for healthy older adults. These generally include:
    - ▪ Immunizations against diphtheria, tetanus, pertussis, varicella, seasonal influenza, herpes zoster, and pneumococcal infections.
    - ▪ Immunizations against measles, mumps, rubella, hepatitis A and B, and meningococcal infections for high-risk individuals.
  - ○ Recommendations change periodically, so check them often.
- Health Screenings
  - ○ Older adults should follow age-related guidelines for screening.
  - ○ Other screenings
    - ▪ Dual-energy x-ray absorptiometry (DEXA) scanning for osteoporosis
    - ▪ Eye examination for glaucoma and other disorders every 2 to 3 years or annually
    - ▪ Mental health screening for depression
- Nutrition
  - ○ In addition to gastrointestinal alterations, other factors influence nutrition in older adults.
    - ▪ Difficulty getting to and from the supermarket to shop for food
    - ▪ A low income
    - ▪ Impaired mobility
    - ▪ Depression or dementia
    - ▪ Social isolation (preparing a meal for one person and eating alone)
    - ▪ Medications that alter taste or appetite

- Prescribed diets that are unappealing
- Incontinence that may cause the person to limit fluid intake
- Constipation

○ Metabolic rates and activity decline as individuals age; therefore, total caloric intake should decrease to maintain a healthy weight. With the reduction of total calorie intake, it becomes even more important that the calories older adults consume be of good nutritional value.

○ Go to www.choosemyplate.gov for nutritional recommendations.

○ Nutritional recommendations for older adults

- Increasing the intake of vitamins D, B$_{12}$, E, folate, fiber, and calcium
- Increasing fluid intake to minimize the risk of dehydration and prevent constipation
- Taking a low-dose multivitamin along with mineral supplementation
- Limiting sodium intake

- Psychosocial interventions to improve self-concept and alleviate social isolation for older adults

○ Therapeutic communication

○ Touch

○ Reality orientation

○ Validation therapy

○ Reminiscence therapy

○ Attending to physical appearance

○ Assistive devices (canes, walkers, hearing aids)

- Injury Prevention

○ Install bath rails, grab bars, and handrails on stairways.

○ Remove throw rugs.

○ Eliminate clutter from walkways and hallways.

○ Remove extension and phone cords from walkways and hallways.

○ Instruct clients about how to properly use ambulation-assistive devices (walkers, canes).

○ Teach clients about safe medication use.

○ Ensure adequate lighting.

○ Remind clients to wear eyeglasses and hearing aids.

○ Avoid drugs, including alcohol. Prevent substance use disorders.

○ Avoid driving a vehicle during or after drinking alcohol or taking drugs that impair sensory and motor functions.

○ Wear a seat belt when operating a vehicle.

○ Wear a helmet while bike riding, skiing, and other recreational activities that increase the risk of head injury.

○ Install smoke and carbon monoxide detectors in the home.

○ Secure firearms in a safe location.

APPLICATION EXERCISES

1. A nurse is counseling an older adult who describes having difficulty dealing with several issues. Which of the following problems verbalized by the client should the nurse identify as the priority?

    A. "I spent my whole life dreaming about retirement, and now I wish I had my job back."

    B. "It's been so stressful for me to have to depend on my son to help around the house."

    C. "I just heard my friend Al died. That's the third one in 3 months."

    D. "I keep forgetting which medications I have taken during the day."

2. A nurse is admitting an older adult client who has lost 4.5 kg (9.9 lb) since his last admission 6 months ago. Which of the following questions should the nurse ask to investigate the source of his weight loss? (Select all that apply.)

    _____ A. "Do you eat alone or with someone?"

    _____ B. "Do you watch television while eating your meals?"

    _____ C. "Have you started any new medications in the past 6 months?"

    _____ D. "What foods have you eaten within the past 24 hours?"

    _____ E. "Are you on a fixed income?"

3. A nurse is planning a presentation to a group of older adults at a senior community center about the essential screening tests and preventive procedures during this stage of life. Which of the following should the nurse include? (Select all that apply.)

    _____ A. Human papilloma virus (HPV) immunization

    _____ B. Pneumococcal immunization

    _____ C. Eye examination

    _____ D. Mental health screening

    _____ E. Dual-energy x-ray absorptiometry (DEXA) scanning

4. A nurse is talking with an older adult client about improving her nutritional status. Which of the following interventions should the nurse recommend? (Select all that apply.)

_____ A. Increase iron intake to prevent anemia.

_____ B. Decrease fluid intake to prevent urinary incontinence.

_____ C. Increase calcium intake to prevent osteoporosis.

_____ D. Limit sodium intake to prevent edema.

_____ E. Increase fiber intake to prevent constipation.

5. A nurse is collecting data from an older adult client as part of a comprehensive physical examination. Which of the following findings should the nurse expect as changes associated with aging? (Select all that apply.)

_____ A. Skin thickening

_____ B. Decreased height

_____ C. Increased saliva production

_____ D. Nail thickening

_____ E. Decreased bladder capacity

6. A nurse is reviewing safety precautions for older adults with a group of home health care nursing assistants. Use the ATI Active Learning Template: Growth and Development to complete this item. Under Injury Prevention, list at least 10 safety recommendations for older adults.

APPLICATION EXERCISES KEY

1. A. INCORRECT: The client is at risk for social isolation and loss of independence because of retirement. However, another issue is the priority.

    B. INCORRECT: The client is at risk for loss of independence and reduced self-esteem due to dependence upon his son. However, another issue is the priority.

    C. INCORRECT: The client is at risk for social isolation due to the loss of a friend. However, another issue is the priority.

    D. **CORRECT:** The greatest risk to this client is injury from overdosing or underdosing his medications due to loss of short-term memory. The priority issue for the nurse is to assist the client to implement safe medication strategies. The nurse should assist the client to use a pill organizer to help him remember to take his medications and to keep a list of all current medications.

    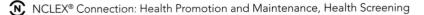 NCLEX® Connection: Health Promotion and Maintenance, Developmental Stages and Transitions

2. A. **CORRECT:** Clients who eat alone are more likely to skip or skimp on meals.

    B. INCORRECT: Determining if the client watches TV while eating is not relevant in this situation.

    C. **CORRECT:** Many medications affect the senses of taste and smell, as well as the abilities to tolerate food and to absorb nutrients.

    D. **CORRECT:** Asking about food the client ate within the last 24 hr will provide a basis to determine what he typically eats in a 24-hr period.

    E. **CORRECT:** Clients who receive a fixed income may not have enough money to buy food.

    NCLEX® Connection: Health Promotion and Maintenance, Health Screening

3. A. INCORRECT: HPV typically affects people in their teens and early 20s, so it is not a recommendation for older adults.

    B. **CORRECT:** Older adults are especially susceptible to pneumococcal infections, so this is an essential preventive measure for this stage of life.

    C. **CORRECT:** Screening for glaucoma via regular eye examinations is essential for older adults.

    D. **CORRECT:** Screening for depression via mental health assessments is essential for older adults.

    E. **CORRECT:** Screening for osteoporosis via DEXA scanning is essential for older adults.

    NCLEX® Connection: Health Promotion and Maintenance, Health Promotion/Disease Prevention

4.　A.　INCORRECT: Older adult women do not need as much iron as they did when they were menstruating.

　　B.　INCORRECT: Older adults should increase fluid intake to prevent dehydration and constipation.

　　C.　**CORRECT:** Older adults are at risk for osteoporosis. Increasing calcium intake is one way to help prevent it.

　　D.　**CORRECT:** Older adults are at risk for edema and hypertension. Limiting sodium intake is one way to help prevent them.

　　E.　**CORRECT:** Older adults should increase fiber intake to prevent constipation.

　　Ⓝ NCLEX® Connection: Basic Care and Comfort, Nutrition and Oral Hydration

5.　A.　INCORRECT: Aging brings decreases in skin turgor, subcutaneous fat, and connective tissue (dermis), which leads to wrinkles and dry, thin, transparent skin.

　　B.　**CORRECT:** With aging, height decreases due to the thinning of intervertebral disks.

　　C.　INCORRECT: Saliva production diminishes with age, making xerostomia (dry mouth) a common problem.

　　D.　**CORRECT:** Aging brings thickening of the nails of the fingers and toes, and also changes their shape, color, and growth rate.

　　E.　**CORRECT:** While young adults have a bladder capacity of about 500 to 600 mL, older adults have a capacity of about 250 mL.

　　Ⓝ NCLEX® Connection: Health Promotion and Maintenance, Developmental Stages and Transitions

6.　*Using the ATI Active Learning Template: Growth and Development*
　　• Injury Prevention
　　　○ Install bath rails, grab bars, and handrails on stairways.
　　　○ Teach clients about safe medication use.
　　　○ Remove throw rugs.
　　　○ Eliminate clutter from walkways and hallways.
　　　○ Remove extension and phone cords from walkways and hallways.
　　　○ Instruct about how to use ambulation-assistive devices (walkers, canes).
　　　○ Ensure adequate lighting.
　　　○ Remind clients to wear eyeglasses and hearing aids.
　　　○ Avoid drugs, including alcohol, to prevent substance use disorders.
　　　○ Avoid driving a vehicle during or after drinking alcohol or taking drugs that impair sensory and motor functions.
　　　○ Wear a seat belt when operating a vehicle.
　　　○ Wear a helmet while bike riding, skiing, and other recreational activities that increase head-injury risk.
　　　○ Install smoke and carbon monoxide detectors in the home.
　　　○ Secure firearms in a safe location.

　　Ⓝ NCLEX® Connection: Safety and Infection Control, Accident/Error/Injury Prevention

UNIT 2   Health Promotion

SECTION: HEALTH ASSESSMENT

› Data Collection and General Survey
› Vital Signs
› Head and Neck
› Thorax, Heart, and Abdomen
› Integumentary and Peripheral Vascular Systems
› Musculoskeletal and Neurosensory Systems

NCLEX® CONNECTIONS

When reviewing the chapters in this unit, keep in mind the relevant sections of the NCLEX® outline, in particular:

Client Needs: Health Promotion and Maintenance	Client Needs: Management of Care	Client Needs: Reduction of Risk Potential

› Relevant topics/tasks include:
 » Aging Process
   › Provide care and education that meets the special needs of the adult client ages 19 to 64 years.
 » Developmental Stages and Transitions
   › Compare the client's development to expected age/developmental stage and report any deviations.
 » Health and Wellness
   › Encourage the client's participation in appropriate behavior modification programs related to health and wellness.
	› Relevant topics/tasks include:
	 » Confidentiality/Information Security
	   › Maintain the client's confidentiality/privacy.
		› Relevant topics/tasks include:
		 » System Specific Assessment
		   › Perform a focused assessment and reassessment.

chapter 26

Overview

- Data collection includes obtaining subjective and objective information from clients.

- The health history provides subjective data.

- The physical assessment and diagnostic tests provide objective data.

Interviewing Techniques

- Standardized formats are a framework for obtaining information about clients' physical, developmental, emotional, intellectual, social, and spiritual dimensions.

- Therapeutic techniques for health assessment foster communication and create an environment conducive to an optimal health assessment experience.

- Therapeutic communication helps develop rapport with clients. The techniques encourage a trusting relationship, whereby clients feel comfortable telling their stories. Begin with the purpose of the interview, gather information, and then conclude the interview by summarizing the findings.

  ○ Introduce yourself and the various parts of the assessment.

  ○ Determine what the client wants you to call them.

  ○ Allow more time for responses from older adults.

  ○ Make sure the client is comfortable (room temperature, chair).

  ○ When possible, start by asking for the health history, performing the general survey, and measuring vital signs to build rapport prior to moving on to more sensitive parts of the examination.

  ○ Reduce environmental noises (TV, radio, visitors talking) to enhance communication and eliminate distractions.

  ○ Ensure understanding by obtaining interpretive services for clients who have language or other communication barriers.

  ○ Use therapeutic communication techniques including:

    ▪ Active listening – Shows clients that they have your undivided attention.

    ▪ Open-ended questions – Use initially to encourage clients to tell their story in their own way. Use terminology clients can understand.

- Clarifying – Question clients about specific details in greater depth or directing them toward relevant parts of the history.
  - Back channeling – Use active listening phrases such as "Go on" and "Tell me more" to convey interest and to prompt disclosure of the entire story.
  - Probing – Ask more open-ended questions such as "What else would you like to add to that?" to help obtain comprehensive information.
  - Closed-ended questions – Ask questions that require yes or no answers to clarify information, such as "Do you have any pain when you cannot sleep?"
  - Summarizing – Validate the accuracy of the story.
- Avoid using medical jargon, giving advice, ignoring feelings, and offering false reassurance.

Components of the Health History

- The health history provides subjective data about health status.

HEALTH HISTORY	
Demographic information	› Identifying data include: » Name, address, contact information » Birth date, age » Gender » Race, ethnicity » Marital status » Occupation, employment status » Insurance » Emergency contact information » Family, others living at home » Advance directives
Source of history	› Client, family members, other medical records, other providers › Reliability of the historian
Chief concern	› A brief statement in the client's own words of why he is seeking care
History of present illness	› A detailed, chronological description of why the client seeks care › Details about the symptom(s), such as location, quality, quantity, setting, timing, alleviating or aggravating factors, associated phenomena
Past health history and current health status	› Childhood illnesses, both communicable and chronic › Medical, surgical, obstetrical, gynecological, psychiatric history including time frames, diagnoses, hospitalizations, treatments › Current immunization status, dates and results of any screening tests › Allergies to medication, environment, food › Current medications including prescription, over-the-counter, vitamins, supplements, herbal remedies, time of last dose(s)
Family history	› Health information of immediate relatives such as grandparents, parents, siblings, children, grandchildren › Current ages or age at death, acute and chronic disorders in family members
Psychosocial history	› Relationships, support systems, concerns about living or work situations, financial status, ability to perform activities of daily living, spiritual health
Health promotion behaviors	› Exercise/activity, diet, sun exposure, wearing of safety equipment, substance use, environmental exposures, stress, sleep patterns, related coping measures › Awareness of risks for heart disease, cancer, diabetes mellitus, cerebrovascular accident

Review of Systems

- An extensive review of systems ascertains information about the functioning of all body systems and related or other health problems

SYSTEM	QUESTIONS TO ASK
Integumentary	› Do you have any skin diseases? › Do you have any itching, bruising, lumps, hair loss, nail changes, or sores? › Do you have any allergies? › How do you care for your hair, skin, and nails? › Do you use lotions, soaps, or sunscreen or wear protective clothing?
Head and neck	› Do you get headaches? If so, how often? (Ask about and note onset, duration, character, pattern, and associated symptoms.) » What do you do to relieve the pain? › Have you ever had a head injury? › Can you move your head and shoulders with ease? › Are any of your lymph nodes swollen? (If so, rule out recent colds or viral infections.) › Have you noticed any unusual facial movements? › Does anyone in your family have thyroid disease?
Eyes	› How is your vision? › Have you noticed any changes in your vision? › Do you ever have any thick fluid draining from your eyes? › Do you wear glasses? Contact lenses? › When was your last eye examination? › Does anyone in your family have any eye disorders? › Do you have diabetes?
Ears, nose, mouth, and throat	› How well do you hear? › Have you noticed any changes in your hearing? › Have other people commented that you aren't hearing what they say? › Do you wear hearing aids? › Do you ever have ringing or buzzing in your ears, drainage, dizziness, or pain? › Have you had ear infections? › How do you clean your ears? › Are you having any pain, stuffiness, or fluid draining from your nose? › Do you have nosebleeds? › Have you noticed any change in your sense of smell or taste? › How often do you go to the dentist? › Do you have dentures or retainers? › Do you have any problems with your gums, like bleeding or soreness? › Do you have any difficulty swallowing or problems with hoarseness or a sore throat? › Do you have allergies? › Do you use nasal sprays? › Do you snore?

SYSTEM	QUESTIONS TO ASK
Breasts	› Do you perform breast self-examinations? For women: What time of the month do you perform it? › Do you have any tenderness, lumps, thickening, pain, drainage, distortion, or change in breast size, or any retraction or scaling of the nipples? › Has anyone in your family had breast cancer? › Are you aware of breast cancer risks? › For clients over 40: How often do you get a mammogram?
Respiratory	› Do you have any difficulties breathing? › Do you breathe easier in any particular position? › Are you ever short of breath? › Have you recently been around anyone who has a cough, cold, or influenza? › Do you receive an influenza vaccine every year? › Have you had the pneumonia vaccine? › Do you smoke? If yes, for how long and how much? Are you interested in quitting? › Are you exposed to second-hand smoke? › Do you have environmental allergies? › Has anyone in your family had lung cancer or tuberculosis? › Have you been exposed to tuberculosis? › Have you had a tuberculosis test?
Cardiovascular	› Do you have any problems with your heart? › Do you take any medications for your heart? › Do you ever have pain in your chest? Do you also feel it in your arms, neck, or jaw? › Do you have high cholesterol or high blood pressure? › Do you have any swelling in your feet and ankles? › Do you cough frequently? › Are you familiar with the risk factors for heart disease?
Gastrointestinal	› Do you have any problems with your stomach, such as nausea, vomiting, heartburn, or pain? › Do you have any problems with your bowels, such as diarrhea or constipation? › When was your last bowel movement? › Do you ever use laxatives or enemas? › Have you had any black or tarry stools? › Do you take aspirin or ibuprofen? If so, how often? › Do you have any abdominal or lower back pain or tenderness? › Have you had any recent weight changes? › Do you have any swallowing difficulties? › Do you drink alcohol? If so, how much? › For clients over 50: Have you had a colonoscopy? › Do you know the signs and symptoms of colon cancer? › What is your typical day's intake of food and fluid? › Do you have any dietary restrictions, food intolerances, or special practices?

SYSTEM	QUESTIONS TO ASK
Genitourinary	› Do you have any difficulties with urination, such as burning, leakage or loss of urine, urgency, frequency, waking up at night to urinate, or hesitancy? › Have you noticed any change in the color of your urine? › Have you noticed any changes in your menstrual cycle? › Have you had pain during intercourse? › Have you had any sexual problems? › Have you had any pain in your scrotum or testes?
Musculoskeletal	› Have you noticed any pain in your joints or muscles? › Do you have any weakness or twitching? › Have you had any recent falls? › Are you able to care for yourself? › Do you exercise or participate in sports? › For postmenopausal women: What was your maximum height? › For postmenopausal women: Do you take calcium supplements?
Neurological	› Have you noticed any change in your vision, speech, ability to think clearly, or loss of or change in memory? › Do you have any dizziness or headaches? › Do you ever have seizures? If so, what triggers them? › Do you ever have any weakness, tremors, numbness, or tingling anywhere? If so, where?
Mental health	› Is there anything stressful going on at work or at home? › Are you having any problems with depression or changes in mood? › Have you had any recent losses? › Are you having any problems concentrating?
Endocrine	› Have you noticed any change in urination patterns? › Have you noticed any change in your energy level? › Have you noticed any change in your ability to handle stress? › Have you had any change in weight or appetite? › Have you had any visual disturbances? › Have you had any palpitations?
Allergic/ immunologic	› Do you have any allergies to medications, foods, or environmental substances? › Have you ever received a blood transfusion? If so, did you have any adverse reactions?

Physical Assessment Techniques

- During a physical assessment:
  - Ensure adequate lighting.
  - Maintain a quiet and comfortable environment.
  - Provide privacy, using a gown or draping the client with a sheet and visualizing only one section of the body at a time.

- ○ Explain the various assessment techniques you will use.
- ○ Look and observe before touching.
- ○ Keep nails short, and hands and stethoscope warm.
- ○ Do not feel or listen through clothing. (Clothing can obscure or create sounds.)
- ○ Have necessary equipment ready.
- ○ Use standard precautions when in contact with body fluids, wound drainage, and open lesions.
- Ⓖ • Additional guidelines for performing a physical assessment of older adults include:
  - ○ Allow enough time for position changes.
  - ○ Perform assessments in several shorter segments to avoid overtiring older adults.
  - ○ Make sure older adults who use sensory aids (eyeglasses, hearing aids) have them available for use.
  - ○ Invite the client to use the bathroom before beginning the physical examination.
- Inspect, palpate, percuss, and auscultate in that order. The exception is the abdomen; inspect, auscultate, percuss, and palpate in that order to avoid altering bowel sounds.
- Inspection
  - ○ Inspection, the first step, begins with the first interaction and continues throughout the examination.
  - ○ A penlight, an otoscope, an ophthalmoscope, or another lighted instrument may enhance the process.
  - ○ Inspection involves using the senses of vision, smell (olfaction), and hearing to observe and detect any expected or unexpected findings. Inspect for size, shape, color, symmetry, and position.
- Palpation is touching to determine the size, consistency, texture, temperature, location, and tenderness of an organ or body part. Palpate tender areas last.
  - ○ Use light palpation (less than 1 cm [0.4 in]) for most body surfaces. Use deeper palpation (4 cm [1.6 in]) to assess abdominal organs or masses.
  - ○ Various parts of the hands detect different sensations.
    - The dorsal surface is the most sensitive to temperature.
    - The palmar surface and base of the fingers are sensitive to vibration.
    - Fingertips are sensitive to pulsation, position, texture, size, and consistency.
    - The fingers and thumb are useful for grasping an organ or mass.
  - ○ Starting with light palpation, be systematic, calm, and gentle. Proceed to deep palpation if necessary.
- Percussion involves tapping body parts with fingers, fists, or small instruments to evaluate size, location, tenderness, and presence or absence of fluid or air in body organs, and to detect any abnormalities. The denser the tissue, the quieter the sound.
  - ○ Techniques for percussion include:
    - Direct percussion, which involves striking the body to elicit sounds.
    - Indirect percussion, which involves placing a hand flatly on the body, as the striking surface, for sound production.
    - Fist percussion, which helps assess for tenderness over the kidneys, liver, and gallbladder.

- Auscultation is listening to sounds the body produces. Some sounds are loud enough to hear unaided, but most sounds require a stethoscope or a Doppler technique (heart sounds, air moving through the respiratory tract, blood moving through blood vessels). The examiner must learn to isolate the various sounds to make accurate assessments.

  ○ Evaluate sounds for amplitude or intensity (loud or soft), pitch or frequency (high or low), duration (time the sound lasts), and quality (what it sounds like).

  ○ Use the diaphragm of the stethoscope to listen to high-pitched sounds (heart sounds, bowel sounds, lung sounds).

    ▪ Place the diaphragm firmly on the body part.

  ○ Use the bell of the stethoscope to listen to low-pitched sounds (unexpected heart sounds, bruits).

    ▪ Place the bell lightly on the body part.

Equipment

- Equipment for a screening examination includes:
  ○ Gown
  ○ Drapes
  ○ Scale with height measurement
  ○ Thermometer
  ○ Stethoscope with diaphragm and bell
  ○ Sphygmomanometer
  ○ Reading/eye chart
  ○ Otoscope, ophthalmoscope, and nasal speculum
  ○ Penlight (or ophthalmoscope)
  ○ Cotton balls
  ○ Sharp and dull objects
  ○ Tuning fork
  ○ Glass of water
  ○ Items to test smell and taste
  ○ Clean gloves
  ○ Tongue depressor
  ○ Reflex hammer
  ○ Pulse oximeter
  ○ Marking pen
  ○ Measuring tape and clear, flexible ruler with measurements in centimeters
  ○ Watch or clock to measure time in seconds

General Survey

- The general survey is a written summary of impressions of overall health. Gather this information from the first encounter with the client and continue to make observations throughout the assessment process. Assess:
  - Physical appearance
    - Age
    - Gender and race
    - Level of consciousness
    - Color of skin
    - Facial features
    - Signs of distress (pallor, labored breathing, guarding, anxiety)
    - Signs of possible physical abuse or neglect
    - Signs of substance use disorders
  - Body structure
    - Body build, stature, height, and weight
    - Nutritional status
    - Symmetry of body parts
    - Posture and usual position
    - Gross abnormalities (skin lesions, amputations)
  - Mobility
    - Gait
    - Range of motion
    - Motor activity
  - Behavior
    - Facial expression and mannerisms
    - Mood and affect
    - Speech
    - Dress, hygiene, grooming, and odors (body and breath)
  - Vital signs
    - Temperature
    - Pulse
    - Respiration
    - Blood pressure
    - Oxygen saturation

Sample Documentation

- Client – 16-year-old male, alert and oriented x 3. No distress. Personal hygiene and grooming slightly unkept but appropriate for age. Weight appropriate for height, erect posture, and steady gait. Full range of motion. Does not maintain eye contact. Volunteers no information but answers questions appropriately. No gross abnormalities.

APPLICATION EXERCISES

1. A nurse is introducing herself to a client as the first step of a comprehensive physical examination. Which of the following strategies should the nurse use with this client? (Select all that apply.)

_____ A. Address the client with the appropriate title and her last name.

_____ B. Use a mix of open- and closed-ended questions.

_____ C. Reduce environmental noise.

_____ D. Have the client complete a printed history form.

_____ E. Perform the general survey before the examination.

2. A nurse in a provider's office is documenting his findings following an assessment he performed for a client new to the practice. Which of the following parameters should he include as part of the general survey? (Select all that apply.)

_____ A. Posture

_____ B. Skin lesions

_____ C. Speech

_____ D. Allergies

_____ E. Immunization status

3. A nurse is collecting data for a client's comprehensive physical examination. After the nurse inspects the client's abdomen, which of the following skills of the physical examination process should she perform next?

A. Olfaction

B. Auscultation

C. Palpation

D. Percussion

4. A nurse is performing a comprehensive physical examination for an older adult. Which of the following interventions should the nurse use in consideration of the client's age? (Select all that apply.)

_____ A. Perform the assessments in one continuous session.

_____ B. Plan to allow plenty of time for position changes.

_____ C. Make sure the client has any essential sensory aids in place.

_____ D. Tell the client to take her time answering questions.

_____ E. Invite the client to use the bathroom before beginning the examination.

5. A nurse in a family practice clinic is performing a physical examination of an adult client. Which part of her hands should she use during palpation for optimal assessment of the client's skin temperature?

A. Palmar surface

B. Fingertips

C. Dorsal surface

D. Base of the fingers

6. A nurse is reviewing the data to collect from a client for a comprehensive health history prior to the systems review. Use the ATI Active Learning Template: Basic Concept to complete this item. Under Related Content, list at least six general categories to cover and the essential data to include in each category.

APPLICATION EXERCISES KEY

1. A. INCORRECT: The nurse should ask the client what she wants the nurse to call her.

    B. **CORRECT:** Open-ended questions help the client tell her story in her own way. Closed-ended questions are useful for clarifying and verifying information the nurse gathers from the client's story.

    C. **CORRECT:** A quiet, comfortable environment eliminates distractions and helps the client focus on the important aspects of the interview.

    D. INCORRECT: Having the client fill out a printed history form might deter the establishment of a therapeutic relationship. When the nurse asks about her history, the client might feel they are wasting time because she already wrote that information on the form.

    E. **CORRECT:** The general survey is noninvasive and, along with the health history and vital sign measurement, can help put the client at ease before the more sensitive parts of the assessment, such as the examination.

    Ⓝ NCLEX® Connection: Health Promotion and Maintenance, Techniques of Physical Assessment

2. A. **CORRECT:** Posture is part of the body structure or general appearance portion of the general survey.

    B. **CORRECT:** Skin lesions are part of the body structure or general appearance portion of the general survey.

    C. **CORRECT:** Speech is part of the behavior portion of the general survey.

    D. INCORRECT: Allergies are part of the health history, not the general survey.

    E. INCORRECT: Immunization status is part of the health history, not the general survey.

    Ⓝ NCLEX® Connection: Health Promotion and Maintenance, Techniques of Physical Assessment

3. A. INCORRECT: Olfaction is the use of the sense of smell to detect any unexpected findings that the nurse cannot detect via other means, such as a fruity breath odor. Unless there is an open lesion on the client's abdomen, this is not the next step in an abdominal examination.

   B. **CORRECT:** Because palpation and percussion can alter the frequency and intensity of bowels sounds, the nurse should auscultate the abdomen next – and before using those two techniques.

   C. INCORRECT: Palpation is the next step in examining other areas of the body, but not the abdomen.

   D. INCORRECT: Percussion is important for detecting gas, fluid, and solid masses in the abdomen, but it is not the next step in an abdominal assessment.

   Ⓝ NCLEX® Connection: Reduction of Risk Potential, System Specific Assessments

4. A. INCORRECT: The nurse should perform the various parts of the assessment in several shorter segments to avoid overtiring the client.

   B. **CORRECT:** Because many older adults have mobility challenges, the nurse should plan the session to allow extra time for position changes.

   C. **CORRECT:** The nurse should make sure older adults who use sensory aids have them available for use. The client has to be able to hear the nurse and see well enough to avoid injury.

   D. **CORRECT:** Some older clients need more time to collect their thoughts and answer questions, but most are reliable historians. Feeling rushed can hinder communication.

   E. **CORRECT:** This is a courtesy for all clients, to avoid discomfort during palpation of the lower abdomen for example, but this is especially important for older clients who might have a diminished bladder capacity.

   Ⓝ NCLEX® Connection: Health Promotion and Maintenance, Techniques of Physical Assessment

5. A. INCORRECT: The palmar surface of the hands is especially sensitive to vibration, not temperature.

   B. INCORRECT: The fingertips are sensitive to pulsation, position, texture, size, and consistency, not temperature.

   C. **CORRECT:** The dorsal surface of the hand is the most sensitive to temperature.

   D. INCORRECT: The base of the fingers is especially sensitive to vibration, not temperature.

   Ⓝ NCLEX® Connection: Reduction of Risk Potential, System Specific Assessments

6. *Using the ATI Active Learning Template: Basic Concept*
   - Related Content
     - Demographic information
       - Name, address, contact information
       - Birth date, age
       - Gender
       - Race, ethnicity
       - Marital status
       - Occupation, employment status
       - Insurance
       - Family, others living at home
     - Source of history
       - Client, family members, other medical records, other providers
       - Reliability of the historian
     - Chief concern
       - A brief statement in the client's own words of why he is seeking care
     - History of present illness
       - A detailed, chronological description of why the client seeks care
       - Details about the symptom(s), such as location, quality, quantity, setting, timing, alleviating or aggravating factors, associated phenomena
     - Past health history and current health status
       - Childhood illnesses, both communicable and chronic
       - Medical, surgical, obstetrical, gynecological, psychiatric history including time frames, diagnoses, hospitalizations, treatments
       - Current immunization status, dates and results of any screening tests
       - Allergies to medication, environment, food
       - Current medications including prescription, over-the-counter, vitamins, supplements, herbal remedies, time of last dose(s)
     - Family history
       - Health information of immediate relatives such as grandparents, parents, siblings, children, grandchildren
       - Current ages or age at death, acute and chronic disorders in family members
     - Social history
       - Relationships, support systems, concerns about living or work situations, financial status, ability to perform activities of daily living, spiritual health
     - Health promotion behavior
       - Exercise/activity, diet, sun exposure, wearing of safety equipment, substance use, environmental exposures, stress, related coping measures
       - Awareness of risks for heart disease, cancer, diabetes mellitus, and cerebrovascular accident

Ⓝ NCLEX® Connection: Health Promotion and Maintenance, Techniques of Physical Assessment

chapter 27

Overview

- Vital signs are measurements of the body's most basic functions and include temperature, pulse, respiration, and blood pressure. Many health care facilities also consider pain and oxygen saturation vital signs. (See the chapters on *Pain Management* and *Airway Management*.)

  - Temperature reflects the balance between heat the body produces and loses.

  - Pulse is the measurement of heart rate and rhythm. Pulse corresponds to the bounding of blood flowing through various points in the circulatory system.

  - Respiration is the body's mechanism for exchanging oxygen and carbon dioxide between the atmosphere and the cells of the body, which is accomplished through breathing and recorded as the number of breaths per minute.

  - Blood pressure (BP) reflects the force the blood exerts against the walls of the arteries during contraction (systole) and relaxation (diastole) of the heart.

    - Systolic BP (SBP) occurs during ventricular systole of the heart, when the ventricles force blood into the aorta, and represents the maximum amount of pressure exerted on the arteries.

    - Diastolic BP (DBP) occurs during ventricular diastole of the heart, when the ventricles relax and exert minimal pressure against arterial walls, and represents the minimum amount of pressure exerted on the arteries.

TEMPERATURE

- Physiological Responses

  - The neurological and cardiovascular systems work together to regulate body temperature. Disease or trauma of the hypothalamus or spinal cord will alter temperature control.

  - The rectum, tympanic membrane, and urinary bladder are core temperature measurement sites.

  - The skin, mouth, and axillae are surface temperature measurement sites.

- Expected temperature ranges are as follows:

  - An oral temperature range of 36° to 38° C (96.8° to 100.4° F) is acceptable. The average is 37° C (98.6° F).

  - Rectal temperatures are usually 0.5° C (0.9° F) higher than oral temperatures.

  - Axillary and tympanic temperatures are usually 0.5° C (0.9° F) lower than oral temperatures.

  - Temporal temperatures are close to rectal, but they are nearly 0.5° C (1° F) higher than oral, and 1° C (2° F) higher than axillary temperatures.

  - A client's usual temperature serves as a baseline for comparison.

- Heat production results from increases in basal metabolic rate, muscle activity, thyroxine output, and sympathetic stimulation, which increases heat production.

- Heat loss from the body occurs through:

    ○ Conduction – Transfer of heat from the body directly to another surface (when the body is immersed in cold water).

    ○ Convection – Dispersion of heat by air currents (wind blowing across exposed skin).

    ○ Evaporation – Dispersion of heat through water vapor (sweating and diaphoresis).

    ○ Radiation – Transfer of heat from one object to another object without contact between them (heat lost from the body to a cold room).

    ○ Diaphoresis – Visible perspiration on the skin.

- Newborns have a large surface-to-mass ratio; therefore, they lose heat rapidly to the environment. Newborns' temperatures should be between 36.5° and 37.5° C (97.7° and 99.5° F).

- Older adult clients experience a loss of subcutaneous fat that results in lower body temperatures and feeling cold. Their average body temperature is 36° C (96.8° F). Older adult clients are more likely to develop adverse effects from extremes in environmental temperatures (heat stroke, hypothermia). It also takes longer for body temperature to register on a thermometer due to changes in temperature regulation.

- Hormonal changes may influence temperature. In general, temperature rises slightly with ovulation and menses. With menopause, intermittent body temperature may increase by up to 4° C (7.2° F).

- Exercise, activity, and dehydration can contribute to the development of hyperthermia.

- Illness and injury can cause with elevations in temperature. Fever is the body's response to infectious and inflammatory processes.

- Recent food or fluid intake and smoking can interfere with accurate measurement of body temperature, so it is best to wait 20 to 30 min before measuring temperature.

- Circadian rhythm, stress, and environmental conditions can also affect body temperature.

Nursing Interventions

- Equipment

    ○ Electronic thermometers use a probe to measure oral, rectal, or axillary temperature. Place a disposable probe cover on the probe, insert the probe, and when you hear the signal, note the digital reading then discard the probe cover. Tympanic temperatures require a device specifically for measuring temperature at the tympanic membrane (eardrum).

    ○ Disposable, single-use thermometers are for oral or axillary temperature measurement. They reduce the risk of cross-infection.

    ○ Health care facilities no longer use glass, mercury-filled thermometers due to the risk of mercury exposure. If you find one in a client's home, encourage the client to replace it with a safer device and discard it according to community guidelines for hazardous waste disposal.

- Procedure
  - Perform hand hygiene, provide privacy, and apply clean gloves.

TECHNIQUES FOR TAKING TEMPERATURE

Oral

› Gently place the thermometer (with an oral probe) under the tongue in the posterior sublingual pocket lateral to the center of the lower jaw.

› Leave it in place until you hear the signal.

› Age-specific: Use this site for clients who are 4 years of age and older.

› Note: Do not use this site for clients who breathe through their mouth or have experienced trauma to the face or mouth.

Rectal

› Provide privacy.

› Assist the client to Sims' position with the upper leg flexed. Wearing gloves, expose the anal area while keeping other body areas covered. Spread the buttocks to expose the anal opening.

› Ask the client to breathe slowly and relax when placing a lubricated thermometer (with a rectal probe) into the anus in the direction of the umbilicus 2.5 to 3.5 cm (1 to 1.5 in) for an adult. If you encounter resistance, remove it immediately. Once inserted, hold the thermometer in place until you hear the signal.

› Clean the anal area to remove feces or lubricant.

› Safety measure: Do not use for clients who have diarrhea, are on bleeding precautions (such as those who have a low platelet count), or have rectal disorders.

› Age-specific: A rectal measurement of temperature is more accurate than axillary. However, because of the risk of rectal perforation, the American Academy of Pediatrics recommends screening infants 3 months old and younger by measuring axillary temperature initially.

› Use the rectal site to obtain a second measurement if the temperature is above 37.2° C (99° F).

› Note: Stool in the rectum can cause inaccurate readings.

Axillary

› Provide privacy.

› Place the thermometer (with an oral probe) in the center of the client's clean, dry axilla. Lower the arm over the probe.

› Hold the arm down, keeping the thermometer in position until you hear the signal.

Tympanic

› Pull the ear up and back (for an adult) or down and back (for a child who is younger than 3 years old).

› Place the thermometer probe snugly into the client's outer ear canal and press the scan button.

› Leave it in place until you hear the signal.

› Carefully remove the thermometer from the ear canal and read the temperature.

› Age-specific: The American Academy of Pediatrics advises against the use of electronic ear thermometers for infants 3 months old and younger due to the inaccuracy of readings.

› Note: Excess earwax can alter the reading. If noted, use the other ear or select another appropriate site for temperature assessment.

› Ambient temperature can also affect readings.

TECHNIQUES FOR TAKING TEMPERATURE
Temporal
› Remove the protective cap and wipe the lens of the scanning device with alcohol to make sure it is clean.
› While pressing the scan button, hold the probe flat against the forehead while moving it gently across the forehead over the temporal artery, and then touch the skin behind the earlobe.
› Release the scan button to display the temperature reading.
› Note: Depending on facility policy, either use disposable probe covers or clean the probe with a disinfectant wipe between clients.

Complications and Nursing Interventions

- Fever – Fever is usually not harmful unless it exceeds 39° C (102.2° F).
- Hyperthermia is an abnormally elevated body temperature.
  - Obtain specimens for blood cultures.
  - Assess/monitor white blood cell counts, sedimentation rates, and electrolytes.
  - Administer antibiotics (after obtaining specimens for blood culture).
  - Provide fluids and rest. Minimize activity. Use a cooling blanket.
  - Children and older adults are at particular risk for fluid volume deficit.
  - Provide antipyretics (aspirin, acetaminophen [Tylenol], ibuprofen [Advil]). Do not give aspirin to manage fever in children and adolescents who may have a viral illness (influenza, chickenpox) due to the risk of Reye syndrome.
  - Prevent shivering as this increases energy demand.
  - Offer blankets during chills and remove them when the client feels warm.
  - Provide oral hygiene and dry clothing and linens.
  - Keep environmental temperature between 21° and 27° C (70° to 80° F).
- Hypothermia is a body temperature below 35° C (below 95° F).
  - Provide a warm environmental temperature, heated humidified oxygen, a warming blanket, friction to the extremities, and/or warmed oral or IV fluids.
  - Keep the head covered.
  - Provide continuous cardiac monitoring.
  - Have emergency resuscitation equipment on standby.

PULSE

- Physiologic Responses
  - ○ The autonomic nervous system controls the heart rate. The parasympathetic nervous system lowers the heart rate, and the sympathetic nervous system raises the heart rate.
- Assess the wave-like sensations or impulses you feel in a peripheral arterial vessel or over the apex of the heart as a gauge of cardiovascular status.
  - ○ Rate – The number of times per minute you feel or hear the pulse.
  - ○ Rhythm – The regularity of impulses. A premature or late heartbeat can result in an irregular interval between impulses and can indicate abnormal electrical activity of the heart. Typically, you should detect an impulse at regular intervals.
  - ○ Strength (amplitude) – Reflects the volume of blood ejected against the arterial wall with each heart contraction and the condition of the arterial vascular system. The strength of the impulse should be the same from beat to beat. Grade strength on a scale of 0 to 4.
    - ■ Interpret this scale as follows:
      - □ 0 = Absent, unable to palpate
      - □ 1+ = Diminished, weaker than expected
      - □ 2+ = Brisk, expected
      - □ 3+ = Increased, strong
      - □ 4+ = Full volume, bounding
  - ○ Equality – Peripheral pulse impulses should be symmetrical in quality and quantity from the right side of the body to the left. Assess strength and equality to evaluate the adequacy of the vascular system.
- The expected reference range for a pulse of an adult client is 60 to 100/min at rest.
  - ○ Tachycardia – A rate above the expected range or faster than 100/min.
  - ○ Bradycardia – A rate below the expected range or slower than 60/min.
- Dysrhythmia – An irregular heart rhythm, generally with an irregular radial pulse.
- A pulse deficit – The difference between the apical rate and the radial rate. With dysrhythmias, the heart may contract ineffectively, resulting in a beat at the apical site with no pulsation at the radial pulse point. To determine the pulse deficit accurately, two clinicians should measure the apical and radial pulse rates simultaneously.
- Age – For infants, the expected pulse rate is 120 to 160/min. The rate gradually decreases as the child grows older. The average pulse for a 12- to 14-year-old child is 80 to 90/min. The strength of the pulsation may weaken in older adult clients due to poor circulation or cardiac dysfunction, which makes the peripheral pulses more difficult to palpate.

FACTORS LEADING TO TACHYCARDIA	FACTORS LEADING TO BRADYCARDIA
› Exercise	› Long-term physical fitness
› Fever, heat exposure	› Hypothermia
› Medications – epinephrine, levothyroxine (Synthroid), beta₂-adrenergic agonists (albuterol [Proventil])	› Medications – digoxin (Lanoxin), beta-blockers (propranolol [Inderal]), calcium channel blockers (verapamil [Calan])
› Changing position from lying down to sitting or standing	› Changing position from standing or sitting to lying down
› Acute pain	› Chronic severe pain
› Hyperthyroidism	› Hypothyroidism
› Anemia, hypoxemia	› Relaxation
› Stress, anxiety, fear	
› Hypovolemia, shock, heart failure	

Nursing Interventions

- Equipment
  - A watch or clock that allows for counting seconds
  - Stethoscope
- Procedure

  - Perform hand hygiene and provide privacy.
  - Locate the radial pulse on the radial- or thumb-side of the forearm at the wrist.
    - Place the index and middle finger of one hand gently but firmly over the pulse. Assess the pulsation for rate, rhythm, amplitude, and quality.
    - If the peripheral pulsation is regular, count the rate for 30 sec and multiply by 2. If the pulsation is irregular, count for a full minute and compare the result to the apical pulse rate.
  - Locate the apical pulse at the fifth intercostal space at the left midclavicular line. Use this site for assessing the heart rate of an infant, rapid rates (faster than 100/min), irregular rhythms, and rates prior to the administration of cardiac medications.
    - Place the stethoscope on the chest at the fifth intercostal space at the left midclavicular line. Always count an apical pulse rate for 1 min if the pulse is irregular or the client is taking cardiovascular medications.

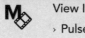
View Images
> Pulse Points

> Apical Pulse

Complications and Nursing Interventions

- Tachycardia
  - Assess/monitor for pain, anxiety, restlessness, fatigue, low blood pressure, and low oxygen saturation.
  - Assess/monitor for potential side/adverse effects of medications.
  - Prevent injury.
- Bradycardia
  - Assess/monitor for hypotension, chest pain, syncope, diaphoresis, dyspnea, and altered mental state.
  - Assess/monitor for potential side/adverse effects of medications.
  - Prevent injury.

RESPIRATIONS

- Physiological Responses
  - Chemoreceptors in the carotid arteries and the aorta primarily monitor carbon dioxide (CO_2) levels of the blood. Rising CO_2 levels trigger the respiratory center of the brain to increase the respiratory rate. The increased respiratory rate rids the body of excess CO_2. For clients with chronic obstructive pulmonary disease (COPD), a low oxygen level becomes the primary respiratory drive.
- The processes of respiration includes:
  - Ventilation – The exchange of oxygen and carbon dioxide in the lungs. Measure ventilation with the respiratory rate, rhythm, and depth.
  - Diffusion – The exchange of oxygen and carbon dioxide between the alveoli and the red blood cells. Measure diffusion with pulse oximetry.
  - Perfusion – The flow of blood to and from the pulmonary capillaries. Measure perfusion with pulse oximetry.
- Accurate assessment of respiration involves observing the rate, depth, and rhythm of chest-wall movement during inspiration and expiration. Do not inform the client that you are measuring respirations.
  - Rate – The number of full inspirations and expirations in 1 min. Determine this by observing the number of times the client's chest rises and falls. The expected reference range for adults is 12 to 20/min.
  - Depth – The amount of chest wall expansion that occurs with each breath. Altered depths are deep or shallow.
  - Rhythm – The observation of breathing intervals. For adults, expect a regular rhythm (eupnea) with an occasional sigh.
- Pulse Oximetry
  - This is a noninvasive, indirect measurement of the oxygen saturation (SaO_2) of the blood. The expected reference range is 95% to 100%, although acceptable levels for some clients range from 91% to 100%. Some illness states may even allow for an SaO_2 of 85% to 89%.

- Age – Respiratory rate decreases with age. Newborns have rates of 30 to 60/min. School-age children have respiratory rates of 20 to 30/min.

- Men and children are diaphragmatic breathers, and abdominal movements are more noticeable. Women use more thoracic muscles, and chest movements are more pronounced when they breathe.

- Pain in the chest wall area may decrease the depth of respirations. At the onset of acute pain, the respiration rate increases but stabilizes over time.

- Anxiety increases the rate and depth of respirations.

- Smoking causes the resting rate of respirations to increase.

- Body position – Upright positions allow the chest wall to expand more fully.

- Medications such as opioids, sedatives, bronchodilators, and general anesthetics decrease the respiratory rate and depth. Respiratory depression can be a serious adverse effect. Amphetamines and cocaine increase rate and depth.

- Neurological injury to the brainstem decreases respiratory rate and rhythm.

- Illnesses can affect the shape of the chest wall, change the patency of passages, impair muscle function, and diminish respiratory effort. With these conditions, the use of accessory muscles and the respiratory rate increase.

- Impaired oxygen-carrying capacity of the blood that occurs with anemia or at high altitudes results in increases in the respiratory rate and alterations in rhythm to compensate.

Nursing Interventions

- Respiratory Rate
  - Equipment
    - A watch or clock that allows for counting seconds.
  - Procedure
    - Perform hand hygiene and provide privacy.
    - Place the client in semi-Fowler's position, being sure the chest is visible.
    - Have the client rest an arm across the abdomen, or place a hand directly on the client's abdomen.
    - Observe one full respiratory cycle, look at the timer, and then begin counting the rate.
    - Count a regular rate for 30 seconds and multiply by 2. Count the rate for 1 min if irregular, faster than 20/min, or slower than 12/min. Note depth (shallow, normal, or deep) and rhythm (regular or irregular).

- Oxygen Saturation
  - Equipment
    - Pulse oximeter
  - Procedure
    - When the readout on the pulse oximeter is stable, record this value as the client's oxygen saturation.

BLOOD PRESSURE

Q
EBP

- Physiological responses
  - The principal determinants of blood pressure (BP) are cardiac output (CO) and systemic vascular resistance (SVR).
  - BP = CO x SVR.

CO	SVR
› CO is determined by: » Heart rate » Contractility » Blood volume » Venous return	› Systemic (peripheral) vascular resistance (SVR) reflects the amount of constriction or dilation of the arteries.
› Increases in any of these increase CO and BP › Decreases in any of these decrease CO and BP	› Increases in SVR increase BP › Decreases in SVR decrease BP

- Classifications of BP according to the Seventh Report of the Joint National Committee on Prevention, Detection, Evaluation, and Treatment of High Blood Pressure:

BP CLASSIFICATION	SYSTOLIC BP (SBP) IN MM HG	DIASTOLIC BP (DBP) IN MM HG
Normal	< 120	and < 80
Prehypertension	120 to 139	or 80 to 89
Stage 1 hypertension	140 to 159	or 90 to 99
Stage 2 hypertension	≥ 160	or ≥ 100

- Base the classification on the highest reading. A client with a BP of 124/92 mm Hg has stage 1 hypertension because the DBP places the client in that category. A client with a BP of 146/82 mm Hg also has stage 1 hypertension because the SBP places the client in that category.

- If the client has a SBP of > 140 mm Hg and a DBP of > 90 mm Hg that are averages of two or more BP measurements, he should return for two or more visits for additional readings. If the readings are elevated on at least three separate occasions over several weeks, the client has hypertension.

- Hypotension is a BP that is below normal (systolic < 90 mm Hg) and can be a result of fluid depletion, heart failure, or vasodilation.

- Pulse pressure is the difference between the systolic and the diastolic pressure readings.

- Postural (orthostatic) hypotension is a BP that falls when a client changes position from lying to sitting or standing, and it may result from various causes (peripheral vasodilation, medication side effects, fluid depletion, anemia, prolonged bed rest).
  - Assess orthostatic changes by taking the client's BP and HR in the supine position. Next, have the client change to the sitting or standing position, wait 1 to 3 min, and reassess the BP and HR. The client has orthostatic hypotension if the SBP decreases more than 20 mm Hg and/or the DBP decreases more than 10 mm Hg with a 10% to 20% increase in the heart rate (HR).

- Age

  - Infants have a low BP that gradually increases with age.

  - Older children and adolescents have varying BP based on body size. Larger children have a higher BP.

  - Adults' BP tends to increase with age.

  - Older adult clients may have a slightly elevated systolic pressure due to decreased elasticity of blood vessels.

- Circadian (diurnal) rhythms affect BP, with BP usually lowest in the early morning hours and peaking during the later part of the afternoon or evening.

- Stress associated with fear, emotional strain, and acute pain can increase BP.

- Ethnicity – African Americans have a higher incidence of hypertension in general and at earlier ages.

- Gender – Adolescent to middle-age men have higher BPs than their female counterparts. Postmenopausal women have higher BPs than their male counterparts.

- Medications such as opiates, antihypertensives, and cardiac medications can lower BP. Cocaine, smoking, cold medications, oral contraceptives, and antidepressants can raise BP.

- Exercise can cause a decrease in BP for several hours afterward.

- Obesity is a contributing factor to hypertension.

Nursing Interventions

- Equipment

  - The auscultatory method uses a:

    - Sphygmomanometer with a pressure manometer (aneroid or mercury) and an appropriately sized cuff. The width of the cuff should be 40% of the arm circumference at the point where the cuff is wrapped. The bladder (inside the cuff) should surround 80% of the arm circumference of an adult and the whole arm for a child. Cuffs that are too large give a falsely low reading, and cuffs that are too small give a falsely high reading.

    - Stethoscope

  - Use automatic BP devices when available for monitoring clients who require frequent evaluation. Measure BP first using the auscultatory method to make sure the automatic device readings are valid.

- Procedure (Auscultatory Method)

  - Perform hand hygiene and provide privacy.

  - Initially measure BP in both arms. If the difference is more than 10 mm Hg, use the arm with the higher reading for subsequent measurements. This difference may indicate a vascular problem.

THE CLIENT SHOULD
› Not smoke or drink any caffeine for 30 min prior to measurement.
› Rest for 5 min before measurement.
› Sit in a chair, with the feet flat on floor, the back and arm supported, and the arm at heart level.

THE NURSE SHOULD
› Use the auscultatory method with a properly calibrated and validated instrument.
› Not measure BP in an arm with an IV infusion in progress or on the side where the client had a mastectomy or an arteriovenous shunt or fistula.
› Average two or more readings, taken at least 2 min apart. (If they differ by more than 5 mm Hg, obtain additional readings and average them.)
› After initial readings, measure BP and pulse with the client standing.

- ○ Apply the BP cuff 2 cm above the antecubital space with the brachial artery in line with the marking on the cuff.

- ○ Use lower extremity if the brachial artery is not accessible.

- ○ Estimate systolic pressure by palpating the radial pulse and inflating the cuff until the pulse disappears. Inflate the cuff another 30 mm Hg, and slowly release the pressure to note when the pulse is palpable again (the estimated systolic pressure).

- ○ Deflate the cuff and wait 1 min.

- ○ Position the stethoscope over the brachial artery.

- ○ Close the pressure bulb by turning the valve clockwise until tight.

- ○ Quickly inflate the cuff to 30 mm Hg above the palpated systolic pressure.

- ○ Release the pressure no faster than 2 to 3 mm Hg per second.

- ○ The level at which you hear the first clear sounds is the systolic pressure.

- ○ Continue to deflate the cuff until the sounds muffle and disappear and note the diastolic pressure.

- ○ Record the systolic over the diastolic pressure (110/70 mm Hg).

- Unexpected BP Readings

  - ○ It is helpful to measure the BP again near the end of an encounter with the client. Earlier pressures may be higher due to the stress of the clinical setting.

  - ○ Recheck BPs when you use an automatic device.

  - ○ Deflate the cuff completely between attempts. Wait at least 1 full min before reinflating the cuff. Air trapped in the bladder can cause a falsely high reading.

Complications and Nursing Interventions

- Orthostatic (Postural) Hypotension
  - Assess/monitor the client's BP.
  - Assess for dizziness, weakness, and fainting.
  - Instruct the client to activate the call light and not to get out of bed without assistance.
  - Have the client sit at the edge of the bed for at least 1 min before standing up.
  - Assist with ambulation.
  - Home care instructions include:
    - Warning the client that lightheadedness and dizziness can occur.
    - Advising the client to sit or lie down if these symptoms occur.
    - Suggesting that the client get up slowly when lying or sitting and avoid sudden changes in position.
- Hypertension
  - Assess/monitor the client for tachycardia, bradycardia, pain, and anxiety. Primary hypertension is usually asymptomatic.
  - Assess for identifiable causes of hypertension (renal disease, thyroid disease, medication).
  - Administer pharmacological therapy.
  - Assess for risk factors.
  - Encourage lifestyle modifications, which include:
    - Smoking cessation
    - Dietary modifications – DASH (Dietary Approaches to Stop Hypertension) diet
      - Restrict sodium intake.
      - Consume adequate potassium, calcium, and magnesium. These minerals help lower BP.
      - Restrict cholesterol and saturated fat intake.
    - Weight control
    - Modification of alcohol intake
    - Physical activity
    - Stress reduction
  - Encourage the client to follow up with the provider.

APPLICATION EXERCISES

1. A nurse is caring for an 82-year-old client in the emergency department who has an oral body temperature of 38.3° C (101° F), a pulse rate of 114/min, and a respiratory rate of 22/min. He is restless and his skin is warm. Which of the following are appropriate nursing interventions for this client? (Select all that apply.)

_____ A. Obtain culture specimens before initiating antimicrobials.

_____ B. Restrict the client's oral fluid intake.

_____ C. Encourage the client to limit activity and rest.

_____ D. Allow the client to shiver to dispel excess heat.

_____ E. Assist the client with oral hygiene frequently.

2. A nurse is instructing an assistive personnel (AP) in caring for a client who has a low platelet count as a result of chemotherapy. Which of the following is the nurse's priority instruction for measuring vital signs for this client?

A. "Do not measure the client's temperature rectally."

B. "Count the client's radial pulse for 30 seconds and multiply it by 2."

C. "Do not let the client know you are counting her respirations."

D. "Let the client rest for 5 minutes before you measure her blood pressure."

3. A nurse is instructing a group of nursing students in measuring a client's respiratory rate. Which of the following guidelines should the nurse include? (Select all that apply.)

_____ A. Place the client in semi-Fowler's position.

_____ B. Have the client rest an arm across the abdomen.

_____ C. Observe one full respiratory cycle before counting the rate.

_____ D. Count the rate for 1 min if it is regular.

_____ E. Count and report any sighs the client demonstrates.

4. A nurse who is admitting a client who has a fractured femur obtains a blood pressure (BP) reading of 140/94 mm Hg. The client denies any history of hypertension. Which of the following actions should the nurse take next?

   A. Request a prescription for an antihypertensive medication.

   B. Ask the client if she is having pain.

   C. Request a prescription for an anti-anxiety medication.

   D. Return in 30 min to recheck the client's BP.

5. A nurse is performing an admission assessment on a client. When measuring her vital signs, the nurse finds that her radial pulse rate 68/min and her simultaneous apical pulse rate is 84/min. What is the client's pulse deficit?

6. A nurse is explaining to a group of nursing students the various factors that can affect a client's heart rate. Use the Basic Concept ATI Active Learning Template to complete this item. Under Underlying Principles, list at least five factors that can cause tachycardia and at least five factors that can cause bradycardia.

APPLICATION EXERCISES KEY

1. A. **CORRECT:** The provider may prescribe cultures to identify any infectious organisms causing the fever. The nurse should obtain culture specimens before antimicrobial therapy to prevent interference with the detection of the infection.

    B. INCORRECT: The nurse should increase oral fluid intake to replace the loss of body fluids from the diaphoresis and increased metabolic rate the fever can cause.

    C. **CORRECT:** Rest helps conserve energy and decreases metabolic rate. Activity can increase heat production.

    D. INCORRECT: The nurse should provide interventions to prevent shivering, because shivering increases energy demands.

    E. **CORRECT:** Oral hygiene helps prevent cracking of dry mucous membranes of the mouth and lips.

     NCLEX® Connection: Reduction of Risk Potential, Changes/Abnormalities in Vital Signs

2. A. **CORRECT:** The greatest risk to a client with a low platelet count is an injury that results in bleeding. Using a thermometer rectally poses a risk of injury to the rectal mucosa; therefore, the low platelet count contraindicates the use of the rectal route for this client. Of these instructions, this is the nurse's priority.

    B. INCORRECT: It is important for the AP to count the radial pulse, unless it is irregular, for 30 seconds and then multiply by 2 to obtain the number of pulsations per minute; however, there is a higher priority instruction among these options.

    C. INCORRECT: It is important for the AP to avoid letting the client know about counting respirations as this awareness can sometimes alter the respiratory rate; however, there is a higher priority instruction among these options.

    D. INCORRECT: It is important for the AP to let the client rest for 5 min before measuring blood pressure as activity can alter the reading; however, there is a higher priority instruction among these options.

    NCLEX® Connection: Reduction of Risk Potential, Changes/Abnormalities in Vital Signs

3. A. **CORRECT:** Having the client sit upright facilitates full ventilation and gives the students a clear view of chest and abdominal movements.

    B. **CORRECT:** With the client's arm across the abdomen or lower chest, it is easier for the students to see respiratory movements.

    C. **CORRECT:** Observing for one full respiratory cycle before starting to count assists the students in obtaining an accurate count.

    D. INCORRECT: The students should count the rate for 1 min if it is irregular.

    E. INCORRECT: An occasional sigh is an expected finding in adults. It helps expand small airways. Students needn't count nor report sighs.

     NCLEX® Connection: Reduction of Risk Potential, Changes/Abnormalities in Vital Signs

4. A. INCORRECT: If the client's BP remains elevated after the nurse implements other interventions to reduce it, it might be appropriate to request a prescription for an antihypertensive medication. However, there is a higher priority action among these options.

    B. **CORRECT:** The greatest risk to a client with a fracture is unrelieved pain, which can cause multiple complications, including elevated BP. Therefore, the nurse's priority is to perform a pain assessment. If the client's BP is still elevated after pain interventions, the nurse should report this finding to the provider. Of these instructions, this is the nurse's priority.

    C. INCORRECT: If the client's BP remains elevated after the nurse implements other interventions to reduce it, it might be appropriate to request a prescription for an anti-anxiety medication. However, there is a higher priority action among these options.

    D. INCORRECT: If the client's BP remains elevated after the nurse implements other interventions to reduce it, it is appropriate to recheck the client's BP in 30 min and periodically thereafter. However, there is a higher priority action among these options.

     NCLEX® Connection: Reduction of Risk Potential, Changes/Abnormalities in Vital Signs

5. **16/MIN:** The pulse deficit is the difference between the apical and radial pulse rates. It reflects the number of ineffective or nonperfusing heartbeats that do not transmit pulsations to peripheral pulse points. 84 – 68 = 16

     NCLEX® Connection: Reduction of Risk Potential, Changes/Abnormalities in Vital Signs

6. *Using the Basic Concept ATI Active Learning Template*

- Underlying Principles
  - ○ Tachycardia
    - ▪ Exercise
    - ▪ Fever
    - ▪ Medications – epinephrine, levothyroxine (Synthroid), beta2-adrenergic agonists (albuterol [Proventil])
    - ▪ Changing position from lying down to sitting or standing
    - ▪ Acute pain
    - ▪ Hyperthyroidism
    - ▪ Anemia, hypoxemia
    - ▪ Stress, anxiety, fear
    - ▪ Hypovolemia, shock, heart failure
  - ○ Bradycardia
    - ▪ Long-term physical fitness
    - ▪ Hypothermia
    - ▪ Medications – digoxin (Lanoxin), beta-blockers (propranolol [Inderal]), calcium channel blockers (verapamil [Calan])
    - ▪ Changing position from standing or sitting to lying down
    - ▪ Chronic, severe pain
    - ▪ Hypothyroidism

(N) NCLEX® Connection: Reduction of Risk Potential, Changes/Abnormalities in Vital Signs

chapter 28

Overview

- This examination includes the head, neck, eyes, nose, mouth, and throat.

HEAD AND NECK

Overview

- This examination includes the skull, face, hair, neck, shoulders, lymph nodes, thyroid gland, trachea position, carotid arteries, and jugular veins.
- Use the techniques of inspection, palpation, and auscultation to examine the head and neck.
- Unexpected findings include decreased palpability of a mass, limited range of motion of the neck, and enlarged lymph nodes.
- Equipment includes a stethoscope.
- Test the following cranial nerves during the head and neck examination:

ASSESSMENT	CRANIAL NERVES
› Assess the face for strength and sensation.	› CN V (trigeminal)
› Assess the face for symmetrical movement.	› CN VII (facial)
› Assess the head and shoulders for strength.	› CN XI (spinal accessory)

Health History – Review of Systems

- Questions to ask include:
  - Do you get headaches? If so, how often? Would you point to the exact location? Do you have any other symptoms related to your headaches, such as nausea and vomiting?
    - What do you do to relieve the pain?
  - Have you ever had a head injury?
  - Do you have any pain in your neck?
  - Can you move your head and shoulders with ease?
  - Have you noticed any unusual facial movements?
  - Are any of your lymph nodes swollen?
  - Does anyone in your family have thyroid disease?

Inspection and Palpation

- Head: expected findings
  - Skull
    - Size (normocephalic)
    - No depressions, deformities, masses, tenderness
    - Deformities
    - Masses
    - Tenderness
    - Overall contour and symmetry
  - Face
    - Symmetry of facial features
    - Symmetry of expressions
    - No involuntary movements
    - Proportionate features (no thickening as with acromegaly)
    - CN V
      - Motor – Test the strength of the muscle contraction by asking the client to clench her teeth while you palpate the masseter and temporal muscles, and then the temporomandibular joint. Joint movement should be smooth.
      - Sensory – Test light touch by having the client close her eyes while you touch her face gently with a wisp of cotton. Ask her to tell you when she feels the touch.
    - CN VII
      - Motor – Test facial movement by having the client smile, frown, puff out her cheeks, raise her eyebrows, close her eyes tightly, and show her teeth.
- Neck: expected findings
  - Muscles of the neck symmetric.
  - Shoulders equal in height and with average muscle mass.
    - Range of motion (ROM) – Moving her head smoothly and without distress in the following directions:
      - Chin to chest (flexion).
      - Ear to shoulder bilaterally (lateral flexion).
      - Chin up (hyperextension).
    - CN XI – Place your hands on the client's shoulders and ask her to shrug her shoulders against resistance.

- Lymph nodes – Chains of lymph nodes extend from the lower half of the head down into the neck. Palpate each node for enlargement, in the following sequence:

LYMPH NODE	LOCATION
Occipital nodes	› Base of the skull
Postauricular nodes	› Over the mastoid
Preauricular nodes	› In front of the ear
Tonsillar (retropharyngeal) nodes	› Angle of the mandible
Submandibular nodes	› Along the base of the mandible
Submental nodes	› Midline under the chin
Anterior cervical nodes	› Along the sternocleidomastoid muscle
Posterior cervical nodes	› Posterior to the sternocleidomastoid muscle
Supraclavicular nodes	› Above the clavicles

- ○ Lymph nodes are usually difficult to palpate and not tender or visible.
- ○ Use the pads of the index and middle fingers and move the skin over the underlying tissue in a circular motion to try to detect enlarged nodes. Compare from side to side.
- ○ Evaluate any enlarged nodes for location, tenderness, size, shape, consistency, mobility, discreteness, and warmth.
- The thyroid gland has two lobes and is fixed to the trachea. It lies in front of the trachea and extends to both sides. Examine the gland by:
  - ○ First, inspecting the lower half of the neck to see any enlargement of the gland. An average-size thyroid gland is not visible. Having the client hyperextend the neck helps makes the skin taut and allows better visualization.
  - ○ Instructing the client to take a sip of water and feeling the thyroid gland as it moves up with the trachea.
  - ○ Palpating the thyroid gland on both sides of the trachea for size, masses, and smoothness.
- Trachea – Inspect and palpate the trachea for any deviation from midline. Masses in the neck or mediastinum and pulmonary abnormalities cause lateral displacement.

Auscultation

- If the thyroid is enlarged, auscultate the gland using a stethoscope. A bruit indicates an increase in blood flow to the area, possibly due to hyperthyroidism.

EYES

Overview

- This examination includes the external and internal anatomy of the eye, visual pathways, fields, and reflexes.
- The primary technique for examination of the eyes is inspection, with a limited amount of palpation that requires gloves.
- Unexpected findings include loss of visual fields, asymmetric corneal light reflex, periorbital edema, conjunctivitis, and corneal abrasion.
- Perform the eye examination in the following sequence, using the appropriate equipment.

TEST	EQUIPMENT
Visual acuity	› Distant vision – Snellen and Rosenbaum charts, eye cover, Ishihara test for color blindness › Near vision – hand-held card
Extraocular movements (EOMs)	› Penlight or ophthalmoscope light › Eye cover
Visual fields	› Eye cover
External structures	› Penlight or ophthalmoscope light › Gloves
Internal structures	› Ophthalmoscope

- Test cranial nerves during the eye examination.

ASSESSMENT	CRANIAL NERVES (CN)
Visual acuity	› CN II (optic)
Extraocular movements	› CN III (oculomotor), CN IV (trochlear), CN VI (abducens)
Visual fields	› CN II (optic)
Corneal light reflex Pupillary reaction to light	› CN II (optic), CN III (oculomotor)

Health History – Review of Systems

- Questions to ask include:
  - How is your vision? Have you noticed any changes?
  - Do you ever have blurry or double vision? Do you ever see spots or halos?
  - Do you have any eye pain, sensitivity to light, burning, itching, dryness, or excessively watery eyes?
  - Do you ever have drainage or crusting from your eyes?

○ Do you wear eyeglasses? Contact lenses?

○ When was your last eye examination?

○ Does anyone in your family have any eye disorders?

○ Do you have diabetes mellitus?

Inspection

- Visual Acuity – CN II

  ○ Have the client stand 20 ft from the Snellen (E) chart.

  ○ Evaluate both eyes and then each eye separately with and without correction.

  ○ For each eye, cover the opposite eye.

  ○ Ask the client to read the smallest line of print visible.

  ○ Note the smallest line the client can read correctly.

  ○ The first number is the distance (in feet) the client stands from the chart. The second number is the distance at which a visually unimpaired eye can see the line clearly.

- Use the Snellen chart to screen for myopia (impaired far vision).

- Hold the Rosenbaum eye chart 14 inches from the client's face to screen for presbyopia (impaired near vision or farsightedness). Readings correlate with the Snellen chart.

- Assess for color vision using the Ishihara test. The client should be able to identify the various shaded shapes.

- Extraocular movements (EOMs) – Assess EOMs to determine the coordination of the eye muscles using three different tests (CN III, CN IV, CN VI).

 M View Image: Extraocular Movements

  ○ Test the corneal light reflex by directing a light onto the eyes and looking to see if the reflection is symmetric on the corneas.

  ○ Screen for strabismus with the cover/uncover test. While covering one eye, ask the client to look in another direction. Remove the cover and expect both eyes to be gazing in the same direction.

  ○ The six cardinal positions of gaze require the client to follow your finger with his eyes without moving his head. Move your finger in a wide "H" pattern about 20 to 25 cm (7.9 to 9.8 in) to from the client's eyes. Expect smooth, symmetric eye movements with no jerky or tremor-like movements (nystagmus).

- Evaluate visual fields (CN II) by facing the client at a distance of 60 cm (2 ft). The client covers one eye while you cover your direct opposite eye (client's right eye and your left eye). Ask the client to look at you and report when she can see the fingers on your outstretched arm coming in from four directions (up, down, temporally, nasally). The expected finding is that the client sees your fingers at the same time you do.

- External Structures: expected findings

  ○ Eyes parallel to each other without bulging (exophthalmos) or crossing (strabismus)

  ○ Eyebrows symmetric from the inner to the outer canthus

  ○ Eyelids closing completely and opening to show the lower border and most of the upper portion of the iris without ptosis (the upper eyelid covering the pupil)

- Eyelashes curving outward with no inflammation around any of the hair follicles
- No edema or redness in the area of the lacrimal glands
- Conjunctivae
  - Palpebral pink
  - Bulbar transparent
- Sclerae white, light yellow in clients who have dark skin
- Corneas clear
- Lenses clear, cloudy with cataracts
- PERRLA (CN II, CN III)
  - P – Pupils clear
  - E – Equal and between 3 to 7 mm in diameter
  - R – Round
  - RL – Reactive to light both directly and consensually when you direct light into one pupil and then the other
  - A – Accommodation of the pupils when they dilate to look at an object far away and then converge and constrict to focus on a near object
- Irises round and illuminating fully when you shine a light across from the side. A partially illuminated iris indicates glaucoma. Note the color of the irises.
- Internal Examination Technique and Expected Findings
  - Darken the room.
  - Turn on the ophthalmoscope, and use the lens selector disc to find the large white disc.
  - The diopter is set at 0. You can change the setting to bring structures into focus during the examination.
  - Use your right eye to examine the client's right eye and vice versa.
  - Instruct the client to stare at a point somewhere behind you.
  - Start slightly lateral and 25 to 30 cm from the client, finding and following the red reflex, to within a distance of 2 to 3 cm of the client's eye.
  - Expected findings
    - The optic disc is light pink or more yellow than the surrounding retina.
    - The retina is without lesions. The color will be dark pink in those with a dark complexion and light pink in those who have fair skin.
    - The arteries and veins have a 2-to-3 ratio with no nicking.
    - Without pupil dilation, you might only glimpse the macula briefly when the client looks directly at the light.

Palpation

- Palpate the lacrimal apparatus to assess for tenderness and to express any discharge from the lacrimal duct. Expected findings include no tenderness, no discharge, and clear fluid (tears).

EARS, NOSE, MOUTH, AND THROAT

Overview

- This examination includes the external, middle, and internal ear; evaluation of hearing; the nose and sinuses; and the mouth and throat.
- Use the techniques of inspection and palpation to examine the ears, nose (sinuses), mouth, and throat.
- Unexpected findings include otitis externa, osteoma, polyp, retracted drum, decreased hearing acuity, and lateralization.
- Equipment
  - Otoscope
  - Wristwatch or clock to measure time in seconds
  - Tuning fork
  - Nasal speculum
  - Tongue blade
  - Penlight
  - Gauze square
  - Cotton-tipped applicators
- Test the following cranial nerves during the ears, nose, mouth, and throat examination.

ASSESSMENT	CRANIAL NERVES (CN)
› Assess the ears for hearing.	› CN VIII (auditory)
› Assess the nose for smell.	› CN I (olfactory)
› Assess the mouth for taste.	› CN VII (facial) and CN IX (glossopharyngeal)
› Assess the tongue for movement and strength.	› CN XII (hypoglossal)
› Assess the mouth for movement of the soft palate and the gag reflex. Assess swallowing and speech.	› CN IX (glossopharyngeal) and CN X (vagus)

Health History – Review of Systems

- Questions to ask include:
  - How well do you hear?
  - Have you had any injuries to your nose?
  - Have you noticed any changes in your hearing? Do you wear hearing aids?
  - Have other people commented that you aren't hearing what they say?
  - Do you ever have ringing or buzzing in your ears, drainage, dizziness, or pain? Do you have a history of ear infections?
  - How do you clean your ears?
  - Do you ever have pain, stuffiness, or fluid draining from your nose?
  - Do you ever have nosebleeds?
  - Have you noticed any change in your senses of smell or taste?

- ○ Do you use nasal sprays?
- ○ Do you snore?
- ○ How often do you go to the dentist? Do you have dentures? Retainers? Do you have any problems with your gums?
- ○ Do you have any difficulty swallowing or problems with a hoarseness or sore throat?

Inspection and Palpation

- Ears
  - ○ External ear: expected findings
    - ■ Alignment – The top of the auricles meeting an imaginary horizontal line that extends from the outer canthus of the eye
    - ■ Ear color matching face color
    - ■ No lesions or tenderness
    - ■ No foreign bodies or discharge
    - ■ No cerumen
  - ○ Internal ear
    - ■ Straighten the ear canal by pulling the auricle up and back for adults and older children, and down and back for younger children. Using the otoscope, insert the speculum slightly down and forward 1 to 1.5 cm (0.4 to 0.6 in) following, but not touching, the ear canal to visualize:
      - □ Tympanic membranes that are pearly gray and intact, free from tears.
      - □ A light reflex that is visible and in a well-defined cone shape.
      - □ Umbo and manubrium landmarks that are readily visible.
      - □ Ear canals that are pink with fine hairs.
  - ○ Auditory screening tests

TEST	TECHNIQUE	EXPECTED FINDING
Whisper test (CNV III)	› Occlude one ear and test the other to see if the client can hear whispered sounds without seeing your mouth move. › Repeat with the other ear.	› The client can hear you whisper softly from 30 to 60 cm (1 to 2 ft) away.
Rinne test	› Place a vibrating tuning fork firmly against the mastoid bone and note the time. › Have the client state when he can no longer hear the sound, note the time, and then move the tuning fork in front of the ear canal. When the client can no longer hear the tuning fork, note the time.	› Air conduction (AC) greater than bone conduction (BC); 2-to-1 ratio.
Weber test	› Place a vibrating tuning fork on top of the client's head. Ask whether the client can hear the sound best in the right ear, the left ear, or both ears equally.	› The client hears sound equally in both ears (negative Weber test).

View Images
  › Rinne Test   › Weber Test

- Nose: expected findings
  - The nose is midline, symmetrical, and the same color as the face.
  - Each naris (nostril) is patent without excessive flaring. The structure of the nose is firm and stable.
  - To examine internal structures, insert a nasal speculum just barely into each naris as the client tips his head back.
    - Septum is midline and intact.
    - Mucous membranes are deep pink and moist with no discharge or lesions.
  - Assess smell (CN I) by asking the client to close his eyes, occlude one naris at a time, and identify a familiar smell with the eyes closed.
- Mouth and Throat: expected findings
  - Lips are darker pigmented skin than the face and are moist, symmetric, smooth, soft with no lesions, and nontender.
  - Gums are coral pink and tight against the teeth with no bleeding on gloves from palpation.
  - Mucous membranes are pink and moist with no lesions.
  - Tongue – Use a gauze pad to hold the tip and move the tongue from side to side. The dorsal surface is pink, with the presence of papillae, and symmetric. The underside of the tongue is smooth with a symmetric vascular pattern. Assess taste (CN VII, CN IX) by having the client close his eyes and identify foods you place on his tongue. Ask the client to move his tongue up, down, and side to side. Test strength (CN XII) by applying resistance against each cheek while the client sticks his tongue into each cheek.
    - The tongue is midline, moist, free of lesions, and moves freely.
  - Teeth are shiny, white, and smooth. Check for malocclusions by asking the client to clench his teeth. Note any missing or loose teeth, as well as any discoloration.
  - The hard palate is whitish, intact, symmetric, firm, and concave.
  - The soft palate is light pink, intact, smooth, symmetric, and moves with vocalization (CN IX, CN X).
  - The uvula is pink, midline, intact, and moves with vocalization.
  - Tonsils are the same color as the surrounding mucosa and vary in size and visibility:
    - +1 – Barely visible
    - +2 – Halfway to the uvula
    - +3 – Touching the uvula
    - +4 – Touching each other or midline
  - Elicit the gag reflex by using a tongue blade to stimulate the back of the throat (CN IX, CN X). Explain the procedure to the client prior to performing this assessment.
  - Speech is clear and articulate.

Palpation of Sinuses

- Technique
  - Palpate the frontal sinuses by pressing upward with the thumbs from just below the eyebrows on either side of the bridge of the nose.
  - Palpate the maxillary sinuses by pressing upward at the skin crevices that run from the sides of the nose to the corner of the mouth.
- Expected finding – nontender

Expected Changes with Aging

AREA OF THE BODY	EXPECTED FINDINGS
Eyes	› Decreased visual acuity, decreased peripheral vision, diminishing ability to see close objects or read small print (presbyopia), decreased ability to accommodate extreme changes in light (glare, darkness), difficulty distinguishing colors, intolerance to glare, delayed pupillary reaction to light, yellowing of the lens, thin gray-white ring surrounding the cornea, loss of lateral third of eyebrows
Ears	› Hearing loss, loss of acuity for high-frequency tones (presbycusis), cerumen accumulation in the ear canal, thickening of the tympanic membrane
Mouth	› Decreased sense of taste, reduced number of taste buds, tooth loss, pale gums, gum disease due to inadequate oral hygiene
Voice	› Rise in pitch, loss of power and range
Nose	› Decreased sense of smell

Sample Documentation

Client reports no pain in head or neck region.

Skull normocephalic, symmetrical, and nontender. Symmetric facial features, movements. Trachea midline. Thyroid lobes palpable but not enlarged; no nodules. Neck supple with no palpable lymph nodes. Full range of motion of the neck.

Visual acuity 20/30 in the left eye, 20/20 in the right eye, 20/20 in both eyes without correction. EOMs symmetric with no strabismus or nystagmus. Peripheral fields full bilaterally. Eyebrows evenly distributed. Eyelids close completely with no ptosis. No discharge. Bulbar conjunctivae clear, palpebral conjunctivae pink, sclerae white, irises blue bilaterally. Corneas and lenses clear. PERRLA intact bilaterally. Red reflex bilaterally. Retinas yellowish orange with no nicking or hemorrhaging of vessels.

No lesions or tenderness on external ears. Top of ears align with outer canthus of eyes. Tympanic membranes pearly gray and translucent with well-defined cone of light. Light yellow cerumen in ear canals bilaterally. Auditory acuity intact to whispered voice bilaterally. Negative Weber test and AC > BC bilaterally. Nose midline, symmetrical. Nares patent. Nasal mucosa pink, septum intact and midline, no discharge. No sinus tenderness. Lips darker pink and intact, symmetric. Oral mucosa pink, no dental caries, no missing teeth. Tongue pink and midline. Papillae on dorsum, symmetrical vascular pattern on the underside of the tongue. Gums tight against the teeth with no bleeding. Hard and soft palates intact with no lesions. Uvula midline. Gag reflex present. Tonsils +1 bilaterally. Taste and smell sensations intact. Speech clear. CN I through XII intact.

APPLICATION EXERCISES

1. A nurse in a provider's office is preparing to test a client's cranial nerve function. Which of the following directions should she include when testing cranial nerve V? (Select all that apply.)

_____ A. "Close your eyes."

_____ B. "Tell me what you can taste."

_____ C. "Clench your teeth."

_____ D. "Raise your eyebrows."

_____ E. "Tell me when you feel a touch."

2. A client asks the nurse what her Snellen eye test results mean. Her visual acuity is 20/30. Which of the following responses is appropriate?

A. "Your eyes see at 20 feet what visually unimpaired eyes see at 30 feet."

B. "Your right eye can see the chart clearly at 20 feet, and your left eye can see the chart clearly at 30 feet."

C. "Your eyes see at 30 ft what visually unimpaired eyes see at 20 ft."

D. "Your left eye can see the chart clearly at 20 feet, and your right eye can see the chart clearly at 30 feet."

3. A nurse is assessing a client's thyroid gland as part of a comprehensive physical examination. Which of the following findings should the nurse expect? (Select all that apply.)

_____ A. Palpating the thyroid in the lower half of the neck

_____ B. Visualizing the thyroid on inspection of the neck

_____ C. Hearing a bruit when auscultating the thyroid

_____ D. Feeling the thyroid ascend as the client swallows

_____ E. Finding symmetric extension of the trachea on both sides of the midline

4. A nurse is assessing an adult client's internal ear canals with an otoscope as part of a head and neck examination. Which of the following actions are appropriate? (Select all that apply.)

_____ A. Pull the auricle down and back.

_____ B. Insert the speculum slightly down and forward.

_____ C. Insert the speculum 2 to 2.5 cm (0.8 to 1 in).

_____ D. Make sure the speculum does not touch the ear canal.

_____ E. Use the light to visualize the tympanic membrane in a cone shape.

5. A nurse is performing a head and neck examination for an older adult client. Which of the following age-related findings should the nurse expect? (Select all that apply.)

_____ A. Reddened gums

_____ B. Lowered vocal pitch

_____ C. Tooth loss

_____ D. Glare intolerance

_____ E. Thickened eardrums

6. A nurse is assessing a client's lymph nodes as part of a comprehensive physical examination. Use the ATI Active Learning Template: Nursing Skill to complete this item. Under Nursing Actions, list the nine chains of lymph nodes and the location of each, in the appropriate sequence for palpating them.

APPLICATION EXERCISES KEY

1. A. **CORRECT:** Testing cranial nerve V, the trigeminal nerve, involves testing light touch by having the client tell the nurse when he feels a gentle touch on his face from a wisp of cotton.

    B. INCORRECT: Testing cranial nerve VII, the facial nerve, involves testing the mouth for taste sensations.

    C. **CORRECT:** Testing cranial nerve V, the trigeminal nerve, involves testing the strength of muscle contraction by asking the client to clench his teeth while the nurse palpates the masseter and temporal muscles, and then the temporomandibular joint.

    D. INCORRECT: Testing cranial nerve VII, the facial nerve, involves testing for a range of facial expressions by having the client smile, raise his eyebrows, puff out his cheeks, and perform other facial movements.

    E. **CORRECT:** The first step of testing cranial nerve V, the trigeminal nerve, is to have the client close his eyes.

     NCLEX® Connection: Reduction of Risk Potential, Diagnostic Tests

2. A. **CORRECT:** The first number is the distance (in feet) the client stands from the chart. The second number is the distance at which a visually unimpaired eye can see the line clearly.

    B. INCORRECT: Each eye has its own visual acuity, which includes both numbers.

    C. INCORRECT: The numerator of visual acuity results is a constant. It does not change with a client's ability to see clearly.

    D. INCORRECT: Each eye has its own visual acuity, which includes both numbers.

     NCLEX® Connection: Reduction of Risk Potential, Therapeutic Procedures

3. A. **CORRECT:** The thyroid gland lies in the anterior portion of the lower half of the neck, just in front of the trachea.

    B. INCORRECT: An average-size thyroid gland is not visible on inspection.

    C. INCORRECT: A bruit indicates increased blood flow, possibly due to hyperthyroidism.

    D. **CORRECT:** When the client swallows a sip of water, the nurse should feel the thyroid move upward with the trachea.

    E. **CORRECT:** The thyroid gland lies in front of the trachea and extends symmetrically to both sides of the midline.

     NCLEX® Connection: Reduction of Risk Potential, System Specific Assessments

4.   A.   INCORRECT: The nurse should pull the auricle up and back for adults and down and back for children younger than 3 years.

     B.   **CORRECT:** Inserting the speculum slightly down and forward follows the natural shape of the ear canal.

     C.   INCORRECT: The nurse should insert the speculum 1 to 1.5 cm (0.4 to 0.6 in).

     D.   **CORRECT:** The lining of the ear canal is sensitive. Touching it with the speculum could cause pain.

     E.   **CORRECT:** Due to the angle of the ear canal, the nurse can only visualize the light reflecting off of the tympanic membrane as a cone shape rather than a circle.

     Ⓝ NCLEX® Connection: Reduction of Risk Potential, Diagnostic Tests

5.   A.   INCORRECT: The nurse should expect an older adult's gums to be pale.

     B.   INCORRECT: The nurse should expect an older adult's vocal pitch to rise.

     C.   **CORRECT:** Tooth loss and gum disease are common in older adults.

     D.   **CORRECT:** Older adults tend to become intolerant of glaring lights and also lose some ability to distinguish colors.

     E.   **CORRECT:** Tympanic membranes (eardrums) thicken in older adults, and they tend to accumulate cerumen in their ear canals.

     Ⓝ NCLEX® Connection: Physiological Adaptations, Pathophysiology

6.   *Using the ATI Active Learning Template: Nursing Skill*
     • Nursing Actions
       ○ Occipital nodes: base of the skull
       ○ Postauricular nodes: over the mastoid
       ○ Preauricular nodes: in front of the ear
       ○ Tonsillar (retropharyngeal) nodes: angle of the mandible
       ○ Submandibular nodes: along the base of the mandible
       ○ Submental nodes: midline under the chin
       ○ Anterior cervical nodes: along the sternocleidomastoid muscle
       ○ Posterior cervical nodes: posterior to the sternocleidomastoid muscle
       ○ Supraclavicular nodes: above the clavicles

     Ⓝ NCLEX® Connection: Health Promotion and Maintenance, Techniques of Physical Assessment

chapter 29

Overview

- This examination includes the thorax (breast and lungs), heart, and abdomen.

BREASTS

Overview

- For clients who have had a mastectomy, breast augmentation, or reconstruction, palpate the incisional lines. Look for lymphedema in clients who have impaired lymphatic drainage on the affected side.

- Instruct clients who do not perform monthly breast self-examination (BSE) to inspect their breasts in front of a mirror and palpate them during a shower. The optimal time is 2 or 3 days after menstruation ends. Clients who are postmenopausal should perform BSE on the same day of each month.

- Perform breast examinations on female and male clients.

- Use the techniques of inspection and palpation to examine the breasts.

  - Equipment

    - Gloves

    - Drape

    - Small pillow or folded towel

- Documentation of nodules includes:

  - Location (quadrant or clock method)

  - Size (actual centimeters)

  - Shape

  - Consistency (soft, firm, or hard)

  - Discreteness (well-defined borders of mass)

  - Tenderness

  - Erythema

  - Dimpling or retraction over the mass

  - Lymphadenopathy

  - Mobility

Health History – Review of Systems

- Questions to ask include:
  - Do you perform breast self-examinations? How often?
  - Have you noticed any tenderness or lumps? For women: Does this change with your menstrual cycle?
  - Do you have any thickening, pain, drainage, distortion, or change in breast size, or any retraction or scaling of the nipples?
  - For clients over 40: How often are you having mammograms?
  - Has anyone in your family had breast cancer?
  - Are you aware of the risks for breast cancer?

Inspection

FEMALE	MALE
› Four positions (sitting or standing)	› In sitting or lying position (with arms at the side only)
» Arms at the side	
» Arms above the head	
» Hands on the hips pressing firmly	
» Leaning forward (arms out in front or on hips)	

- Inspect for:
  - Size, symmetry (One breast is often slightly larger than the other.)
  - Shape (convex, conical, pendulous)
  - Symmetric venous patterns and consistency of skin color
  - No lesions, edema, erythema (Rashes and ulcerations are unexpected findings.)
  - Round or oval shape of areola
  - Darker-pigmented areola and nipple
  - Direction of nipples (Nipples are usually everted; recent inversion is unexpected.)
  - For women with large breasts, check for excoriation under the breasts.

Palpation

- Palpate axillary and clavicular lymph nodes with the client sitting with her arms at her sides. Expect them to be nonpalpable with no tenderness.
- Breast examination – Wear gloves if skin is not intact. Feel for lumps using the finger pads of your three middle fingers. The best position is for the client to be lying down with the arm up by her head and a small pillow or folded towel under the shoulder of the side you are examining. This position spreads the breast tissue more evenly over the chest wall, allowing for easier palpation.
  - Palpate each breast from the sternum to the posterior axillary line, and from the clavicle to the bra line (including the areola, nipple, and tail of Spence) using one of three techniques:
    - Circular pattern
    - Wedge pattern
    - Vertical strip pattern

- Compress the nipples carefully between your thumb and index finger to check for discharge (unexpected in nonlactating women). Note the color, consistency, and odor of any discharge.
- For pendulous breasts, use one hand to support the lower portion of the breast while using your other hand to palpate breast tissue against the supporting hand.

	EXPECTED FINDINGS	UNEXPECTED FINDINGS
Female	› Breasts firm, dense, elastic, and without lesions or nodules › Breast tissue granular or lumpy bilaterally in some women	› Fibrocystic breast disease: tender cysts often more prominent during menstruation
Male	› No edema, masses, nodules, or tenderness › Areolas round and darker pigmented	› Unilateral or bilateral (but asymmetrical) gynecomastia in adolescent boys or bilateral gynecomastia in older adult males

THORAX AND LUNGS

Overview

- This examination includes the anterior and posterior thorax and lungs.
- Use the techniques of inspection, palpation, percussion, and auscultation.
- Equipment
  - Stethoscope
  - Centimeter ruler
  - A wristwatch or clock that allows for counting seconds
- Positioning – Assess the posterior thorax with the client sitting or standing. Assess the anterior thorax with the client sitting, lying, or standing.
- Anatomical reminder: The right lung has three lobes; the left lung has two lobes. Auscultate the right middle lobe via the axillae.
- Use the following vertical chest landmarks to perform assessments and describe findings.
  - The midsternal line is through the center of the sternum.
  - The midclavicular line is through the midpoint of the clavicle.
  - The anterior axillary line is through the anterior axillary folds.
  - The midaxillary line is through the apex of the axillae.
  - The posterior axillary line is through the posterior axillary fold.
  - The right and left scapular lines are through the inferior angle of the scapula.
  - The vertebral line is along the center of the spine.

 View Animation: Lung Landmarks

- Percussion and auscultatory sites are in the intercostal spaces (ICSs). The number of the ICSs corresponds to the rib above it.

  - Posterior thorax – The sites are between the scapula and the vertebrae on the upper portion of the back. Below the scapula, the sites are along the right and left scapular lines.

  - Anterior thorax – The sites are along the midclavicular lines bilaterally, with several sites at the anterior/midaxillary lines bilaterally in the lower portions of the chest wall and on either side of the sternum following along the rib cage.

    - Observe for accessory muscle use.

  - Percussing and auscultating in a systemic pattern allows side-to-side comparisons.

  - Maximize sounds by:

    - Having the client take deep breaths with an open mouth each time you move the stethoscope.

    - Placing the stethoscope directly on the skin to prevent muffling or distortion of sounds.

    - Facilitating breathing by medicating for pain, giving clear directions, and assisting the client to a sitting position.

Health History – Review of Systems

- Questions to ask include:

  - Do you have any chronic lung conditions such as asthma or emphysema? Do you take any medications for your respiratory problems?

  - Have you ever had pneumonia? If so, when?

  - Do you get coughs and colds frequently?

  - Do you have environmental allergies?

  - Do you ever have shortness of breath or difficulty breathing with activity?

  - Do you have a cough now? Do you cough up sputum? If so, what does it look like?

  - Do you currently or have you ever smoked? If you no longer smoke, when did you quit? How long did you smoke? If you do currently smoke, when did you start and how much do you smoke? Are you interested in quitting?

  - Are you exposed to secondhand smoke?

  - Has anyone in your family had lung cancer or tuberculosis? Have you had any exposure to tuberculosis?

  - Do you receive an influenza vaccine every year?

Inspection

- Shape – The anteroposterior diameter is half of the transverse diameter.

- Symmetry – The chest is symmetric with no deformities of the ribs, sternum, scapula, or vertebrae, and equal movements during respiration.

- ICS – No excessive retractions.

- Respiratory Effort
  - Rate and pattern – 12 to 20/min and regular
  - Character of breathing (diaphragmatic, abdominal, thoracic)
  - Use of accessory muscles
  - Chest wall expansion
  - Depth of respirations – unlabored, quiet breathing
- Cough – If productive, note the color and consistency of sputum.
- Trachea is midline.

Palpation

- Surface characteristics include tenderness, lesions, lumps, and deformities. Tenderness is an unexpected finding. Avoid deep palpation if the client reports pain or tenderness.
- Chest excursion or expansion of the posterior thorax
  - With thumbs aligned parallel along the spine at the level of the tenth rib, and the hands flattened around the client's back, instruct the client to take a deep breath. Move your thumbs outward approximately 5 cm (2 in) when the client takes a deep inspiration.
- Vocal (tactile) fremitus
  - Palpate the chest wall using the palms of both hands, comparing side to side from top to bottom.
  - Ask the client to say "99" each time you move your hands.
  - Expected findings – Vibration is symmetric and more pronounced at the top, near the level of the tracheal bifurcation.

Percussion

- Compare sounds from side to side.
- Percussion of the thorax elicits resonance.
- Unexpected Findings and Significance
  - Dullness – In fluid or solid tissue, this can indicate pneumonia or a tumor.
  - Hyperresonance – In the presence of air, this can indicate pneumothorax or emphysema.

Auscultation

- Expected Sounds
  - Bronchial – loud, high-pitched, expiration longer than inspiration over the trachea
  - Bronchovesicular – medium pitch and intensity with equal inspiration and expiration times over the larger airways
  - Vesicular – soft, low-pitched, inspiration three times longer than expiration over most of the peripheral areas of the lungs

- Unexpected or Adventitious Sounds

  - Crackles or rales – fine to coarse popping (not cleared with coughing) as air passes through fluid or re-expands collapsed small airways

  - Wheezes – high-pitched whistling, musical sounds as air passes through narrowed or obstructed airways, usually louder on expiration

  - Rhonchi – coarse sounds during either inspiration or expiration resulting from fluid or mucus, may clear with coughing

  - Pleural friction rub – grating sound as the inflamed visceral and parietal pleura rub against each other during inspiration or expiration

  - Absence of breath sounds from collapsed or surgically removed lobes.

HEART

Overview

- This examination includes measuring heart rate and blood pressure, examining the jugular veins, and auscultating heart sounds.

- Equipment

  - Stethoscope

  - Blood pressure cuff

  - A wristwatch or clock that allows for counting seconds

  - Two rulers

- Cardiac Cycle and Heart Sounds

  - Closure of the mitral and tricuspid valves signals the beginning of ventricular systole (contraction) and produces the S1 sound (lub). Place the diaphragm of the stethoscope at the apex.

  - Closure of the aortic and pulmonic valves signals the beginning of ventricular diastole (relaxation) and produces the S2 sound (dub). Place the diaphragm of the stethoscope at the aortic area.

  - An S3 sound (ventricular gallop) indicates rapid ventricular filling and can be an expected finding in children and young adults. Use the bell of the stethoscope.

  - An S4 sound reflects a strong atrial contraction and can be an expected finding in older and athletic adults and children. Use the bell of the stethoscope.

  - Murmurs are audible when blood volume in the heart increased or its flow is impeded or altered. Use the bell of the stethoscope to hear the characteristic blowing or swishing sound.

    - Systolic murmurs occur just after S1.

    - Diastolic murmurs occur just after S2.

  - Thrills are a palpable vibration that can accompany murmurs or cardiac malformation.

  - Bruits are blowing or swishing sounds that indicate obstructed peripheral blood flow. Use the bell of the stethoscope.

- Auscultatory Sites for the Heart

 View Image: Cardiac Landmarks

- Aortic – just right of the sternum at the second ICS
- Pulmonic – just left of the sternum at the second ICS
- Erb's point – just left of the sternum at the third ICS
- Tricuspid – just left of the sternum at the fourth ICS
- Apical/mitral – left midclavicular line at the fifth ICS

Health History – Review of Systems

- Questions to ask include:
  - Do you have any problems with your heart? Do you take any medications for your heart?
  - Do you have high blood pressure or high cholesterol?
  - Do your feet and ankles ever swell?
  - Do you cough frequently?
  - Do you have chest pain? When? How long does it last? How often does it occur? Describe the pain. Do you also feel it in your arms, neck, or jaw?
  - What are you doing before the pain begins?
  - Do you have any other symptoms with the pain (nausea, shortness of breath, sweating, dizziness)?
  - What have you tried to relieve the pain? Does it work?
  - Describe your energy level. Are you frequently tired? Do you have unusual fatigue?
  - Do you have fainting spells or dizziness? If so, how often? When was the last time?
  - Are you familiar with the risk factors for heart disease?

Inspection and Palpation

- Vital signs – Pulse and blood pressure reflect cardiovascular status.
- Peripheral Vascular System
  - Inspect jugular veins with the client in bed with the head of the bed at a 30° to 45° angle to assess for right-sided heart failure.
    - Appearance – no neck vein distention
    - Jugular venous pressure (JVP) – Measure at less than 2.5 cm (1 in) above the sternal angle using the following technique:
      - Place one ruler vertically at the sternal angle.
      - Locate the pulsation in the external jugular vein and place the straight edge of another ruler parallel to the floor at the level of the pulsation.
      - Line up the two rulers as a T square, keeping the horizontal ruler at the level of pulsation.
      - Measure JVP at the level where the horizontal ruler intersects the vertical ruler.
        - Examine one carotid artery at a time. If you occlude both arteries simultaneously during palpation, the client loses consciousness as a result of inadequate circulation to the brain.

- Heart

  - Apical pulse or point of maximal impulse (PMI)

    - May be visible just medial to the left midclavicular line at the fourth or fifth ICS. With female clients, displace the breast tissue.

    - Palpate where you visualized it. Otherwise, try to palpate the location to feel the pulsations.

  - Heaves (or lifts) are unexpected, visible elevations of the chest wall that indicate heart failure, and are often along the left sternal border or at the PMI.

  - Thrills – Use the palm of the hand to feel for vibration similar to that of a purring kitten. This is an unexpected finding.

Auscultation

- Heart

  - Positioning the client in three different ways allows for optimal assessment of heart sounds, as some positions amplify extra or abnormal sounds.

    - Sitting, leaning forward

    - Lying supine

    - Turned toward the left side (best position for auscultating extra heart sounds or murmurs)

  - Use both the diaphragm and the bell of the stethoscope in a systematic manner to listen at all of the auscultatory sites.

  - To measure the heart rate, listen and count for 1 min. Determine if the rhythm is regular. If a dysrhythmia exists, check for a pulse deficit (radial pulse slower than apical pulse). Report a difference in pulse rates to the provider immediately.

- Assess the peripheral vascular system for bruits. Locations to assess for bruits include:

  - Carotid arteries – over the carotid pulses

  - Abdominal aorta – just below the xiphoid process

  - Renal arteries – midclavicular lines above the umbilicus on the abdomen

  - Iliac arteries – midclavicular lines below the umbilicus on the abdomen

  - Femoral arteries – over the femoral pulses

ABDOMEN

Overview

- This examination includes observing the shape of the abdomen, palpating for masses, and auscultating for vascular sounds.

- Use the techniques of inspection, auscultation, percussion, and palpation. Note that this changes the usual order of assessment techniques. Auscultate just after inspection, because percussion and palpation can alter bowel sounds.

- Equipment
  - Stethoscope
  - Tape measure or ruler
  - Marking pen
- Ask the client to urinate before the abdominal examination. Have the client lie supine with his arms at his sides and with his knees slightly bent.
- Imagine vertical and horizontal lines through the umbilicus to divide the abdomen into four quadrants with the xiphoid process as the upper boundary and the symphysis pubis as the lower boundary:

 View Image: Abdominal Assessment

  - Right upper quadrant (RUQ)
  - Left upper quadrant (LUQ)
  - Right lower quadrant (RLQ)
  - Left lower quadrant (LLQ)

Health History – Review of Systems

- Questions to ask include:
  - Do you ever have nausea or vomiting?
  - Have you had any change in your appetite? Do you have any food intolerances? Any recent weight changes?
  - Do you have any swallowing difficulties?
  - Do you have any problems with your bowels? Do you get diarrhea? Constipation? When was your last bowel movement? Do you often use laxatives or enemas?
  - Have you had any black or tarry stools?
  - Do you take aspirin or ibuprofen? If so, how often?
  - Do you ever have heartburn? When? How often?
  - Have you had any low abdominal or back pain? Any tenderness in these areas?
  - Have you had any abdominal surgery, injuries, or diagnostic tests in this area?
  - Has anyone in your family had colon cancer?
  - For clients over 50: Do you have routine colonoscopies?
  - Are you aware of the warning signs of colon cancer?
  - Do you drink alcohol? If so, how much?
  - What do you eat and drink on a typical day?
  - Do you have any dietary restrictions or special practices?

Inspection

- Note any guarding or splinting of the abdomen.
- Assess the skin for:
  - Lesions – bruising, rashes, or other primary lesions
  - Scars – location and length
  - Silver striae or stretch marks (expected findings)
  - Dilated veins – an unexpected finding possibly reflecting cirrhosis or inferior vena cava obstruction
  - Jaundice, cyanosis, or ascites – possibly reflecting cirrhosis
- Shape or contour
  - Flat – in a horizontal line from the xiphoid process to the symphysis pubis
  - Convex – rounded
  - Concave – a sunken appearance
  - Distended – a large protrusion of the abdomen due to fat, fluid, or flatus
    - Fat – The client has rolls of fat tissue along her sides, and the skin does not look taut.
    - Fluid – The flanks also protrude, and when the client turns onto her side, the protrusion moves to the dependent side.
    - Flatus – The protrusion is mainly midline, and there is no change in the flanks.
    - Hernias – Protrusions through the abdominal muscle wall are visible, especially when the client raises her head.
- Movement of the abdominal wall as:
  - Peristalsis – Wavelike movements visible in thin adults or in clients who have intestinal obstructions.
  - Pulsations – Regular beats of movement midline above the umbilicus are expected findings in thin adults, but a pulsating mass is unexpected.
- Inspect the umbilicus for position, shape, color, inflammation, discharge, and masses.

Auscultation

- Bowel sounds result from the movement of air and fluid in the intestines. The most appropriate time to auscultate bowel sounds is in between meals.
  - Technique – Listen with the diaphragm of the stethoscope in all four quadrants.
  - Expected sounds – High-pitched clicks and gurgles 5 to 35 times/min. To make the determination of absent bowel sounds, you must hear no sounds after listening for a full 5 min.
  - Unexpected sounds – Loud, growling sounds (borborygmi) are hyperactive sounds and indicate increased gastrointestinal motility. Possible causes include diarrhea, anxiety, bowel inflammation, and reactions to some foods.
- Friction rubs result from the rubbing together of inflamed layers of the peritoneum.
  - Listen with the diaphragm over the liver and spleen.
  - Ask the client to take a deep breath while you listen for any grating sounds (like sandpaper rubbing together).

Percussion

- Expect to hear tympany over most of the abdomen. A lower-pitch tympany over the gastric bubble in the left upper quadrant is common.
- Expect dullness over the liver or a distended bladder.
- The liver span is a measurement of liver size at the right midclavicular line.
  - ○ Establish the lower border of the liver by percussing upward from below the umbilicus at the right midclavicular line until tympany turns to dullness.
  - ○ Make a mark.
  - ○ Establish the upper border by percussing downward, starting at the right midclavicular line over the lung until resonance turns to dullness.
  - ○ Make a mark.
  - ○ Measure the distance between the two marks for the size of the liver span.
  - ○ The expected finding is 6 to 12 cm (2.4 to 4.7 in).
- Assess for kidney tenderness by fist percussion over the costovertebral angles at the scapular lines on the back. The expected finding is no tenderness.

Palpation

- Palpate tender areas last.
- Light
  - ○ Use the finger pads on one hand to palpate to a depth of 1.3 cm (0.5 in) in each quadrant.
  - ○ Expect softness, no nodules, and no guarding.
  - ○ The bladder is palpable if full; otherwise, it is nonpalpable.
- Deep
  - ○ Two-handed approach – The top hand depresses the bottom hand 2.5 to 7.5 cm (1 to 3 in) in depth. The bottom hand assesses for organ enlargement or masses.
  - ○ Expected findings:
    - The stool may be palpable in the descending colon.
- Rebound tenderness (Blumberg's sign) is an indication of irritation or inflammation somewhere in the abdominal cavity. Use the following technique in all four quadrants.
  - ○ Apply firm pressure for 4 seconds with the hand at a 90° angle and with the fingers extended.
  - ○ After releasing the pressure, observe the client's response to see if releasing the pressure caused pain.
  - ○ Ask about pain and tenderness.
  - ○ Never palpate an abdominal mass, tender organs, or surgical incisions deeply.

Expected Changes with Aging

AREA OF BODY	EXPECTED CHANGES
Breasts	› With menopause, glandular tissue atrophies. Adipose tissue replaces it, making it feel softer and more pendulous. The atrophied ducts may feel like thin strands. › Nipples no longer have erectile ability and may invert.
Lungs	› Chest shape changes so that the AP diameter becomes similar to the transverse diameter (barrel chest), resulting in decreased vital capacity. › Chest excursion or expansion diminishes. › Cough reflex diminishes. › Cilia ineffectively removes dust and irritants from the airways. › Alveoli dwindle, airway resistance increases, and the risk of pulmonary infection increases. › Kyphosis, an increased curvature of the thoracic spine due to osteoporosis and weakened cartilage, results in vertebral collapse and impairment of respiratory effort.
Cardiovascular system	› Systolic hypertension (widened pulse pressure) is a common finding with atherosclerosis. › The PMI becomes more difficult to palpate because the AP diameter of the chest widens. › Coronary blood vessel walls thicken and become more rigid with a narrowed lumen. › Cardiac output decreases and strength of contraction leads to poor activity tolerance. › Heart values stiffen due to calcification. › The left ventricle thickens. › Pulmonary vascular tension increases. › Systolic blood pressure rises. › Peripheral circulation diminishes.
Abdomen	› Weaker abdominal muscles declining in tone and more adipose tissue result in a rounder, more protruding abdomen. › Peritoneal inflammation is more difficult to detect due to less pain, guarding, fever, and rebound tenderness. › Saliva, gastric secretions, and pancreatic enzymes decrease. › Esophageal peristalsis and small-intestine motility decrease.

Sample Documentation

- Breasts conical, symmetric in size, and without masses or lesions. Nipples and areolae darker pigmented and symmetric. Everted nipples without discharge. No palpable axillary or clavicular lymph nodes. No pain or tenderness.

- Respiratory rate 16/min and regular. Respirations easy and unlabored. Thorax has a greater transverse than AP diameter. No chest wall deformities. Trachea midline. Movement symmetric with 5 cm of expansion. Equal tactile fremitus. Resonant sounds throughout. Vesicular sounds primarily over the bases bilaterally. No adventitious sounds. No cough, shortness of breath, difficulty breathing.

- Heart rhythm and rate regular at 72/min. Blood pressure 118/76 mm Hg. No thrills or heaves. PMI approximately 1 cm at the fifth ICS left midclavicular line. S1 louder at the apex than S2. S2 loudest in the pulmonary area on inspiration. No extra heart sounds, murmurs, or bruits. JVP 2 cm bilaterally. No chest pain or discomfort.

- Abdomen flat with active bowel sounds every 10 to 20 seconds in all four quadrants. No bruits or friction rubs. Abdomen soft, nontender, and without masses or enlargement of spleen or liver. Liver span 8 cm. No rebound or costovertebral tenderness. Bladder not palpable. No pain or discomfort in abdominal region.

APPLICATION EXERCISES

1. A nurse in a provider's office is preparing to perform a breast examination for an older adult who is postmenopausal. Which of the following findings should the nurse expect? (Select all that apply.)

_____ A. Smaller nipples

_____ B. Less adipose tissue

_____ C. Nipple discharge

_____ D. More pendulous

_____ E. Nipple inversion

2. A nurse in a provider's office is preparing to auscultate and percuss a client's thorax as part of a comprehensive physical examination. Which of the following findings should the nurse expect? (Select all that apply.)

_____ A. Rhonchi

_____ B. Crackles

_____ C. Resonance

_____ D. Tactile fremitus

_____ E. Bronchovesicular sounds

3. During an abdominal examination, a nurse in a provider's office determines that a client has abdominal distention. The protrusion is at midline, the skin over the area is taut, and the nurse notes no involvement of the flanks. Which of the following possible causes of distention should the nurse suspect?

A. Fat

B. Fluid

C. Flatus

D. Hernias

4. During a cardiovascular examination, a nurse in a provider's office places the diaphragm of the stethoscope on the left midclavicular line at the fifth intercostal space. Which of the following heart sounds is the nurse attempting to auscultate? (Select all that apply.)

_____ A. Ventricular gallop

_____ B. Closure of the mitral valve

_____ C. Closure of the pulmonic valve

_____ D. Closure of the tricuspid valve

_____ E. Murmur

5. A nurse in a provider's office is preparing to auscultate and percuss a client's abdomen as part of a comprehensive physical examination. Which of the following findings should the nurse expect? (Select all that apply.)

_____ A. Tympany

_____ B. High-pitched clicks

_____ C. Borborygmi

_____ D. Friction rubs

_____ E. Bruits

6. A nurse is teaching a group of nursing students about identifying chest landmarks to help them find the optimal locations for auscultation of the thorax. Use the ATI Active Learning Template: Basic Concept to complete this item. Under Underlying Principles, list the seven key chest landmarks, along with their location on the thorax.

APPLICATION EXERCISES KEY

1. A. **CORRECT:** In older adulthood, the nipples become smaller and flatter.

    B. INCORRECT: Older adults have more adipose tissue and less glandular tissue in their breasts.

    C. INCORRECT: Older adults have no nipple discharge, unless there is some underlying pathophysiology.

    D. **CORRECT:** In older adulthood, the breasts become softer and more pendulous.

    E. **CORRECT:** Nipple inversion is common among older adults, due to fibrotic changes and shrinkage.

     NCLEX® Connection: Physiological Adaptations, Pathophysiology

2. A. INCORRECT: Rhonchi are coarse sounds that result from fluid or mucus in the airways.

    B. INCORRECT: Crackles are fine to coarse popping sounds that result from air passing through fluid or re-expanding collapsed small airways.

    C. **CORRECT:** Resonance is the expected percussion sound over the thorax. It is a hollow sound that indicates air inside the lungs.

    D. **CORRECT:** Tactile fremitus is an expected vibration the nurse can expect to feel as the client vocalizes. Speech creates sound waves, the vibrations of which travel from the vocal cords through the lungs and to the chest wall.

    E. **CORRECT:** Bronchovesicular sounds are expected breath sounds of medium pitch and intensity and of equal inspiration and expiration time. The nurse can expect to hear them over the larger airways.

     NCLEX® Connection: Physiological Adaptations, Pathophysiology

3. A. INCORRECT: With fat, there are rolls of adipose tissue along the sides, and the skin does not look taut.

    B. INCORRECT: With fluid, the flanks also protrude, and when the client turns onto one side, the protrusion moves to the dependent side.

    C. **CORRECT:** With flatus, the protrusion is mainly midline, and there is no change in the flanks.

    D. INCORRECT: With hernias, protrusions through the abdominal muscle wall are visible, especially when the client raises her head.

     NCLEX® Connection: Physiological Adaptations, Pathophysiology

4. A. INCORRECT: To auscultate a ventricular gallop (an S3 sound), the nurse places the bell of the stethoscope at each of the auscultatory sites.

    B. **CORRECT:** To auscultate the closure of the mitral valve, the nurse places the diaphragm of the stethoscope over the apex, or apical/mitral site, which is on the left midclavicular line at the fifth intercostal space.

    C. INCORRECT: To auscultate the closure of the pulmonic valve, the nurse places the diaphragm of the stethoscope over the aortic area, which is just to the right of the sternum at the second intercostal space.

    D. **CORRECT:** To auscultate the closure of the tricuspid valve, the nurse places the diaphragm of the stethoscope over the apex, or apical/mitral site, which is on the left midclavicular line at the fifth intercostal space.

    E. INCORRECT: To auscultate a murmur, the nurse places the bell of the stethoscope at various auscultatory sites.

     NCLEX® Connection: Physiological Adaptations, Pathophysiology

5. A. **CORRECT:** Tympany is the expected drumlike percussion sound over the abdomen. It indicates air in the stomach.

    B. **CORRECT:** Typical bowel sounds are high-pitched clicks and gurgles occurring about 35 times/min.

    C. INCORRECT: Borborygmi are unexpected loud, growling sounds that indicate increased gastrointestinal motility. Possible causes include diarrhea, anxiety, bowel inflammation, and reactions to some foods.

    D. INCORRECT: Friction rubs result from the rubbing together of inflamed layers of the peritoneum and are unexpected findings.

    E. INCORRECT: Bruits indicate narrowed blood vessels and are unexpected findings.

     NCLEX® Connection: Physiological Adaptations, Pathophysiology

6. *Using the ATI Active Learning Template: Basic Concept*
    - Underlying Principles
        ○ Midsternal line: through the center of the sternum
        ○ Midclavicular line: through the midpoint of the clavicle
        ○ Anterior axillary line: through the anterior axillary folds
        ○ Midaxillary line: through the apex of the axillae
        ○ Posterior axillary line: through the posterior axillary fold
        ○ Right and left scapular lines: through the inferior angle of the scapula
        ○ Vertebral line: along the center of the spine

     NCLEX® Connection: Health Promotion and Maintenance, Techniques of Physical Assessment

chapter 30

Overview

- Assess the integumentary and peripheral vascular systems at the same time.

- Examine the upper extremities while the client is sitting or recumbent. Remove stockings/socks, and drape the client to expose the entire lower extremity at once.

- Make side-to-side comparisons to evaluate for any variations.

- Examine lesions individually.

- Use the Braden scale or a similar assessment tool to predict pressure-ulcer risk.

- Inspect and palpate simultaneously.

- Equipment includes:

  - Adequate lighting

  - Gloves for palpating open or draining lesions

  - A flexible ruler or tape measure to measure the size and depth of lesions in centimeters

Health History – Review of Systems

- Integumentary and Peripheral Vascular Systems

  - Questions to ask include:

    - Have you noticed any changes in your skin color? If so, is the change widespread or just in one area?

    - Do you have a rash? Where? Does it itch? How long have you had it? What have you used to treat the rash?

    - Is your skin excessively dry or oily? Does this change with the seasons? Do you use anything to treat it?

    - Have you developed any new moles or lesions? Have any of the moles or lesions changed in any way (color, borders, size)?

    - How often are you out in the sun? Do you use sunscreen or wear protective clothing and a hat?

    - Do you have any swelling? If in your legs, is it in both legs? Does the swelling cause pain? What do you do to relieve the swelling? Does it occur at any particular time of day?

Inspection and Palpation

- Assess the color of the hair, nails, and skin for uniformity. Hair color may vary due to dyes or from aging changes. Typically, skin color varies from ivory to ruddy to deep brown. Color changes are more difficult to notice in dark-skinned clients.

COLOR CHANGE	DESCRIPTION	INDICATION
Pallor	› Loss of color – face, conjunctivae, nail beds, palms	› Anemia or lack of blood flow
Cyanosis	› Bluish – nail beds, lips, mouth, skin	› Hypoxia or impaired venous return
Jaundice	› Yellow to orange – skin, sclera, mucous membranes	› Liverdysfunction, red blood-cell destruction
Erythema	› Redness – face, trauma and pressure sore areas	› Inflammation, localized vasodilation

- Note cleanliness of the hair, skin, and nails, as well as any odors. Expect firm nail bases. Note the curvature of the nail plate in relationship to the tissue just before the cuticle. Expect angles less than 160°. Clubbing is an unexpected curvature of the nail with an angle greater than 160°. This can result from chronic low oxygen saturation (emphysema, chronic bronchitis).

- Note hair distribution patterns. Expect symmetric hair loss, as with male pattern baldness. Note any infestations of the hair or skin. Alopecia can result from endocrine disorders and poor nutrition.

- Expect pink, symmetric nail beds. Capillary refill assesses circulation to the periphery. Blanching the nail bed with firm pressure and then quick release should result in a brisk return of color (within 2 seconds).

 View Video: Capillary Refill

- Expect skin color of the extremities to be symmetric and similar to that of the rest of the body.
  - ○ Brown pigmentation changes with venous insufficiency.
  - ○ Shiny and translucent skin without hair on the toes and foot indicates arterial insufficiency.

- Palpate the temperature of the skin with the dorsal part of the hand; check for symmetry, and expect warmth. Changes reflect circulation impairment or environmental temperature. Slightly cooler temperatures of the hands or feet are acceptable.

- Expect smooth, soft, even skin and smooth, firm nails. Expect smooth and coarse or fine hair. Thicker skin of the palms and soles of the feet is an expected finding.

- Assess skin turgor by lifting and releasing a fold of skin on the forearm or sternum to verify that it returns quickly into place. Tenting is a delay in the skin returning to its usual place. Poor turgor indicates dehydration or aging and increases the risk for skin breakdown.

 View Video: Skin Turgor

- Moisture in the axillae is an expected finding. Otherwise, the skin should be dry. Note diaphoresis, oiliness, or excessive dryness with flaking or scaling.

- Peripheral Arteries
  - Palpate the peripheral pulses for strength (amplitude) and equality (symmetry).
    - Strength (amplitude) – the same from beat to beat
    - Grade strength as:
      - 0 = Absent, unable to palpate
      - 1+ = Diminished, weaker than expected
      - 2+ = Brisk, expected
      - 3+ = Increased
      - 4+ = Full volume, bounding
    - Equality – symmetric in quality and quantity from the right side of the body to the left
  - With the exception of the carotid arteries, palpate pulse sites bilaterally to make comparisons.
    - Carotid pulse – on either side of the trachea, just medial to the sternocleidomastoid muscle on the neck
    - Radial pulse – on the radial side of each wrist
    - Brachial pulse – in the antecubital fossa above the elbow
    - Femoral pulse – midway between the symphysis pubis and the anterosuperior iliac spine
    - Popliteal pulse – behind the knee, deep in the popliteal fossa, just lateral to midline
    - Dorsalis pedis pulse – on the top of the foot, along a line with the groove between the first toe and the extensor tendons of the great toe
    - Posterior tibial pulse – behind and below the medial malleolus of the ankles
  - Inspect peripheral veins for varicosities, redness, and swelling.
- Edema is fluid in the tissues causing swollen, tight, and shiny skin surfaces, most often from direct trauma or impaired venous return. Assess the swelling for discoloration, location, and tenderness. In the extremities, measure the circumference of the swollen body area and compare both sides.
  - Evaluate pitting by compressing the skin for at least 5 seconds over a bony prominence (behind the medial malleolus, the dorsum of foot, or over the shin) and then assess. The depth of pitting reflects the degree of edema.

FOUR-POINT SCALE	DEGREE	RESPONSE
1+	2 mm – trace	Rapid
2+	4 mm – mild	10 to 15 seconds
3+	6 mm – moderate	1 to 2 min
4+	8 mm – severe	2 to 5 min

- Examine lesions for size, color, shape, consistency, elevation, location, distribution, configuration, tenderness, fluid, and drainage. Measure the height, width, and depth of lesions.

  ○ Primary lesions arise from healthy skin tissue. Common examples include:

LESIONS	DESCRIPTIONS	EXAMPLES
Macule	› Nonpalpable, skin color change, smaller than 1 cm	› Freckle
Papule	› Palpable, circumscribed , smaller than 1 cm	› Elevated nevus
Nodule/tumor	› Palpable, circumscribed, deep, firm, 1 to 2 cm	› Wart
Vesicle	› Serous fluid-filled, smaller than 1 cm	› Blister, herpes simplex, varicella
Pustule	› Pus-filled	› Acne
Tumor	› Solid mass, deep, larger than 1 to 2 cm	› Epithelioma
Wheal	› Palpable, irregular borders, edematous	› Insect bite

  ○ Secondary lesions result from a change in a primary lesion. Common examples include:

LESIONS	DESCRIPTIONS	EXAMPLES
Erosion	› Lost epidermis, moist surface, no bleeding	› Ruptured vesicle
Crust	› Dried blood, serum, or pus	› Scab
Scale	› Flakes of skin that exfoliate	› Dandruff or psoriasis
Fissure	› Linear crack	› Tinea pedis
Ulcer	› Loss of epidermis and dermis with possible bleeding, scarring	› Venous stasis ulcer, pressure ulcer

- Common examples of skin lesions in various age groups include:

CHILDREN	ADULTS	OLDER ADULTS
› Diaper dermatitis	› Primary contact dermatitis	› Lentigines (liver spots)
› Intertrigo	› Tinea pedis (ringworm of the foot)	› Seborrheic keratosis
› Impetigo	› Psoriasis	› Acrochordons (skin tags)
› Atopic dermatitis (eczema)	› Labial herpes simplex (cold sores)	› Sebaceous hyperplasia

○ Vascular lesions result from aging changes or blood-vessel damage in or near the skin. Common examples include:

LESIONS	DESCRIPTIONS
Spider angioma	› Red center with radiating red legs, up to 2 cm, possibly raised
Cherry angioma	› Red, 1 to 3 cm, round, possibly raised
Spider vein	› Bluish, spider-shaped or linear, up to several inches in size
Petechia/purpura	› Deep reddish purple, flat, petechiae 1 to 3 mm, purpura larger than 3 mm
Ecchymosis	› Purple fading to green or yellow over time, variable in size, flat
Hematoma	› Raised ecchymosis

Expected Changes with Aging

SYSTEM	CHANGES
Integumentary	› Skin thin and translucent, dry, flaky, tears easily, loss of elasticity and wrinkling › Thinning of hair › Slow growth of nails with thickening › Decline in glandular structure and function (less oil, moisture, sweat) › Uneven pigmentation › Slow wound healing › Little subcutaneous tissue over bony prominences
Peripheral vascular	› Thicker, more rigid peripheral blood vessel walls with a narrowed lumen leading to poor peripheral circulation › Higher systolic blood pressure

Sample Documentation

• Skin pink, warm, and dry. Turgor brisk, skin elastic. Rough, thickened skin over heels, elbows, and knees; otherwise, smooth. A 0.5 cm brown papule on right forearm and a 2.5 cm scar on left knee. Scalp dry with slight dandruff. Hair brown, clean, smooth, straight, evenly distributed on the head. Axillary and pubic hair evenly distributed with no infestations. Nails short and firm with no clubbing. Capillary refill < 3 seconds. No edema. Pulses palpable and equal bilaterally.

APPLICATION EXERCISES

1. A nurse in a provider's office is preparing to assess a client's skin as part of a comprehensive physical examination. Which of the following findings should the nurse expect? (Select all that apply.)

_____ A. Capillary refill in 2 seconds

_____ B. 1+ pitting edema in both feet

_____ C. Pale nail beds in both hands

_____ D. Thick skin on the soles of the feet

_____ E. Numerous light brown macules on the face

2. A nurse's assessment of an older adult client identifies significant tenting of the skin over his forearm. Which of the following can explain this finding? (Select all that apply.)

_____ A. Thin, parchment-like skin

_____ B. Loss of adipose tissue

_____ C. Dehydration

_____ D. Diminished skin elasticity

_____ E. Excessive dryness and wrinkling

3. A nurse is caring for a client who is postoperative following knee surgery. Which of the following should the nurse examine to assess the client's peripheral vascular system? (Select all that apply.)

_____ A. Range of motion

_____ B. Skin color

_____ C. Edema

_____ D. Skin lesions

_____ E. Skin temperature

4. A nurse is reviewing the various types of lesions nursing students might encounter when performing integumentary assessments for their clients. Which of the following lesions should the nursing students recognize as vesicles? (Select all that apply.)

_____ A. Acne

_____ B. Warts

_____ C. Psoriasis

_____ D. Herpes simplex

_____ E. Varicella

5. A nurse is instructing a group of nursing students in the priorities of care in performing an integumentary assessment for their clients. Which of the following findings should the students recognize as requiring immediate intervention?

A. Pallor

B. Cyanosis

C. Jaundice

D. Erythema

6. A nurse is reviewing the questions to ask when interviewing clients as part of an integumentary and peripheral vascular assessment. Use the ATI Active Learning Template: Basic Concept to complete this item. Under Nursing Interventions, compose an appropriate series of questions to ask prior to beginning the inspection and palpation portions of the assessment.

APPLICATION EXERCISES KEY

1. A. **CORRECT:** Capillary refill in less than 2 seconds is an expected finding.

   B. INCORRECT: Pitting edema is an unexpected finding that reflects excess fluid that has accumulated in body tissues.

   C. INCORRECT: Pallor in the nail beds is an unexpected finding that reflects anemia or impaired circulation.

   D. **CORRECT:** Thicker skin on the palms of the hands and the soles of the feet is an expected finding.

   E. **CORRECT:** Light brown macules on the face are likely to be freckles, which are an expected finding.

   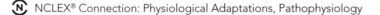 NCLEX® Connection: Physiological Adaptations, Pathophysiology

2. A. INCORRECT: Aging skin does become thin and translucent, but this typically does not affect tenting.

   B. **CORRECT:** Tenting is a delay in the skin returning to its normal place after pinching. It can be a sign of aging skin and loss of subcutaneous tissue that provides recoil in younger skin.

   C. **CORRECT:** Tenting is a delay in the skin returning to its normal place after pinching. It can be a sign of dehydration, which easily develops in older adult clients for many reasons.

   D. **CORRECT:** Tenting is a delay in the skin returning to its normal place after pinching. It can be a sign of aging skin and its loss of elasticity.

   E. INCORRECT: Aging skin does become dry and wrinkled, but this typically does not affect tenting.

   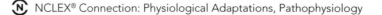 NCLEX® Connection: Physiological Adaptations, Pathophysiology

3. A. INCORRECT: Determining range of motion helps the nurse evaluate joint function, not circulation.

   B. **CORRECT:** Assessing the peripheral vascular system to verify adequate circulation to the client's legs includes skin color. Pallor and cyanosis reflect inadequate circulation.

   C. **CORRECT:** Assessing the peripheral vascular system to verify adequate circulation to the client's legs includes edema. Edema reflects inadequate venous circulation.

   D. INCORRECT: Inspecting for skin lesions is part of an integumentary assessment, but it does not evaluate circulation. Some skin lesions do reflect inadequate circulation, but they would not have developed in the immediate postoperative period.

   E. **CORRECT:** Assessing the peripheral vascular system to verify adequate circulation to the client's legs includes skin temperature. Coolness of the extremity compared with the nonoperative extremity indicates inadequate circulation.

   NCLEX® Connection: Pharmacological and Parenteral Therapies, Expected Actions/Outcomes

4. A. INCORRECT: Acne lesions are pustules, not vesicles.

    B. INCORRECT: Warts are nodules, not vesicles.

    C. INCORRECT: Psoriasis lesions are scales, not vesicles.

    D. **CORRECT:** Herpes simplex lesions are vesicles, which are circumscribed fluid-filled skin elevations. Eczema and impetigo also cause vesicles to appear on the skin.

    E. **CORRECT:** Varicella (chickenpox) lesions are vesicles, which are circumscribed fluid-filled skin elevations. Eczema and impetigo also cause vesicles to appear on the skin.

    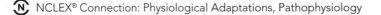 NCLEX® Connection: Physiological Adaptations, Pathophysiology

5. A. INCORRECT: Pallor can indicate anemia or circulation difficulties. These are important and require intervention, but there is a higher priority among these options.

    B. **CORRECT:** The priority finding when using the airway, breathing, circulation (ABC) approach to care delivery is one that affects the client's airway. Cyanosis can reflect hypoxia (inadequate oxygenation), so nurses must take immediate action to report the finding and improve the client's oxygenation.

    C. INCORRECT: Jaundice can indicate liver dysfunction or red blood cell destruction. These are important and require intervention, but there is a higher priority among these options.

    D. INCORRECT: Erythema usually indicates inflammation. This is important and requires intervention, but there is a higher priority among these options.

    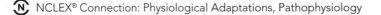 NCLEX® Connection: Physiological Adaptations, Pathophysiology

6. *Using the ATI Active Learning Template: Basic Concept*
    - Nursing Interventions
      ○ Have you noticed any changes in your skin color? If so, is the change widespread or just in one area?
      ○ Do you have a rash? Where? Does it itch? How long have you had it? What have you used to treat the rash?
      ○ Is your skin excessively dry or oily? Does this change with the seasons? Do you use anything to treat it?
      ○ Have you developed any new moles or lesions? Have any of the moles or lesions changed in any way (color, borders, size)?
      ○ How often are you out in the sun? Do you use sunscreen or wear protective clothing and a hat?
      ○ Do you have any swelling? If in your legs, is it in both legs? Does the swelling cause pain? What do you do to relieve the swelling? Does it occur at any particular time of day?

    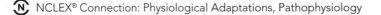 NCLEX® Connection: Reduction of Risk Potential, System Specific Assessments

FUNDAMENTALS FOR NURSING

chapter 31

Overview

- This examination includes muscles, joints, range of motion, mental status, cranial nerves, and motor and sensory function.

MUSCULOSKELETAL SYSTEM

Overview

- Examination of the musculoskeletal system includes looking at the structure and function of the musculoskeletal system.
- This involves examining each joint and muscle and the surrounding tissues and comparing symmetric parts.
- Use the techniques of inspection and palpation to assess the musculoskeletal system.
- Equipment
  - Tape measure
- Assess
  - Gait
  - Alignment
  - Symmetry, muscle mass
  - Muscle tone
  - Range of motion (ROM)
  - Any involuntary movements
  - Signs of inflammation (redness, swelling, warmth, tenderness, loss of function)
  - Gross deformities
- Expected Range of Motion of Joint Movement
  - Flexion – a movement that decreases the angle
  - Extension – a movement that increases the angle
  - Hyperextension – an extreme extension
  - Supination – the ventral surface facing up
  - Pronation – the ventral surface facing down
  - Abduction – the movement of an extremity away from the midline

- ○ Adduction – the movement of an extremity toward the midline
- ○ Dorsiflexion – flexing the foot and toes upward
- ○ Plantar flexion – bending the foot and toes downward
- ○ Eversion – turning the body part away from midline
- ○ Inversion – turning the body part toward the midline
- ○ External rotation – rotating a joint outward
- ○ Internal rotation – rotating a joint inward

Health History – Review of Systems

- Questions to ask
  - ○ Do you have any pain in your joints or muscles?
  - ○ Do you have any stiffness, weakness, or twitching?
  - ○ Have you fallen recently?
  - ○ Are you able to care for yourself?
  - ○ Do you have any physical problems that limit your activities?
  - ○ Do you exercise or participate in sports on a regular basis?
  - ○ For postmenopausal women: What was your maximum height? Do you take calcium supplements?

Inspection

- Symmetry – Observe and compare both sides of the body for symmetry.
- ⓖ Height – Measure for comparison over time. Gradual height loss is a common finding as a person ages.
- Posture – Observe when the client is unaware. Expected finding: client is standing with head erect. Both shoulders and both hips should be at the same height bilaterally.
- Spine – Inspect from the side. Note the following curvatures:
  - ○ Expected curvatures (posteriorly)
    - Concave cervical spine
    - Convex thoracic spine
    - Concave lumbar spine
    - Convex sacral spine
  - ○ Unexpected findings
    - Kyphosis – exaggerated curvature of the thoracic spine (common among older adults)
    - Lordosis – exaggerated curvature of the lumbar spine (common during the toddler years and pregnancy)
    - Scoliosis – exaggerated lateral curvature

Inspection and Palpation

- Expect equal range of motion (ROM) in the joints bilaterally.

  - Assess passive ROM by moving the client's joints through his full range of movements. Do not move a joint past the point of pain or resistance.

  - Assess active ROM by having the client repeat the movements the nurse demonstrates.

  - Assess joints for warmth, inflammation, edema, stiffness, crepitus, deformities, tenderness, limitations, and instability. Assess the following joints:

    - Temporomandibular joint (TMJ)

    - Shoulders

    - Elbows

    - Wrists and hands

    - Spine (scoliosis)

    - Hips

    - Knees

    - Ankles, feet

- Expect muscles that are firm and symmetric in size and strength. The dominant side is usually slightly larger; less than a 1-cm difference is not significant.

  - Size variations include:

    - Hypertrophy – an enlargement of muscle due to strengthening

    - Atrophy – a decrease in muscle size due to disuse; feels soft and boggy

  - During ROM, assess tone – slight resistance of the muscles during relaxation.

  - Assess the strength of muscle groups by asking the client to push or pull against resistance. Expected finding: strength equal or slightly stronger on the dominant side of the body.

  - Assess for muscle tremors.

- Inspect and palpate the spine from the back for any lateral deviations or scoliosis.

  - Instruct the client to bend at the waist with the arms reaching for the toes.

  - Inspect and palpate down the spine using the thumb and forefinger.

  - Inspect and palpate the spine again with the client standing.

  - Expected finding: no tenderness, with spinal vertebrae that are midline.

NEUROSENSORY SYSTEM

Overview

- A neurological screening examination can evaluate the major indicators of neurological function and assist with recognition of areas of dysfunction.

- Integrate the neurological system with other assessments.

- A neurological screening examination includes:

  ○ Mental status examination to test cerebral function

  ○ Assessment of cranial nerves

  ○ Motor function to test cerebellar function

  ○ Sensory function

  ○ Reflexes

- Equipment

  ○ Snellen and Rosenbaum eye charts

  ○ Aromatic substances

  ○ Tongue blades

  ○ Penlight

  ○ Sugar and salt

  ○ Tuning fork

  ○ Reflex hammer

  ○ Cotton balls

  ○ Two test tubes containing water (one cold, one warm)

  ○ Pencil

  ○ Paper clips

  ○ Key

Health History – Review of Systems

- Questions to ask

  ○ Do you have any dizziness or headaches?

  ○ Do you ever have seizures? If so, what triggers them?

  ○ Have you ever had a head injury or any loss of consciousness?

  ○ Have you noticed any change in your vision, speech, ability to think clearly, loss of memory, or change in memory or behavior?

  ○ Do you have any weakness, numbness, tremors, or tingling? If so, where?

Mental Status

- Describe levels of consciousness and observed behavior with the following terms:
  - Alert – The client is responsive and able to open his eyes and answer questions spontaneously and appropriately.
  - Lethargic – The client is able to open his eyes and respond but is drowsy and falls asleep readily.
  - Obtunded – The client responds to light shaking but may be confused and slow to respond.
  - Stuporous – The client requires painful stimuli (pinching a tendon or rubbing the sternum) to achieve a brief response. The client may not be able to respond verbally.
  - Comatose – There is no response to repeated painful stimuli. Abnormal posturing in clients who are comatose:
    - Decorticate rigidity – Flexion and internal rotation of upper extremity joints and legs
    - Decerebrate rigidity – Neck and elbow extension, with the wrists and fingers flexed
- Assess appearance by observing hygiene, grooming, and clothing choice. Expected findings: client is clean and dressed appropriately for the environment or situation.
- Assess mood by inspecting mannerisms and actions during interactions. Expected findings: client makes eye contact, and emotions correspond to the conversation and situation.
- Assess cognitive and intellectual processes:
  - Assess memory, both recent and remote.
    - Recent – Ask the client to repeat a series of numbers or a list of objects.
    - Remote – Ask the client to state his birth date or mother's maiden name (verifiable).
  - Level and fund of knowledge – Ask the client what he knows about his current hospitalization or illness.
  - Ability for calculation – Ask the client to count backward from 100 in serials of 7.
  - Abstract thinking – Ask the client the interpretation of a cliché such as, "A bird in the hand is worth two in the bush." This demonstrates a higher level of thought processes.
  - Insight – Perform an objective assessment of the client's perception of illness.
  - Judgment – Ask the client about the solution to a specific dilemma. ("What would you do if you locked your keys in your car?")
  - Thought process – Note processing differences, such as a rapid change of topic (flight of ideas) and use of nonsense words ("hipsnippity").
  - Thought content – Note the presence of delusions, hallucinations, and other ideas the client presents during the interview.
- Expect speech and language rate and features, such as quality, quantity, and volume, to be articulate and responses meaningful and appropriate.

- Standardized Screening Tools
  - Use the Mini-Mental State Examination (MME) to assess cognitive status objectively. The tool evaluates:
    - Orientation to time and place
    - Attention and calculation of counting backward by sevens
    - Registration and recalling of objects
    - Language, including naming of objects, following of commands, and ability to write
    - Reading
  - Use the Glasgow Coma Scale to obtain a baseline assessment of the client's level of consciousness and for ongoing assessment.
    - This assessment looks at eye, verbal, and motor response, and assigns a number value based on the client's response. The highest value possible is 15, indicating full consciousness.

Cranial Nerve Function

CRANIAL NERVE (CN)	FUNCTION OF THE NERVE	SYSTEM
I (Olfactory)	› Sensory – smell	› Ears, nose, mouth, and throat
II (Optic)	› Sensory – visual acuity, visual fields	› Eyes
III (Oculomotor), IV (Trochlear), and VI (Abducens)	› Motor PERRLA, six cardinal positions of gaze	› Eyes
V (Trigeminal)	› Sensory – light touch sensation to the face (forehead, cheek, jaw) › Motor – jaw opening, clenching, chewing	› Head and neck
VII (Facial)	› Sensory – taste (salt/sweet) on anterior two thirds of the tongue › Motor – facial movements	› Head and neck
VIII (Auditory)	› Sensory – hearing and balance	› Ears, nose, mouth, and throat
IX (Glossopharyngeal)	› Sensory – taste (sour/bitter) on posterior third of the tongue › Motor – swallowing, speech sounds, gag reflex	› Ears, nose, mouth, throat, neurological
X (Vagus)	› Sensory – gag reflex › Motor – swallowing, speech sounds	› Ears, nose, mouth, and throat
XI (Spinal accessory)	› Motor – turning head, shrugging shoulders	› Head and neck
XII (Hypoglossal)	› Motor – tongue movement	› Ears, nose, mouth, and throat

Motor Function

- Assess coordination by asking the client to extend his arms and rapidly touch his finger to his nose, alternating hands, and then doing it with his eyes closed. Expected findings include smooth, coordinated movements.

- Assess gait when the client is unaware of the assessment. Expected finding: Gait is steady, smooth, and coordinated.

- Assess balance using the following tests:

  ○ Romberg test – Ask the client to stand with his feet together, his arms at his sides, and his eyes closed. Expected finding: The client stands with minimal swaying for at least 5 seconds.

  ○ Heel-to-toe walk – Ask the client to place the heel of one foot in front of the toes of the other foot as he walks in a straight line. Expected finding: The client walks in a straight line without losing his balance.

- Muscle Strength

  ○ Assess the strength of muscle groups by asking the client to push or pull against resistance. Expected finding: Strength is equal or slightly stronger on the dominant side of the body.

Sensory Function

- Perform tests on all four extremities with the client's eyes closed.

  ○ Assess pain sensation by alternating sharp and dull objects on the skin and asking the client to report what he feels.

  ○ Assess temperature by using two test tubes containing water (one warm and one cold), and ask the client to identify which he feels.

  ○ Assess light touch by asking the client to report when and where he feels a cotton ball touching his skin.

  ○ Assess vibration by having the client report when and where he feels the handle of the vibrating tuning fork on his skin.

  ○ Assess position by repositioning the client's appendages and asking him to report whether each is positioned up or down.

  ○ Assess discrimination by using one of the following:

    ▪ Two-point discrimination – Use open paper clips to determine the smallest distance between the two points at which the client can still feel the two points on his skin and not just one. Compare bilaterally. Minimal distance varies with the body part.

    ▪ Stereognosis – Place a familiar object (key, cotton ball) in the client's hand, and ask him to identify it.

    ▪ Graphesthesia – Trace a number on the client's palm with the blunt end of a pencil and ask him to identify it.

Deep-Tendon Reflexes (DTRs)

- Using a reflex hammer, assess DTRs bilaterally and compare results for symmetry as follows:

DTR – SPINAL CORD INNERVATION	TECHNIQUE	EXPECTED RESPONSE
Biceps – C_5 and C_6	› Flex arm 45°. › Place the thumb on the tendon in antecubital fossa. › Strike the thumb with a reflex hammer.	› Flexion of the elbow
Brachioradialis – C_5 and C_6	› Rest a forearm on the examiner's forearm with the wrist slightly pronated. › Strike the tendon 2.5 to 5 cm above the wrist.	› Pronation of the forearm and flexion of the elbow
Triceps – C_7 and C_8	› Support the upper arm with the forearm hanging at a 90° angle. › Strike the tendon above the elbow.	› Extension of the elbow
Patellar – L_2, L_3, and L_4	› With the upper leg supported and the lower leg dangling freely, strike the tendon below the knee.	› Extension of the lower leg
Achilles – S_1 and S_2	› Flex the knee, dorsiflex the foot, and strike the tendon above the heel.	› Plantar flexion of the foot

- Grade DTR responses as:
  - 4+ = Very brisk with clonus
  - 3+ = More brisk than average
  - 2+ = Expected
  - 1+ = Diminished
  - 0 = No response

Expected Changes with Aging

SYSTEM	CHANGES
Musculoskeletal	› Reduced muscle mass › Declines in speed, strength, resistance to fatigue, reaction time, coordination › Osteoporosis (fragility of bones, loss of bone mass and height) › Greater risk of fractures and vertebral compression › Degenerative alterations in joints › Limited range of motion › Flexed elbows, hips, and knees › Thinning intervertebral discs, kyphosis (with height loss), wider stance altering posture
Neurological	› Some short-term memory decline › Diminished/slowed reflex and motor responses, impulse transmission, and reaction times › Altered vibration, position, hearing, vision, smell, and deep pain and temperature sensation › Slower fine finger movement (no change in superficial pain and light touch sensation, standing balance) › Decline in mental function probably related to less cognitive stimulation and solitude › Fewer brain cells, smaller brain volume, deteriorating nerve cells, fewer neurotransmitters › With infection, delirium more common than fever › Greater risk of depression

Sample Documentation

Full range of motion without pain in all joints and spine. No joint deformities, warmth, or swelling. Posture erect. Spine midline with expected cervical, thoracic, and lumbar curvatures. No scoliosis. Muscle strength equal and strong bilaterally.

APPLICATION EXERCISES

1. A nurse in a provider's office is preparing to assess a young adult male client's musculoskeletal system as part of a comprehensive physical examination. Which of the following findings should the nurse expect? (Select all that apply.)

_____ A. A concave thoracic spine posteriorly

_____ B. An exaggerated lumbar curvature

_____ C. A concave lumbar spine posteriorly

_____ D. An exaggerated thoracic curvature

_____ E. Muscles slightly larger on his dominant side

2. A nurse is evaluating a client's neurosensory system. To evaluate stereognosis, she should ask the client to close his eyes and identify which of the following items?

A. A word she whispers 30 cm from his ear

B. A number she traces on the palm of his hand

C. The vibration of a tuning fork she places on his foot

D. A familiar object she places in his hand

3. A nurse is assessing a client who reports pain when the nurse evaluates the internal rotation of her right shoulder. Which of the following activities is this problem likely to affect?

A. Mopping her floors

B. Brushing the back of her hair

C. Fastening her bra behind her back

D. Reaching into a cabinet above her sink

4. A nurse is performing a neurosensory examination for a client. Which of the following tests should the nurse perform to test the client's balance? (Select all that apply.)

_____ A. Romberg test

_____ B. Heel-to-toe walk

_____ C. Snellen test

_____ D. Spinal accessory function

_____ E. Rosenbaum test

5. A nurse is collecting data from an older adult client as part of a neurosensory examination. Which of the following findings should the nurse expect as changes associated with aging? (Select all that apply.)

_____ A. Slower light touch sensation

_____ B. Some vision and hearing decline

_____ C. Slower fine finger movement

_____ D. Some short-term memory decline

_____ E. Slower superficial pain sensation

6. A nurse is reviewing the expected range of motion of joint movement with a group of nursing students. What information should the nurse include in the review? Use the ATI Active Learning Template: Basic Concept to complete this item. Under Related Content, list the 13 common types of motion along with the actions that demonstrate them.

APPLICATION EXERCISES KEY

1. A. **CORRECT:** A convex thoracic spine posteriorly (with the convexity arching toward the back of the body) is an expected finding.

    B. INCORRECT: Although lordosis, an exaggerated lumbar curvature, is common among toddlers and pregnant women, it is an unexpected finding in most adults.

    C. **CORRECT:** A concave lumbar spine posteriorly (with the concavity moving inward from the back of the body) is an expected finding.

    D. INCORRECT: Although kyphosis, an exaggerated lumbar curvature, is common among older adults, it is an unexpected finding in younger adults.

    E. **CORRECT:** Muscle size equal on both sides or slightly larger on the dominant side is an expected finding.

    (N) NCLEX® Connection: Physiological Adaptations, Pathophysiology

2. A. INCORRECT: Identifying a whispered word confirms that CN VIII is intact.

    B. INCORRECT: Identifying a tracing on the palm confirms the client's sense of graphesthesia, which is the ability to use only the sensation of touch to recognize writing on the skin.

    C. INCORRECT: Identifying the vibration of a tuning fork confirms the client's vibratory sense.

    D. **CORRECT:** Identifying a familiar object in the hand confirms the client's sense of stereognosis, which is tactile recognition.

    (N) NCLEX® Connection: Reduction of Risk Potential, System Specific Assessments

3. A. INCORRECT: Mopping the floor requires flexion and extension of the shoulder.

    B. INCORRECT: Brushing the back of the hair requires external rotation of the shoulder.

    C. **CORRECT:** Fastening a bra from behind requires internal rotation of the shoulder, so this activity will elicit pain.

    D. INCORRECT: Reaching for something up high requires external rotation of the shoulder.

    (N) NCLEX® Connection: Pharmacological and Parenteral Therapies, Central Venous Access Devices

4. A. **CORRECT:** For the Romberg test, the client stands with his eyes closed, arms at his side, and feet together. The nurse verifies balance if he can stand with minimal swaying for at least 5 seconds.

    B. **CORRECT:** For the heel-to-toe walk, the client places the heel of one foot in front of the toes of the other foot as he walks in a straight line. The nurse verifies balance if he can walk in a straight line without losing his balance.

    C. INCORRECT: A Snellen eye chart tests visual acuity, not balance.

    D. INCORRECT: Testing spinal accessory function verifies that cranial nerve XI is intact by asking the client to shrug his shoulders and turn his head against resistance.

    E. INCORRECT: A Rosenbaum eye chart tests visual acuity, not balance.

    Ⓝ NCLEX® Connection: Reduction of Risk Potential, Diagnostic Tests

5. A. INCORRECT: With aging, light touch sensation typically remains the same.

    B. **CORRECT:** With aging, losses in vision, hearing, taste, and smell decline.

    C. **CORRECT:** With aging, fine finger movement slows, along with some reflex and motor responses.

    D. **CORRECT:** With aging, some decline in short-term memory is an expected finding. Major cognitive decline is an expected finding.

    E. INCORRECT: With aging, superficial pain sensation typically remains the same.

    Ⓝ NCLEX® Connection: Health Promotion and Maintenance, Developmental Stages and Transitions

6. *Using the ATI Active Learning Template Basic Concept*
    - Related Content
        - Flexion – a movement that decreases the angle
        - Extension – a movement that increases the angle
        - Hyperextension – an extreme extension
        - Supination – the ventral surface facing up
        - Pronation – the ventral surface facing down
        - Abduction – the movement of an extremity away from the midline
        - Adduction – the movement of an extremity toward the midline
        - Dorsiflexion – flexing the foot and toes upward
        - Plantar flexion – bending the foot and toes downward
        - Eversion – turning the body part away from midline
        - Inversion – turning the body part toward the midline
        - External rotation – rotating a joint outward
        - Internal rotating – rotating a joint inward

    Ⓝ NCLEX® Connection: Physiological Adaptations, Pathophysiology

UNIT 3   Psychosocial Integrity

CHAPTERS

> Therapeutic Communication
> Coping
> Self-Concept and Sexuality
> Cultural and Spiritual Nursing Care
> Grief, Loss, and Palliative Care

NCLEX® CONNECTIONS

When reviewing the chapters in this unit, keep in mind the relevant sections of the NCLEX® outline, in particular:

Client Needs: Psychosocial Integrity

> Relevant topics/tasks include:

  » Coping Mechanisms

    > Provide information to the client on stress management techniques.

  » Cultural Diversity

    > Incorporate the client's cultural practices and beliefs when planning and providing care.

  » End-of-Life Care

    > Identify end-of-life needs of the client.

  » Religious and Spiritual Influences on Health

    > Assess and plan interventions that meet the client's emotional and spiritual needs.

  » Therapeutic Communication

    > Allow time to communicate with the client.

UNIT 3   PSYCHOSOCIAL INTEGRITY

CHAPTER 32   Therapeutic Communication

Overview

- Communication is a complex process of sending, receiving, and comprehending messages between two or more people. It is a dynamic and ongoing process that creates a unique experience between the participants.

  - Communicating effectively is a skill that can be developed.

  - Nurses use communication when providing care to demonstrate caring, establish relationships, obtain and deliver information, and assist with changing behavior.

  - Therapeutic communication is foundational to the nurse-client relationship.

  - Effective communication is key to ensuring client safety.

Basic Communication

- Levels of Basic Communication

  - Intrapersonal communication – Communication that occurs within an individual. Also identified as "self-talk." This is the internal discussion that takes place when an individual is thinking but not outwardly verbalizing the thoughts. In nursing, intrapersonal communication allows the nurse to assess clients and/or situations and think critically about the clients/situations before communicating verbally.

  - Interpersonal communication – Communication that occurs between two people. This form of communication is the most common in nursing and requires an exchange of information with an individual or small group.

  - Public communication – Communication that occurs within large groups of people. In nursing, this commonly occurs during educational endeavors during which the nurse is teaching a large group of individuals, such as in a community setting.

  - Transpersonal communication – Communication that addresses spiritual needs and provides interventions to meet these needs.

  - Small group communication – Communication within a group of people, usually working toward a mutual goal.

- Functional Components of Basic Communication

COMPONENT	DESCRIPTION
Referent	› The incentive or motivation for communication to occur between one person and another
Sender	› The person who initiates the message
Receiver	› The person to whom the message is aimed at and received by
Message	› The verbal and/or nonverbal information that is expressed by the sender and intended for the receiver
Channel	› The method of transmitting and receiving a message (received via sight, hearing, and/or touch)
Environment	› The emotional and physical climate in which the communication takes place
Feedback	› May be verbal and/or nonverbal, positive and/or negative › The message that is returned to the sender by the receiver that indicates that the message was received › An essential component of ongoing communication
Interpersonal variables	› Variables that influence communication between the sender and the receiver

- Methods of Communication
  - Verbal Communication

CHARACTERISTICS OF VERBAL COMMUNICATION	IMPACT ON THE COMMUNICATION
› Vocabulary – These are the words used to communicate either a written or spoken message.	› Limited vocabulary or speaking another language may make it difficult for the nurse to communicate with the client. Use of medical jargon may decrease client understanding.
› Denotative/connotative meaning – When communicating, participants must share meanings.	› Words that have multiple meanings may cause miscommunication if interpreted differently.
› Clarity/brevity – The shortest, simplest communication is usually most effective.	› Long and complex communication may be difficult to understand.
› Timing/relevance – Knowing when to communicate allows the receiver to be more attentive to the message.	› Communicating with a client who is in physical discomfort or distracted will make it difficult to convey the message.
› Pacing – The rate of speech can communicate an unintended meaning to the receiver.	› Speaking rapidly may communicate the impression that the nurse is in a rush and does not have time for the client.
› Intonation – The tone of voice can communicate a variety of feelings.	› The nurse can communicate feelings such as acceptance, judgment, and dislike through tone of voice.

○ Nonverbal Communication

▪ Nurses should be aware of how they communicate nonverbally. The nurse should assess the client's nonverbal communication for the meaning being conveyed, remembering that culture impacts interpretation. Attention to the following in both the communicator and the receiver is necessary:

CHARACTERISTICS OF NON-VERBAL COMMUNICATION	IMPACT ON THE COMMUNICATION
Appearance/posture/gait	› Physical characteristics can convey professionalism. Body language and posture may demonstrate comfort and ease in the situation.
Facial expressions/eye contact/gestures	› Facial expressions can reveal feelings that can be misinterpreted by clients. Eye contact typically conveys interest and respect but varies with culture and situation. Gestures can enhance verbal communication or create their own messages.
Sounds	› Crying or moaning can have multiple meanings when accompanied by other nonverbal communication.
Territoriality/personal space	› Lack of awareness of territoriality (right to space) and personal space (the area around an individual) can cause clients to feel threatened and react with defensiveness.

Therapeutic Communication

• Therapeutic communication is the purposeful use of communication to build and maintain helping relationships with clients, families, and significant others.

M View Video: Therapeutic Communication

• The nurse uses interactive, purposeful communication skills to

○ Elicit and attend to the client's thoughts, feelings, concerns, and needs.

○ Express empathy and genuine concern for the client and the family's issues.

○ Obtain information and give feedback about the client's condition.

○ Intervene to promote functional behavior and effective interpersonal relationships.

○ Evaluate the client's progress toward desired goals and outcomes.

• Children and older adults frequently require altered techniques to enhance communication.

• Use of the nursing process depends on therapeutic communication between the nurse, client/family/ significant other, and the interprofessional health care team.

• Characteristics of Therapeutic Communication

○ Client-centered – Not social or reciprocal

○ Purposeful, planned, and goal-directed

Q
PCC
- Essential Components of Therapeutic Communication
  - Time – Plan for and allow adequate time to communicate with others.
  - Attentive behaviors or active listening – A means of conveying interest, trust, and acceptance.
  - Caring attitude – Show concern and facilitate an emotional connection and support between the nurse and the client/family/significant other.
  - Honesty – Be open, direct, truthful, and sincere.
  - Trust – Demonstrate to the client/family/significant other that they can rely on the nurse without doubt, question, or judgment.
  - Empathy – Convey an objective awareness and understanding of the feelings, emotions, and behaviors of the client/family/significant other, including trying to envision what it must be like to be in the client/family/significant other's position.
  - Nonjudgmental attitude – A display of acceptance of the client/family/significant other will encourage open, honest communication.

Nursing Process

- Assessment/Data Collection
  - Determine verbal and nonverbal communication needs.
    - Clients who are hearing impaired, visually impaired, cognitively impaired, unresponsive, non-English speaking, or aphasic
  - Consider physical status.
  - Consider the developmental level, and alter communication accordingly.
    - Children
      - Use simple, straightforward language.
      - Be aware of nonverbal messages because children are sensitive to nonverbal communication.
      - Enhance communication by being at the child's eye level.
      - Incorporate play in interactions.
    - Older adult clients
      - Recognize that the client may require amplification.
      - Minimize distractions, and face the client when speaking.
      - Allow plenty of time for the client to respond.
      - When impaired communication is assessed, ask for input from caregivers or family to determine the extent of the deficits and how best to communicate.
    - Identify any cultural considerations that may affect communication.
      - Provide an interpreter as needed.
      - Address the client directly when the interpreter is present.
      - Provide educational materials and instructions in the client's language.

- Planning
    - Minimize distractions.
    - Provide privacy.
    - Identify mutually agreed-upon client outcomes.
    - Set priorities according to the client's needs.
    - Collaborate with other health care professionals when necessary.
    - Plan adequate time for interventions.
- Implementation
    - Establish a trusting nurse-client relationship. The client feels more at ease during the implementation phase when a helping relationship has been established.
    - Provide empathetic responses and explanations to the client by using observations, giving information, conveying hope, and using humor.

Effective Skills and Techniques

EFFECTIVE COMMUNICATION	INFLUENCE ON COMMUNICATION
Silence	› Silence allows time for meaningful reflection.
Active listening	› The nurse is able to hear, observe, and understand what the client communicates and provide feedback.
Open-ended questions	› This technique facilitates spontaneous responses and interactive discussion. Allows the client to explore feelings and thoughts. Avoids yes/no answers.
Clarifying techniques	› This technique is used to determine whether the message received was accurate: » Restating – Uses the client's exact words » Reflecting – Directs the focus back to the client in order for the client to examine his feelings » Paraphrasing – Restates the client's feelings and thoughts for the client to confirm what has been communicated » Exploring – Allows the nurse to gather more information regarding important topics mentioned by the client
Offering general leads, broad opening statements	› This encourages the client to start and to continue talking.
Showing acceptance and recognition	› This technique acknowledges the nurse's interest and nonjudgmental attitude.
Focusing	› This technique helps the client concentrate on what is important.
Asking questions	› Asking questions is a way to seek additional information.
Giving information	› This technique provides details that the client may need for decision-making.

EFFECTIVE COMMUNICATION	INFLUENCE ON COMMUNICATION
Presenting reality	› This technique is used to help the client focus on what is actually happening and to dispel delusions, hallucinations, or faulty beliefs.
Summarizing	› This technique emphasizes important points and reviews what has been discussed.
Offering self	› This technique demonstrates a willingness to spend time with the client. Limited personal information may be shared, but the focus should return to the client as soon as possible. Relevant self-disclosure by the nurse allows the client to see that his experience is shared by others and understood.
Touch	› If appropriate, touch may communicate caring and provide comfort.

Barriers to Effective Communication

- Asking irrelevant personal questions
- Offering personal opinions
- Giving advice
- Giving false reassurance
- Minimizing feelings
- Changing the topic
- Asking "why" questions or asking for explanations
- Offering value judgments
- Excessive questioning
- Responding approvingly or disapprovingly

APPLICATION EXERCISES

1. A nurse is caring for a client who states, "I have to check with my wife and see if she thinks I am ready to be discharged." The nurse replies, "How do you feel about going home today?" Which clarifying technique is the nurse displaying to enhance communication between the nurse and the client?

    A. Pacing

    B. Reflecting

    C. Paraphrasing

    D. Restating

2. A nurse is caring for a client who is concerned about being discharged home with a new colostomy because he is an avid swimmer. Which of the following statements made by the nurse indicates use of an effective communication technique? (Select all that apply.)

    _____ A. "You will do great! You just have to get used it."

    _____ B. "Why are you worried about going home?"

    _____ C. "Your daily routines will be different when you get home."

    _____ D. "Tell me about your support system when you leave the hospital."

    _____ E. "Let me tell you about a friend of mine with a colostomy who also enjoys swimming."

3. A nurse recognizes that a helping relationship is established with a client if the communication

    A. is equally reciprocal between the nurse and the client.

    B. encourages the client to express his thoughts and feelings.

    C. has no time limits.

    D. occurs spontaneously throughout the nurse-client relationship.

4. A nurse is caring for a school-age child who is seated. In order to facilitate effective communication, the nurse should

    A. touch the child.

    B. sit at eye level with the child.

    C. stand facing the child.

    D. stand with a relaxed posture.

5. Which of the following are behaviors of active listening? (Select all that apply.)

_____ A. Maintaining an open posture

_____ B. Writing down what the client says so that details are not forgotten

_____ C. Establishing and maintaining eye contact

_____ D. Nodding in agreement with the client throughout the conversation

_____ E. Responding positively when giving feedback

6. A nurse manager is reviewing nonverbal communication with the staff. Use the ATI Active Learning Template: Basic Concept to complete this item.

A. Related Content: List at least four examples of nonverbal communication.

B. Underlying Principles: Explain the related effect on the communication.

APPLICATION EXERCISES KEY

1.   A. INCORRECT: Pacing is a characteristic of verbal communication, not a clarifying technique.

   B. **CORRECT:** Reflecting directs the focus of the conversation back to the client so that the client can further explore his own feelings.

   C. INCORRECT: Paraphrasing restates the client's feelings for the client to confirm what has been communicated. In this scenario, the client did not verbalize his feelings to the nurse.

   D. INCORRECT: Restating uses the client's exact words. In this scenario, the nurse did not restate what the client stated.

    NCLEX® Connection: Psychosocial Integrity, Therapeutic Communication

2.   A. INCORRECT: Giving false reassurance and minimizing the client's feelings are both barriers to effective communication.

   B. INCORRECT: Although this may appear to allow the client to open up and discuss his feelings, asking a "why" question is a barrier to effective communication.

   C. **CORRECT:** Presenting reality is an effective communication technique that can help the client focus on what will really happen based on the changes that have occurred.

   D. **CORRECT:** Asking open-ended questions and offering general leads and broad opening statements are effective communication techniques that encourage the client to express feelings through dialogue and offer additional information.

   E. **CORRECT:** Offering self is an effective communication technique that can convey understanding and shared experience to the client. The focus should return to the client as soon as the relevant point is communicated.

    NCLEX® Connection: Psychosocial Integrity, Therapeutic Communication

3.   A. INCORRECT: The communication should not be reciprocal but client-focused.

   B. **CORRECT:** Therapeutic communication facilitates a helping relationship that maximizes the client's ability to openly express his thoughts and feelings.

   C. INCORRECT: Therapeutic communication is limited to the boundaries of the therapeutic relationship.

   D. INCORRECT: Therapeutic communication is planned by a health care professional.

    NCLEX® Connection: Psychosocial Integrity, Therapeutic Communication

4.   A. INCORRECT: Touching may intimidate the child and block communication.

     B. **CORRECT:** The nurse should be at the same eye level as the child to facilitate communication.

     C. INCORRECT: Standing may appear domineering and intimidating.

     D. INCORRECT: Standing may appear domineering and intimidating.

     Ⓝ NCLEX® Connection: Psychosocial Integrity, Therapeutic Communication

5.   A. **CORRECT:** Having an open posture and leaning forward, establishing and maintaining eye contact, and responding positively when giving feedback are ways the nurse can demonstrate active listening.

     B. INCORRECT: Writing down everything the client says will interfere with the nurse's ability to maintain eye contact and an open posture.

     C. **CORRECT:** Having an open posture and leaning forward, establishing and maintaining eye contact, and responding positively when giving feedback are ways the nurse can demonstrate active listening.

     D. INCORRECT: Nodding in agreement throughout the conversation may be interpreted as agreement with what the client is saying when it was only intended to indicate attending to what was being said.

     E. **CORRECT:** Having an open posture and leaning forward, establishing and maintaining eye contact, and responding positively when giving feedback are ways the nurse can demonstrate active listening.

     Ⓝ NCLEX® Connection: Psychosocial Integrity, Therapeutic Communication

6.   *Using ATI Active Learning Template: Basic Concept*

     A. Related Content
        - Appearance, posture, gait
        - Facial expressions, eye contact, gestures
        - Sounds
        - Territoriality, personal space

     B. Underlying Principles
        - Appearance/posture/gait: Physical characteristics convey professionalism, may demonstrate comfort and ease in the situation.
        - Facial expressions: Can reveal feelings that can be misinterpreted by clients.
        - Eye contact: Eye contact conveys interest and respect but varies by culture and situation.
        - Gestures: Can enhance verbal communication or create their own messages.
        - Sounds: Crying or moaning can have multiple meanings when accompanied by other nonverbal communication
        - Territoriality/personal space: Lack of awareness of territoriality (right to space) and personal space (the area around an individual) can cause clients to feel threatened and react with defensiveness.

     Ⓝ NCLEX® Connection: Psychosocial Integrity, Therapeutic Communication

chapter 33

Overview

- Coping describes how an individual deals with problems, such as illness and stress. Factors involved in coping and adaptation include the client's family dynamics, adherence to treatment regimens, and the role an individual may play in important relationships.

STRESS, COPING, ADAPTATION, AND ADHERENCE

Overview

- Stress
  - Stress describes changes in an individual's state of balance in response to stressors, the internal and external forces that disrupt that state of balance. Any stressor, whether it is perceived as "good" or "bad," produces a similar biological response in the body.
  - Stress may be situational (adjusting to a chronic disease or a stressful job change).
  - Stress may be developmental (varying with life stage). Adult stressors can include losing parents, having a baby, and getting married.
  - Stress may be caused by sociocultural factors, including substance use, lack of education, and prolonged poverty.
  - Research has shown that stress not only impairs and weakens the immune system but has been identified as a causal factor in numerous health conditions.
- Coping
  - Coping is a term that describes how an individual deals with problems and issues.
  - Factors influencing an individual's ability to cope include the number, duration, and intensity of the stressors; the individual's past experiences; the current support system; and available resources (financial).
  - Coping strategies are unique to an individual and may vary greatly with each stressor.
  - Caregiver burden results from the accumulated stress that family members experience after caring for a loved one over a period of time. Some responses include fatigue, difficulty sleeping, and illness (increased blood pressure, mental illness).
- Adaptation
  - Coping behavior that describes how an individual handles demands imposed by the environment.

- General Adaptation Syndrome (GAS)
  - Hans Selye developed a theory of adaptation that describes the stress reaction in three stages.
    - Alarm reaction – Body functions are heightened to respond to stressors. Hormones are released, which cause elevated blood pressure and heart rate, heightened mental alertness, increased secretion of epinephrine and norepinephrine, and increased blood flow to muscles.
    - Resistance stage – Body functions normalize while responding to the stressor. The body attempts to cope with the stressor and return to homeostasis.
    - Exhaustion stage – Body functions are no longer able to maintain a response to the stressor. The end of this stage results in recovery or death.
- Adherence
  - The commitment and ability of the client and family to follow a given treatment regimen.
  - Commitment to the regimen increases adherence.
  - Complicated regimen interferes with adherence.
  - Involvement of the client and significant support people in the planning stage increases adherence.
  - Adverse effects of medications diminish adherence.
  - Coping mechanisms, such as denial, can cause nonadherence.
  - Available resources increase adherence.

Assessment/Data Collection

- Ask the client questions related to
  - Current stress, perception of stressors, and ability to cope
  - Support systems
  - Adherence to healthy behaviors and/or the treatment regimen
  - Sleep patterns
  - Altered elimination patterns, changes in appetite, and weight loss or gain
- Observe the client's appearance and eye contact.
- Measure vital signs.
- Observe for irritability, anxiety, and tension.

Patient-Centered Care

- Nursing Care

NURSING INTERVENTIONS FOR STRESS, COPING, AND ADHERENCE	
Stress	› Encourage health promotion strategies, including regular exercise, optimal nutrition, and adequate sleep and rest. › Assist with time management, and determine priority tasks. › Encourage appropriate relaxation techniques, including breathing exercises, massage, imagery, yoga, and meditation. › Listen attentively, and take the time to understand the client's perspective. › Control the environment to reduce the number of external stressors, including noise and breaks in the continuity of care. › Identify available support systems. › Use effective communication techniques to foster the expression of feelings.
Coping	› Be empathetic in communication, and encourage the client to verbalize feelings. › Identify the client's and family's strengths and abilities. › Discuss the client's and family's abilities to deal with the current situation. › Encourage the client to describe coping skills used effectively in the past. › Identify available community resources, and refer the client for counseling if needed.
Adherence	› Put instructions in writing. › Allow the client to give input into the treatment regimen. › Simplify treatment regimens as much as possible. › Follow up with the client to address any questions or problems.

Family Systems and Family Dynamics

- Family is defined by the client. It is typically two or more individuals whose relationships create a bond and influence their mutual development, support, goals, and resources.
- Consider five realms of processes involved in family function during a family assessment.
  - Interactive, developmental, coping, integrity, health.
- Assessment of a family can focus on family as a context, a client, or a system.
- Families and clients are not mutually exclusive; family-centered care creates a holistic approach to nursing care.
- Family dynamics are constantly evolving due to the processes of family life and developmental stages of the family members.
- Current Trends
  - Fastest-growing population – those older than 65 years, leading to caregiver issues
  - Declining economic status of families (increased unemployment)
  - Family violence and its endless cycle
  - Any acute or chronic illness the disrupts the family unit (may include end-of-life care issues)
  - Homelessness – lack of stable environment, financial issues, inadequate access to health care (fastest-growing homeless population is families with children)

- Attributes of Families
  - Structure dictates the family's ability to cope.
    - Rigid structure is dictatorial and strict.
    - Open structure includes few or no boundaries, consistent behavior, or consequences.
    - Either structure may provide positive or negative outcomes.
  - Function describes the course of action the family uses to reach its goals, including members' communication skills, problem-solving abilities, and available resources.

Assessment/Data Collection

- Assess all clients within the context of the family.
- Assess a family by looking at its structure and function.
- Identify who is a family member, what role each family member plays, and the dynamic interactions within the family.
- Listen attentively, and use the therapeutic communication techniques of reflection and restatement to clarify the family's concerns.
- Cultural variables – all of which may differ between and within generations
  - Perception of events
  - Rites and rituals
  - Health beliefs

Patient-Centered Care

- Nursing Care
  - Identify and adapt family strengths to perceived stressor(s).
    - Communication
    - Adaptability
    - Nurturing
    - Crisis as a growth element
    - Parenting skills
    - Resiliency
  - Set realistic goals with the family.
  - Provide information about support networks and community resources.
    - Child and adult day care
    - Caregiver support groups

- ○ Promote family unity.
- ○ Ensure safety for families at risk for violence.
- ○ Encourage conflict resolution.
- ○ Minimize family process disruption effects.
- ○ Remove barriers to health promotion.
- ○ Increase family members' abilities to participate.
- ○ Perform interventions that the family cannot perform.
- ○ Evaluate goals within the context of the family by checking back to ensure that goals were realistic and achievable.

SITUATIONAL ROLE CHANGES

Overview

- • A role is the function a person adopts within his life. Seldom is it limited to one role, but rather is multidimensional and is often relative to the role of others.
  - ○ Grandparent
  - ○ Parent
  - ○ Dependent child
  - ○ Employee/employer
  - ○ Committee member
  - ○ Community activist
- • Stress affects roles in many ways.
- • The presence of stressors delays a client's return to health in the same way that the presence of a foreign body or infection delays the healing of a wound.
- • Illness causes role stress by creating a situation in which roles can and do change simply due to the effect and progression of the illness.
- • Nurses must be aware of a client's roles in life, as well as how the situation of illness might change these roles, either temporarily or permanently.
- • A basic assumption is that a client can either advance or regress in the face of a situational role change.
- • Types of Role Problems
  - ○ Role conflict – This develops when a person must assume opposing roles with incompatible expectations. Role conflicts may be interpersonal (when parents expect adolescents to participate in sports and perform household tasks) or inter-role (when a mother wants to stay at home with her infant, but family finances require her to work).
  - ○ Sick role – Expectations of others and society regarding how one should behave when sick (caring for self and continuing to provide childcare to grandchildren).
  - ○ Role ambiguity – Uncertainty about what is expected when assuming a role.

○ Role strain – The frustration and anxiety that occurs when a person feels inadequate for assuming a role.

○ Role overload – More responsibility and roles than are manageable (assuming the role of student, employee, and parent).

- Situational Role Changes

○ Caused by situations other than physical growth and development (marriage, job changes, divorce)

○ Can disrupt one or more of the client's roles in life (with illness or hospitalization)

○ With resolution, can contribute to healing in the physical, mental, and spiritual realms

▪ Temporary role changes – The client will resume the role when illness resolves.

▪ Permanent role changes – Illness has altered the level of the client's health to a point that previous roles are no longer available.

Assessment/Data Collection

- Identify the roles the client perceives as owning.
- Identify the client's roles as perceived by significant others.
- Validate any discrepancies.
- Identify the effect that the loss or addition of a role is having on the client. The client may grieve the loss of a role.
- Identify who will now take on the client's role while the client cannot. Make referrals as appropriate.

Patient-Centered Care

- Nursing Care

○ Provide short-term care to provide relief for the family caregiver.

○ Provide encouragement during times of stress.

○ Seek congruence among perceived roles.

○ Prepare the client for the anticipated situational crisis.

○ Anticipate role conflict or overload on the client's part.

○ Help the client improve relationships by supplementing specific role behaviors.

○ Explore which roles the client can relinquish.

○ Help the client improve personal judgment of self-worth given the current situational role change.

○ Counsel the client about roles that are permanently altered.

○ Refer the client to community services for outpatient adaptation to lost or new roles.

○ Refer the client to social services for assistance in some roles.

○ Evaluate the client after acceptance of the role change(s) to assess adaptation.

APPLICATION EXERCISES

1. A nurse is caring for a client whose partner passed away 4 months ago and who has been recently diagnosed with diabetes mellitus. He is tearful and states, "How could you possibly understand what I am going through?" Which of the following is an appropriate response by the nurse?

    A. "It takes time to get over the loss of a loved one."

    B. "You are right; I cannot really understand. Perhaps you'd like to tell me more about what you're feeling."

    C. "Why don't you try something to take your mind off your troubles, like watching a funny movie."

    D. "I might not share your exact situation, but I do know what people go through when they deal with a loss."

2. A nurse is caring for a client awaiting transport to the surgical suite for a coronary artery bypass graft. Just as the transport team arrives, the nurse takes the client's vital signs and notes an elevation in blood pressure and heart rate. The nurse should recognize this response as which part of the general adaptation syndrome (GAS)?

    A. Exhaustion stage

    B. Resistance stage

    C. Alarm reaction

    D. Recovery reaction

3. A nurse is caring for a client who has a new diagnosis of type 2 diabetes mellitus. Which of the following nursing interventions for stress, coping, and adherence to the treatment plan would be appropriate at this time? (Select all that apply.)

    _____ A. Suggest coping skills for the client to utilize in this situation.

    _____ B. Allow the client to provide input in the treatment plan.

    _____ C. Assist the client with time management, and address the client's priorities.

    _____ D. Provide extensive instructions on the client's treatment regimen.

    _____ E. Encourage the client in the expression of feelings and concerns.

4. A nurse is caring for a client who has left-sided hemiplegia resulting from a cerebrovascular accident. The client works as a carpenter and is now experiencing a situational role change based on physical limitations. The client is the primary wage earner in the family. Which of the following best describes the client's role problem?

    A. Role conflict

    B. Role overload

    C. Role ambiguity

    D. Role strain

5. Which of the following approaches should the nurse use when working with a family using an open structure for coping with crisis?

     A. Prescribing tasks unilaterally

     B. Delegating care to one member

     C. Speaking to the primary client privately

     D. Convening a family meeting

6. A nurse manager is reviewing coping factors with the members of her team. Use the ATI Active Learning Template: Basic Concept to complete this item to include the following:

     A. Related Content: List at least four factors that influence an individual's ability to cope.

     B. Nursing Interventions: List three interventions the nurse can take to assist the client in coping with a stressful event or situation.

APPLICATION EXERCISES KEY

1. A. INCORRECT: Telling the client it will take more time to heal belittles the client's feelings and gives false reassurance.

    B. **CORRECT:** By stating that she is not in his situation, the nurse is using the therapeutic communication technique of validation, whereby she shows sensitivity to the meaning behind his behavior. She is also creating a supportive and nonjudgmental environment, and inviting him to express his frustrations.

    C. INCORRECT: Telling the client to try a distraction dismisses the client's feelings and gives common advice instead of expert advice.

    D. INCORRECT: Saying she knows what clients feel is presumptive and inappropriate.

    Ⓝ NCLEX® Connection: Psychosocial Integrity, Therapeutic Communication

2. A. INCORRECT: Although the exhaustion stage is a component of GAS, body functions are no longer able to respond to the stressor in this stage.

    B. INCORRECT: Although the resistance stage is a component of GAS, body functions normalize in an attempt to cope with the stressor in this stage.

    C. **CORRECT:** As a component of GAS, body functions, such as blood pressure and heart rate, are heightened in order to respond to the stressor in the alarm stage.

    D. INCORRECT: Although not technically a component of GAS, recovery reaction is an alternative to the exhaustion stage, but it would not account for an elevation in blood pressure and heart rate.

    Ⓝ NCLEX® Connection: Reduction of Risk Potential, Changes/Abnormalities in Vital Signs

3. A. INCORRECT: Although it may seem helpful to suggest specific coping skills for the client, it is best to allow the client to discuss coping skills that have worked in the past.

    B. **CORRECT:** Allowing the client to contribute to the treatment plan allows for greater adherence to the plan.

    C. **CORRECT:** Helping the client to prioritize is an intervention that can reduce levels of stress for the client because many times time management is extremely difficult in times of stress.

    D. INCORRECT: Although it is necessary to provide complete information on treatment plans, simplifying treatment regimens as much as possible allows for greater adherence to the treatment plan.

    E. **CORRECT:** By using effective communication techniques, encouraging the client to verbalize feelings is an intervention for stress, coping, and adherence that allows the client to reduce stress, validate emotions, and start planning for valid concerns.

    Ⓝ NCLEX® Connection: Psychosocial Integrity, Coping Mechanisms

4. A. **CORRECT:** The client is experiencing role conflict because his career is extremely physical, and he can no longer perform his job duties. However, the client is the primary wage earner in the family.

    B. INCORRECT: Although the client may feel overloaded and overwhelmed, role overload occurs when the client is trying to juggle too many roles.

    C. INCORRECT: The client is not experiencing role ambiguity because his job duties and his physical limitations are quite clear.

    D. INCORRECT: The client is not experiencing role strain. That occurs when one feels inadequate for assuming a role.

    (N) NCLEX® Connection: Psychosocial Integrity, Coping Mechanisms

5. A. INCORRECT: Prescribing tasks is too rigid for acceptance by a family with an open structure.

    B. INCORRECT: Delegating care is too rigid for acceptance by a family with an open structure.

    C. INCORRECT: Speaking to the primary client privately excludes the family.

    D. **CORRECT:** An open structure is loose, and convening a family meeting would give all family members input and an opportunity to express their feelings.

    (N) NCLEX® Connection: Psychosocial Integrity, Coping Mechanisms

6. *Using ATI Active Learning Template: Basic Concept*

    A. Related Content
    - Number of stressors
    - Duration of the stressors
    - Intensity of the stressors
    - Individual's past experiences
    - Current support system
    - Available resources (financial)

    B. Nursing Interventions
    - Be empathetic in communication, and encourage the client to verbalize feelings.
    - Identify the client's and family's strengths and abilities.
    - Discuss the client's and family's abilities to deal with the current situation.
    - Encourage the client to describe coping skills used effectively in the past.
    - Identify available community resources, and refer the client for counseling if needed.

    (N) NCLEX® Connection: Psychosocial Integrity, Coping Mechanisms

chapter 34

Overview

- Self-concept is the way individuals feel and view themselves. This involves conscious and unconscious thoughts, attitudes, beliefs, and perceptions.
  - Body image, a component of self-concept, refers to the way individuals perceive their appearance, size, and body structure/function.
- Sexuality and sexual orientation are integrated into individuals' personalities as well as their general health. Sexuality encompasses their sense of maleness and/or femaleness and their physical and emotional connections with others.
- Individuals' sexuality and sexual health are influenced by self-concept, body image, gender identity, and sexual orientation.
- Nurses should assess their own comfort levels with issues related to sexuality because clients usually can sense any discomfort nurses have about these issues.
  - Some of the skills that nurses use in dealing with clients' sexuality issues are a knowledge of sexual growth and development, and an understanding of how health problems and treatments affect sexuality.

Self-Concept

- Self-concept is subjective and includes self-identity, body image, role performance, and self-esteem.
  - Individuals who have high self-esteem are better equipped to cope successfully with life's stressors.
  - Stressors that affect self-concept include unrealistic expectations, surgery, chronic illness, and changes in role performance.
- Individuals who have positive self-concepts tend to feel good about themselves.
- Individuals' self-concepts can be adversely affected by physical, spiritual, emotional, sexual, familial, and sociocultural stressors.
- Body Image
  - Body image changes with growth and development. During adolescence, hormonal changes, including the development of secondary sex characteristics, influence body image. Among older adults, changes in mobility, thinning and graying of hair, and decreased visual and hearing acuity are just a few factors that affect body image.
  - Stressors that affect body image include a loss of body parts due to an amputation, mastectomy, or hysterectomy; a loss of body function due to arthritis, a spinal cord injury, or a stroke; and an unattainable body ideal.
  - External influences (media, others' perceptions and responses, cultural standards) can affect body image.

Sexuality

- Sexuality and sexual health are vital components of general health and part of a nursing assessment.

- Aspects of sexual health include a knowledge of sexual behavior, an understanding of expected growth and development, and access to appropriate health care resources for preventing and treating problems related to sexual health.

- Sexuality is affected by one's developmental stage. For example, during adolescence, primary and secondary sex characteristics develop, menarche occurs, relationships involving sexual activity may develop, and masturbation is common.

- Sexuality is influenced by culture. Various cultures view premarital sex, homosexuality, and polygamy differently.

- Sexuality affects health status. Certain conditions may alter sexual expression. For example, the presence of a sexually transmitted disease may cause fear of transmission to a partner, leading to a decrease in sexual desire.

- Some prescription medications affect sexual functioning. Diuretics decrease vaginal lubrication, cause erectile dysfunction, and reduce sexual desire. Erectile dysfunction can also be caused by antidepressant medications.

Assessment/Data Collection

SUBJECTIVE DATA	OBJECTIVE DATA
› Cultural background	› Posture
› Quality of relationships	› Appearance
› Feelings related to recent body image changes, self-concept, and issues of sexuality	› Demeanor
	› Eye contact
› Coping mechanisms used in the past	› Grooming
› Expectations	› Unusual behavior

Patient-Centered Care

SELF-CONCEPT

> Suggest a healthier lifestyle (exercise, diet, stress management).

> Encourage the client to verbalize fears or anxieties.

> Use therapeutic communication skills to assist the client with self-awareness.

> Encourage the use of effective coping skills.

> Reinforce successes and strengths.

BODY IMAGE

> Establish a therapeutic relationship with the client. A caring and nonjudgmental manner puts the client at ease and fosters meaningful communication.

> Ensure privacy and confidentiality. Let the client know that sensitive issues are safe to discuss.

> Identify individuals who may be at risk for body image disturbances.

> Acknowledge anger, depression, and denial as feelings to be expected when adjusting to body changes.

> Encourage the client to participate in the plan of care.

> Arrange for a visit from a volunteer who has experienced a similar body image change.

SEXUALITY

> Allow the client to discuss issues and concerns related to sexuality.

> Be straightforward with questions. ("Are you, or have you been, concerned about sexual functioning since your surgery?")

> Health promotion: Determine the client's current knowledge base regarding sexuality, and provide education as needed.

> Acute care: Increase awareness by introducing or clarifying information, and referring the client for counseling if necessary.

> Inform the client of available resources and support groups.

> Discuss alternative means of sexual expression if the client experiences a change in body functioning or structure (hugging, cuddling).

APPLICATION EXERCISES

1. A nurse in an ambulatory care clinic is caring for a client who had a mastectomy 6 months ago. The client tells the nurse that she has not had much desire for sexual relations since her surgery, stating, "My body is so different now." Which of the following is an appropriate response by the nurse?

    A. "Really, you look just fine to me. There's no need to feel undesirable."

    B. "I'm interested in finding out more about how your body feels to you."

    C. "Consider an afternoon at a spa. A facial will make you feel more attractive."

    D. "It's still too soon to expect to feel normal. Give it a little more time."

2. A nurse is caring for a group of clients on a medical-surgical unit. Which of the following clients are at high risk for body image disturbances? (Select all that apply.)

    _____ A. 30-year-old male following laparoscopic appendectomy

    _____ B. 45-year-old female following mastectomy

    _____ C. 20-year-old female following left above-the-knee amputation

    _____ D. 65-year-old male following cardiac catheterization

    _____ E. 55-year-old male following stroke with right-sided hemiplegia

3. A nurse is caring for a client who is 3 days postoperative following a below-the-knee amputation as a result of a motor vehicle crash. Which of the following client statements indicates to the nurse that the client has a distorted body image?

    A. "I'll be able to function exactly as I did before the accident."

    B. "I just can't stop crying."

    C. "I am so mad at that guy who hit us. I wish he lost a leg."

    D. "I don't even want to look at my leg. You can check the dressing."

4. A nurse is caring for a client who is recovering from a myocardial infarction and a cardiac catheterization. The client states, "I am concerned that things might be a little, you know, 'different' with my wife when I get home." Which of the following statements is an appropriate response by the nurse?

    A. "Sounds like something you should discuss with her when you get home."

    B. "It sounds like you are concerned about sexual functioning. Let's discuss your concerns."

    C. "Oh, I wouldn't be too concerned. Things will be fine as soon as we get you home."

    D. "Just make sure you take your medication as directed, and you should be fine."

5. A nurse is teaching a group of clients how to care for their colostomies. Which of the following statements should alert the nurse that one of the clients is having an issue with self-concept?

    A. "I was having difficulty with attaching the appliance at first, but my wife was able to help."

    B. "I'll never be able to care for this at home. Can't you just send a nurse to the house?"

    C. "I met a neighbor who also has a colostomy, and he taught me a few things."

    D. "It may take me a while to get the hang of this. I have to admit, I am pretty nervous."

6. A nurse manager is reviewing self-concept assessment findings with her staff. Use the ATI Active Learning Template: Systems Disorder to complete this item. Under Assessment, list at least three examples of subjective data findings and three examples of objective data findings.

APPLICATION EXERCISES KEY

1. A. INCORRECT: Telling the client she looks fine is using the nontherapeutic communication technique of giving an opinion; assuming she feels undesirable is using the nontherapeutic communication technique of interpreting.

    B. **CORRECT:** Showing interest in the client is applying the therapeutic communication technique of offering self; asking more about how the client feels is applying the therapeutic communication technique of encouraging a description of perception.

    C. INCORRECT: Suggesting a facial is using the nontherapeutic communication technique of giving advice.

    D. INCORRECT: Telling her it is too soon to feel normal and to give it more time is belittling the client's feelings and giving false reassurance.

     NCLEX® Connection: Psychosocial Integrity, Coping Mechanisms

2. A. INCORRECT: Based on the concept of body image, an appendectomy would not place a client at high risk for a body image disturbance.

    B. **CORRECT:** Having a mastectomy involves a change in the physical appearance of a woman and can lead to body image disturbances related to femininity and sexuality.

    C. **CORRECT:** Having an above-the-knee amputation involves a change in physical appearance and can lead to body image disturbances related to function, health, and strength.

    D. INCORRECT: Depending on the client's prognosis postcatheterization, the client may experience some limitations. However, in general, a cardiac catheterization would not place a client at high risk for a body image disturbance.

    E. **CORRECT:** Having right-sided hemiplegia involves a change in physical appearance and can lead to body image disturbances related to function, health, and strength.

     NCLEX® Connection: Psychosocial Integrity, Coping Mechanisms

3. A. INCORRECT: Denial is a normal and expected reaction when adjusting to body changes.

    B. INCORRECT: Depression and sadness are normal and expected reactions when adjusting to body changes.

    C. INCORRECT: Anger is a normal and expected reaction when adjusting to body changes.

    D. **CORRECT:** Refusing to look at the leg or the dressing indicates that the client is having difficulty acknowledging the fact that the leg has been amputated. This would imply a distorted body image.

     NCLEX® Connection: Psychosocial Integrity, Coping Mechanisms

4. A. INCORRECT: The nurse should allow the client to discuss issues and concerns related to sexuality and not dismiss his concerns.

    B. **CORRECT:** The nurse is acknowledging and allowing the client to discuss his concerns regarding sexual functioning.

    C. INCORRECT: False reassurance should not be used. The client has valid concerns. The nurse also is dismissing the client's feelings.

    D. INCORRECT: The nurse is not allowing the client to express his feelings and is displaying false reassurance, which should not be used because the client has valid concerns.

     NCLEX® Connection: Psychosocial Integrity, Coping Mechanisms

5. A. INCORRECT: Although the client was having difficulty at first, the client expressed how he was able to use his resources, resulting in a positive outcome, and does not show signs of self-concept issues.

    B. **CORRECT:** This client is displaying a lack of interest in learning how to care for the colostomy and dependence on others to care for him. The nurse should suspect issues with self-concept with this client.

    C. INCORRECT: This client is displaying a positive self-concept by reaching out and using his resources to learn additional information regarding the colostomy.

    D. INCORRECT: Expression of feelings is a sign of positive self-concept even if the client admits being nervous or hesitant regarding caring for the colostomy on his own.

     NCLEX® Connection: Psychosocial Integrity, Coping Mechanisms

6. *Using the ATI Active Learning Template: Systems Disorder*
    - Assessment
        - Subjective Data
            - Cultural background
            - Quality of relationships
            - Feelings related to recent body image changes, self-concept, and issues of sexuality
            - Coping mechanisms used in the past
            - Expectations
        - Objective Data
            - Posture
            - Appearance
            - Demeanor
            - Eye contact
            - Grooming
            - Unusual behavior

     NCLEX® Connection: Psychosocial Integrity, Coping Mechanisms

chapter 35

Overview

- Clients vary widely in their cultural and spiritual backgrounds and belief systems.

- Nurses must examine their own beliefs before providing optimal cultural and spiritual care to their clients.

Culture

- Culture is a collection of learned, adaptive, and socially and intergenerationally transmitted behaviors, values, beliefs, and customs that form the context from which a group interprets the human experience. Culture includes language, communication style, traditions, religions, art, music, dress, health beliefs, and health practices. These components can be shared by members of an ethnic, racial, social, or religious group.

  ○ Ethnicity, the bond or kinship people feel with their country of birth or place of ancestral origin, affects culture.

  ○ Culture influences health beliefs, health practices, and the manifestations of, responses to, and treatment of illness or injury. Culture evolves over time and is shared by members of a group who have similar needs and life experiences.

  ○ Many cultures consider the mind-body-spirit to be a single entity; therefore, no distinction is made between physical and mental illness.

  ○ The predominant culture in the United States is anglicized or English-based, with a general cultural tendency to

    ▪ Express positive and negative feelings freely

    ▪ Prefer direct eye contact when communicating

    ▪ Address people in a casual manner

    ▪ Prefer a strong handshake as a way of greeting

  ○ Culture evolves as

    ▪ Knowledge

    ▪ Values

      ▫ Values are a set of rules by which individuals in a culture live.

      ▫ Values guide decision-making and behavior. For example, if health promotion and maintenance are valued, monthly breast self-examinations are done.

      ▫ Values develop unconsciously during childhood.

- Beliefs
- Morals and law
- Customs and habits
    - Although everyone within a culture shares cultural values, diversity exists, forming subcultures based on age, gender, sexual orientation, marital status, family structure, income, education level, religious views, and life experiences.

Culturally Responsive Nursing Care

- Culturally responsive nursing care involves the delivery of care that transcends cultural boundaries and considers a client's culture as it affects health, illness, and lifestyle. Communication, dietary preferences, and dress are influenced by culture.
- Within the context of culturally responsive nursing care is terminology that describes how nurses approach clients' culture. Culturally sensitive means that nurses are knowledgeable about the cultures prevalent in their area of practice. Culturally appropriate means that nurses apply their knowledge of a client's culture to their care delivery. Culturally competent means that nurses understand and address the entire cultural context of each client within the realm of the care they deliver.
- Culturally responsive nursing care improves communication, fosters mutual respect, promotes sensitive and effective care, and increases adherence with the treatment plan as clients' and families' needs are met.
- Culturally responsive nursing care should encourage client decision-making by introducing self-empowerment strategies.
- A key prerequisite to the delivery of culturally responsive nursing care is the nurses' understanding and awareness of their own culture and any cultural biases that might affect care delivery.
- Nurses should accommodate each client's cultural beliefs and values whenever possible, unless they are in direct conflict with essential health practices.
- Barriers to providing culturally responsive nursing care include the following:
    - Language, communication, and perception of time differences
    - Culturally inappropriate tests and tools that lead to misdiagnosis
    - Ethnic variations in drug metabolism related to genetics
    - Ethnocentrism is the belief that one's culture is superior to others. Ethnocentric ideas interfere with the provision of cultural nursing care.

Spirituality

- Spirituality can also play an important role in clients' abilities to achieve balance in life, to maintain health, to seek health care, and to deal with illness and injury. Hope, faith, and transcendence are integral components of spirituality.
    - Spiritual distress is a challenge to belief systems or spiritual well-being. It often arises as a result of catastrophic events.
    - When faced with health care issues such as acute, chronic, or life-limiting illness, clients often find ways to cope through the use of spiritual practices. Clients who begin to question their belief systems and are unable to find support from those belief systems may experience spiritual distress.

Q
PCC

- ○ Nursing interventions are directed at identification, restoration, and/or reconnection of clients and families to spiritual strength.
- ○ Spirituality implies connectedness.
  - Intrapersonal – within one's self
  - Interpersonal – with others and the environment
  - Transpersonal – with an unseen higher power
- ○ Faith is a belief in something or a relationship with a higher power.
  - Faith can be defined by a culture or a religion.
- ○ Hope is a concept that includes anticipation and optimism and provides comfort during times of crisis.
- ○ Religion is a system of beliefs practiced outwardly to express one's spirituality.
- Spiritual rituals and observances include the following:

BUDDHISM	
Birth rituals and health care decisions	› Buddhists may refuse care on holy days. › Buddhists may refuse analgesics or strong sedatives.
Dietary rituals	› Some are vegetarians. › Those practicing Buddhism may avoid alcohol and tobacco. › Clients may fast on holy days.
Death rituals	› Clients may request a priest to deliver last rites. › Chanting is common. › Brain death is not considered as a requirement for death.
CHRISTIANITY	
Birth rituals and health care decisions	› Some baptize infants at birth.
Dietary rituals	› Some avoid alcohol, tobacco, and caffeine. › Clients may fast during Lent. › Some may wish to receive the Eucharist.
Death rituals	› Some give last rites.
HINDUISM	
Birth rituals and health care decisions	› Those practicing Hinduism do not prolong life. › Personal hygiene and cleanliness is valued.
Dietary rituals	› Some are vegetarians.
Death rituals	› Clients may want to lie on the floor while dying. › A thread is placed around the neck/wrist. › The family pours water into the mouth. › The family bathes the body. › Clients may want to be cremated.

ISLAM	
Birth rituals and health care decisions	› Women must be cared for by female health care providers, especially during childbirth. › Women often must wear head and/or body covering when in the presence of males who are not immediate family. › Have strict rules regarding handwashing. › Must pray five times a day facing Mecca.
Dietary rituals	› Those practicing Islam avoid alcohol and pork. › Clients may fast during Ramadan.
Death rituals	› Dying clients confess their sins. › The body faces Mecca. › The body is washed and enveloped in a white cloth. › A prayer is said.
JEHOVAH'S WITNESSES	
Birth rituals and health care decisions	› May not accept blood transfusions, even in life-threatening situations.
Dietary rituals	› Clients avoid foods having or prepared with blood.
Death rituals	› Clients can choose burial or cremation.
JUDAISM	
Birth rituals and health care decisions	› On the eighth day after birth, males are circumcised.
Dietary rituals	› Some may practice a kosher diet.
Death rituals	› Someone stays with the body. › A burial society prepares the body.
MORMONISM	
Birth rituals and health care decisions	› Children are baptized at age 8 by immersion.
Dietary rituals	› Those practicing Mormonism avoid alcohol, tobacco, and caffeine.
Death rituals	› Last rites are given. › Communion is offered. › Burial is preferred.

Assessment/Data Collection

- To meet a client's cultural needs, a nurse must first perform a cultural assessment to identify those needs.

DATA TO BE COLLECTED	EXAMPLE
Cultural background and the client's acculturation	› The client was born in Central America and has been a resident of New York for 2 years.
Health and wellness beliefs/practices	› The client relies on folk medicine to treat or prevent illness.
Family patterns	› The client is from a patriarchal culture where the oldest male family member makes decisions for all family members.
Verbal and nonverbal communication	› Within the client's culture, it is disrespectful to make direct eye contact.
Space and time orientation	› Within the client's culture, little importance is placed on how past behavior affects future health.
Nutritional patterns	› The client believes that some foods have healing properties.
Meaning of pain	› Within the client's culture, pain is viewed as a punishment for misbehavior or sin.
Death rituals	› Within the client's culture, suicide is acceptable.
Care of ill family members	› The client expects the entire family to remain at the client's bedside during an illness.

- Perform the cultural assessment in a language that is common to both nurse and client, or use a facility-approved medical interpreter.
- Inform the interpreter of questions that may be asked.
  - What do you call the problem you are having now?
  - When did the problem start?
  - What do you think caused the problem?
  - What does the illness do to you? How does it work?
  - What makes it better or worse?
  - How severe is the illness?
  - What treatments have you tried? How do you think it should be treated?
  - What are the chief problems the illness has caused you?
  - What do you fear most about the illness?

- Assess the client's gestures, vocal tones, and inflections.
  - Nonverbal Behavior
    - Culturally competent nurses must understand how nonverbal behaviors vary among cultures.

TONE OF VOICE	
Asian	› Many Asians use a soft tone of voice to convey respect.
Italian and Middle Eastern	› Many Italian and Middle Eastern individuals use a loud tone of voice.
EYE CONTACT	
American	› Americans use direct eye contact. Lack of direct eye contact implies deception or embarrassment.
Middle Eastern	› Middle Eastern individuals usually avoid making direct eye contact with nonrelated members of the opposite gender. Direct eye contact may be seen as rude, hostile, or sexually aggressive.
Asian	› Asians may believe that direct eye contact is disrespectful.
Native American	› Native Americans may believe that direct eye contact leads to soul loss or soul theft.
TOUCH	
American	› Americans may use touch during conversations between intimate partners or family members.
Italian and Latin American	› Italian and Latin American individuals may view frequent touch as a sign of concern, interest, and warmth.
USE OF SPACE	
Anglo-American/North Europeans (English, Swiss, Scandinavian, German)	› Anglo-American/North Europeans tend to keep their distance during communication except in intimate or family relationships.
Italian, French, Spanish, Russian, Latin American, Middle Eastern	› These cultures prefer closer personal contact and less distance between individuals during communication.

- Methods for Assessing Culture
  - Observation
    - Study the client and his environment for examples of cultural relevance.
  - Interview
    - Establish a therapeutic relationship with the client. This may be hindered by misinterpretations of communication.
    - Use focused, open-ended, and nonjudgmental questions.
    - Paraphrasing the client's communication will decrease misinterpretations.
  - Participation
    - Become involved in culturally related activities outside of the health care setting.
    - Awareness of population demographics
      - Number of members in a practice area
      - Average educational and economic levels

- □ Typical occupations
- □ Commonly practiced religious spiritual beliefs
- □ Prevalence of illnesses/health issues
- □ Most commonly held health, wellness, illness, and death beliefs
- □ Social organization
- A spiritual assessment includes several components:
  - ○ Primary – self-reflection (nurses) on personal beliefs and spirituality
  - ○ Initial – identifying the client's religion, if any
  - ○ Focused – ongoing, as nurses identify the clients at risk for spiritual distress
  - ○ Spirituality is a highly subjective area requiring the development of rapport and trust among the client, family, and provider.
  - ○ Assessment of the client includes the following:
    - Faith/beliefs
    - Perception of life and self-responsibility
    - Satisfaction with life
    - Culture
    - Fellowship and the client's perceived place in the community
    - Rituals and practices
    - Incorporation of spirituality within profession or workplace
    - The client's expectations for health care in relation to spirituality (traditional vs. alternative paths, such as shamans, priests, prayer)

Patient-Centered Care

- Death Rituals
  - ○ Death rituals vary among cultures; facilitate such practices and offer appropriate spiritual care whenever possible.
- Pain
  - ○ Recognize that how clients react to, display, and relieve pain varies by culture.
  - ○ Use an alternative to the pain scale (0 to 10) because it may not appropriately reflect pain for all cultures.
  - ○ Explore religious beliefs that influence the meaning of pain.
- Nutrition
  - ○ Provide food choices and preparation consistent with cultural beliefs.
  - ○ When possible, allow the client's family/caregiver to bring in food (as long as it meets the client's dietary restrictions), and allow clients to consume foods that they view as a treatment for illness.
  - ○ Communicate ethnicity-related food intolerances/allergies to the dietary staff.

- Communication
  - Improve nurse-client communication when cultural variations exist.
  - Use facility-approved interpreters when the communication barrier is significant enough to affect the exchange of information between the nurse and the client.
  - Use nonverbal communication with caution because it may have a different meaning for the client than for the nurse.
  - Apologize if cultural traditions or beliefs are violated.
- Family Patterns and Gender Roles
  - Communicate with and include the person who has the authority to make decisions in the family.
- Culture and Life Transitions
  - Assist families as they mark rituals (rites of passage) that symbolize cultural values. Common events expressed with cultural rituals are puberty, pregnancy, childbirth, dying, and death.
- Repatterning
  - Accommodate clients' cultural beliefs and values as much as possible.
  - When a cultural value or behavior hinders a client's health and wellness, attempt to repattern that belief to one that is compatible with health promotion.
  - With knowledge of cultural differences and respect for the client and family, plan and implement appropriate interventions.
- Using an Interpreter
  - Use only a facility-approved medical interpreter. Do not use the client's family or friends or a nondesignated employee to interpret.
  - Inform the interpreter about the reason for and the type of questions that will be asked, the expected response (brief or detailed), and with whom to converse.
  - Allow time for the interpreter and the family to be introduced and become acquainted before starting the interview.
  - Refrain from making comments about the family to the interpreter because the family may understand some of the discussion.
  - Ask one question at a time.
  - Direct the questions to the family, not to the interpreter.
  - Use lay terminology if possible, knowing that some words may not have an equivalent word in the client's language.
  - Do not interrupt the interpreter, the client, or the family as they talk.
  - Do not try to interpret answers.
  - Following the interview, ask the interpreter for any additional thoughts about the interview and the client's and family's responses, both verbal and nonverbal.

- Addressing Spirituality
  - Identify the client's perception of the existence of a higher power.
  - Facilitate growth in the client's abilities to connect with a higher power.
  - Assist the client to feel connected or reconnected to a higher power:
    - Allow time and/or resources for the practice of religious rituals.
    - Provide privacy for prayer, meditation, or the reading of religious materials.
  - Use your facility's pastoral care department if appropriate.
  - Facilitate development of a positive outcome in a particular situation.
  - Provide stability for the person experiencing a dysfunctional spiritual mood.
  - Establish a caring presence in "being with" the client and family rather than merely performing tasks for them.
  - Support all healing relationships:
    - Using a holistic approach to care – seeing the large picture for the client
    - Using client-identified spiritual resources and needs
  - Be aware of diet therapies included in spiritual beliefs.
  - Support religious rituals:
    - Icons
    - Statues
    - Prayer rugs
    - Devotional readings
    - Music
  - Support restorative care:
    - Prayer
    - Meditation
    - Grief work
  - Evaluation of care is ongoing and continuous, with a need for flexibility as the client and family process the current crisis through their spiritual identity.

APPLICATION EXERCISES

1. A nurse is using an interpreter to communicate with a client. Which of the following are appropriate when communicating with a client and his family? (Select all that apply.)

_____ A. Talk to the interpreter about the family while the family is in the room.

_____ B. Ask the family one question at a time.

_____ C. Look at the interpreter when asking the family questions.

_____ D. Use lay terms if possible.

_____ E. Do not interrupt the interpreter and the family as they talk.

2. A nurse is caring for a client who shares the same religious background. The nurse should recognize that

A. members of the same religion share similar feelings about their religion.

B. a shared religious background generates mutual regard for one another.

C. the same religious beliefs may influence individuals differently.

D. they should discuss the differences and commonalities in their beliefs.

3. A nurse is caring for a client who is crying while reading from his devotional book. Which of the following interventions is appropriate for the nurse to take?

A. Contact the hospital's spiritual services.

B. Ask him what is making him cry.

C. Provide quiet times for these moments.

D. Turn on the television for a distraction.

4. A nurse is planning care for a client who is a devout Muslim and is 3 days postoperative following a hip arthroplasty. The client is scheduled for two physical therapy sessions today. Which of the following statements by the nurse indicates culturally appropriate care to the Muslim client?

A. "I will make sure the menu includes kosher options."

B. "I will discuss the daily schedule with the client to make sure the client will have time for prayer."

C. "I will make sure to use direct eye contact when speaking with this client."

D. "I will make sure daily communion is available for this client."

5. A nurse is caring for a client who is a Jehovah's Witness and is scheduled for surgery as a result of a motor vehicle crash. The surgeon tells the client that a blood transfusion is essential. The client tells the nurse that based on his religious values and mandates, he cannot receive a blood transfusion. Which of the following responses by the nurse is appropriate?

    A. "I believe in this case you should really make an exception and accept the blood transfusion."

    B. "I know your family would approve of your decision to have a blood transfusion."

    C. "Why does your religion mandate that you cannot receive any blood transfusions?"

    D. "Let's discuss the necessity for a blood transfusion with your religious and spiritual leaders and come to a reasonable solution."

6. A nurse educator is conducting a class on culturally responsive nursing care. Use the ATI Active Learning Template: Basic Concept to complete this item. Under Related Content, list five examples of subculture categories than can exist within a culture.

APPLICATION EXERCISES KEY

1. A. INCORRECT: Talking to the interpreter about the family while the family is in the room would hinder communication between the family and the nurse/interpreter.

    B. **CORRECT:** Asking the family one question at a time will promote effective communication between the family and the nurse/interpreter.

    C. INCORRECT: Looking at the interpreter instead of the family while the family is in the room would hinder communication between the family and the nurse/interpreter.

    D. **CORRECT:** Using lay terms will promote effective communication between the family and the nurse/interpreter.

    E. **CORRECT:** Not interrupting will promote effective communication between the family and the nurse/interpreter.

    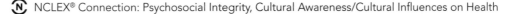 NCLEX® Connection: Psychosocial Integrity, Cultural Awareness/Cultural Influences on Health

2. A. INCORRECT: It would be stereotyping to assume that all members of a specific religion had the same beliefs. Feelings and ideas about religion and spiritual matters may be quite diverse, even within a specific culture.

    B. INCORRECT: Mutual regard does not necessarily follow a shared religious background.

    C. **CORRECT:** Members of any particular religion should be assessed for individual feelings and ideas.

    D. INCORRECT: Due to boundary issues, the nurse's beliefs are not part of a therapeutic client relationship; it is the client's beliefs that are important.

    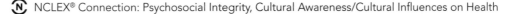 NCLEX® Connection: Psychosocial Integrity, Religious Influences on Health

3. A. INCORRECT: Contacting the hospital's spiritual services presumes there is a problem.

    B. INCORRECT: Asking the client about the crying could be interpreted as discounting or being disrespectful of the client's beliefs.

    C. **CORRECT:** Providing privacy and time for the reading of religious materials supports the client's spiritual health.

    D. INCORRECT: Providing a distraction could be interpreted as discounting or being disrespectful of the client's beliefs.

    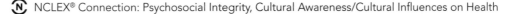 NCLEX® Connection: Psychosocial Integrity, Religious Influences on Health

4. A. **INCORRECT:** Clients of the Jewish culture, not Islam, require their food to be kosher.

    B. **CORRECT:** Devout Muslims pray five times a day. Without proper awareness and planning, the client may refuse necessary treatments such as physical therapy if adequate pray times are not planned for and incorporated into the client's day.

    C. **INCORRECT:** The American culture appreciates direct eye contact. However, in Middle Eastern cultures, direct eye contact may be perceived as rude, hostile, or sexually aggressive.

    D. **INCORRECT:** Daily communion is a ritual to consider for a hospitalized Catholic client, not for a Muslim client.

     NCLEX® Connection: Psychosocial Integrity, Cultural Awareness/Cultural Influences on Health

5. A. **INCORRECT:** The nurse should not impose her opinion to the client and ask him to go against his religious beliefs.

    B. **INCORRECT:** The nurse should not make an assumption on behalf of the client's family.

    C. **INCORRECT:** Asking a "why" question can appear judgmental or accusatory.

    D. **CORRECT:** Involving the client's religious and spiritual leaders is a culturally responsive action at this point. Alternative forms of blood products can be discussed, and a plan acceptable to all can be reached.

     NCLEX® Connection: Psychosocial Integrity, Cultural Awareness/Cultural Influences on Health

6. *Using the ATI Active Learning Template: Basic Concept*
    - Related Content
        - Although everyone within a culture shares cultural values, diversity exists. Forming subcultures is based on
            - Age
            - Gender
            - Sexual orientation
            - Marital status
            - Family structure
            - Income
            - Education level
            - Religious views
            - Life experiences

     NCLEX® Connection: Psychosocial Integrity, Cultural Awareness/Cultural Influences on Health

chapter 36

Overview

- Clients experience loss in many aspects of their lives.
- Grief is the inner emotional response to loss and is exhibited in as many ways as there are individuals.
- Bereavement includes both grief and mourning (the outward display of loss) as the individual deals with the death of a significant individual in his life.
- Palliative or end-of-life care is an important aspect of nursing care and attempts to meet the client's physical, spiritual, emotional, and psychosocial needs.
- End-of-life issues include decision-making in a highly stressful time during which the nurse must consider the desires of the client and the family. Decisions are shared with other health care personnel for a smooth transition during this time of stress, grief, and bereavement.
- Advance directives – legal documents that direct end-of-life issues
    - Living wills – directive documents for medical treatment per the client's wishes
    - Health care proxy, also known as durable power of attorney for health care – a document that appoints someone to make medical decisions when the client is no longer able to do so on his own behalf

Types of Loss

NECESSARY LOSS

› This is a loss related to a change that is part of the cycle of life that is anticipated but still may be intensely felt. This type of loss can be replaced by something different or better.

ACTUAL LOSS

› This is any loss of a valued person, item, or status, such as loss of a job.

PERCEIVED LOSS

› This is any loss defined by the client that is not obvious or verifiable to others.

MATURATIONAL OR DEVELOPMENTAL LOSS

› This is any loss normally expected due to the developmental processing of life. These losses are associated with normal life transitions and help to develop coping skills.

SITUATIONAL LOSS

› This is any unanticipated loss caused by an external event.

Theories of Grief

- Kübler-Ross: Five Stages of Grief

  - Denial – The client has difficulty believing a terminal diagnosis or loss.

  - Anger – The client lashes out at other people or things.

  - Bargaining – The client negotiates for more time or a cure.

  - Depression – The client is overwhelmingly saddened over the inability to change the situation.

  - Acceptance – The client acknowledges what is happening and plans for the future.

  - Stages may not be experienced in order, and the length of each stage varies from person to person.

Factors Influencing Loss, Grief, and Coping Ability

- The individual's current stage of development

- Interpersonal relationships and social support networks

- Type and significance of the loss

- Culture and ethnicity

- Spiritual and religious beliefs and practices

- Prior experience with loss

- Socioeconomic status

- Factors that may increase an individual's risk for dysfunctional grieving

  - Being exceptionally dependent upon the deceased

  - The deceased dying unexpectedly at a young age, through violence, or in a socially unacceptable manner

  - Inadequate coping skills or lack of social supports

  - Lack of hope or preexisting mental health issues, such as depression or substance use disorder

Assessment

MANIFESTATIONS OF GRIEF REACTIONS	
Normal grief	› This grief is considered uncomplicated. › Emotions may be negative, such as anger, resentment, withdrawal, hopelessness, and guilt but should change to acceptance with time. › Some acceptance should be evident by 6 months after the loss. › Somatic complaints can include chest pain, palpitations, headaches, nausea, changes in sleep patterns, and fatigue.
Anticipatory grief	› This grief implies the "letting go" of an object or person before the loss, as in a terminal illness. › Individuals have the opportunity to start the grieving process before the actual loss.
Complicated grief (unresolved or chronic grief is a type of complicated grief)	› This grief involves difficult progression through the expected stages of grief. › Usually, the work of grief is prolonged, the manifestations of grief are more severe, and they may result in depression or exacerbate a preexisting disorder. › The client may develop suicidal ideation, intense feelings of guilt, and lowered self-esteem. › Somatic complaints persist for an extended period of time.
Disenfranchised grief	› This grief entails an experienced loss that cannot be publicly shared or is not socially acceptable, such as suicide.

Nursing Interventions

- Facilitate Mourning

  - Grant time for the grieving process.

  - Identify expected grieving behaviors, such as crying, somatic manifestations, and anxiety.

  - Use therapeutic communication. Name the emotion the client is feeling. For example, the nurse can say, "You sound as though you are angry. Anger is a normal feeling for someone who has lost a loved one. Tell me about how you are feeling."

  - Avoid communication that inhibits the open expression of feelings, such as offering false reassurance, giving advice, changing the subject, and taking the focus away from the grieving individual.

  - Assist the grieving individual to accept the reality of the loss.

  - Support efforts to "move on" in the face of the loss.

  - Encourage the building of new relationships.

  - Provide continuing support; encourage the support of family and friends.

  - Assess for evidence of ineffective coping, such as refusing to leave the home months after the client's spouse died.

  - Share information about mourning and grieving with the client, who may not realize that feelings, such as anger toward the deceased, are expected.

○ Encourage attendance at bereavement or grief support groups. Provide information about available community resources.

○ Initiate referrals for individual psychotherapy for clients who have difficulty resolving grief.

○ Ask the client whether contacting a spiritual advisor would be acceptable, or encourage the client to do so.

○ Participate in debriefing provided by professional grief and mental health counselors.

PALLIATIVE CARE

- The nurse serves as an advocate for the client's sense of dignity and self-esteem by providing palliative care at the end of life.

- Palliative care improves the quality of life of clients and their families facing end-of-life issues.

- Palliative care interventions are primarily used when caring for clients who are dying and family members who are grieving.

- Palliative care interventions focus on the relief of physical manifestations such as pain as well as addressing spiritual, emotional, and psychosocial aspects of the client's life.

- Palliative care may be provided by an interprofessional team of physicians, nurses, social workers, physical therapists, massage therapists, occupational therapists, music/art therapists, touch/energy therapists, and chaplains.

- Hospice care is a comprehensive care delivery system implemented when a client is not expected to live longer than 6 months. Further medical care aimed toward a cure is stopped, and the focus becomes enhancing quality of life and supporting the client toward a peaceful and dignified death.

Assessment/Data Collection

CHARACTERISTICS OF DISCOMFORT		
› Pain	› Dyspnea	› Diarrhea or constipation
› Anxiety	› Nausea or vomiting	› Urinary incontinence
› Restlessness	› Dehydration	› Inability to perform ADLs
CLINICAL MANIFESTATIONS OF APPROACHING DEATH		
› Decreased level of consciousness	› Mucus collecting in large airways	› Pulse weakening and blood pressure dropping
› Muscle relaxation	› Incontinence of bowel and/or bladder	› Cool extremities
› Labored breathing (dyspnea, apnea, Cheyne-Stokes respirations)	› Mottling occurring with poor circulation	› Perspiration
	› Pupils no longer reactive to light	› Decreased urine output
		› Inability to swallow

- Determine the client's sources of strength and hope.

- Identify the desires and expectations of the family and the client for end-of-life care.

Nursing Interventions

- Promote continuity of care and communication by limiting assigned staff changes.
- Assist the client and family to set priorities for end-of-life care.
- Physical Care
  - ○ Give priority to controlling clinical findings.
  - ○ Administer medications that manage pain, air hunger, and anxiety.
  - ○ Perform ongoing assessment to determine the effectiveness of treatment and the need for modifications of the treatment plan, such as lower or higher doses of medications.
  - ○ Manage adverse effects of medications.
  - ○ Reposition the client to maintain airway patency and comfort.
  - ○ Maintain the integrity of skin and mucous membranes.
  - ○ Provide an environment that promotes dignity and self-esteem.
    - ▪ Remove products of elimination as soon as possible to maintain a clean and odor-free environment.
    - ▪ Offer comfortable clothing.
    - ▪ Provide careful grooming for hair, nails, and skin.
    - ▪ Encourage family members to bring in comforting possessions to make the client feel at home.
  - ○ If appropriate, encourage the use of relaxation techniques, such as guided imagery and music.
  - ○ Promote decision-making in food selection, activities, and health care to give the client as much control as possible.
  - ○ Encourage the client to perform ADLs as able and willing to do so.
- Psychosocial Care
  - ○ Use an interprofessional approach.
  - ○ Provide care to the client and family.
  - ○ Use volunteers when appropriate to provide nonmedical care.
  - ○ Use therapeutic communication to develop and maintain a nurse-client relationship.
  - ○ Facilitate the understanding of information regarding disease progression and treatment choices.
  - ○ Facilitate communication between the client, the family, and the provider.
  - ○ Encourage the client to participate in religious practices that bring comfort and strength, if appropriate.
  - ○ Assist the client in clarifying personal values in order to facilitate effective decision-making.
  - ○ Encourage the client to use coping mechanisms that have worked in the past.
  - ○ Be sensitive to comments made in the presence of clients who are unconscious because hearing is the last sensation lost.

- Prevention of Abandonment and Isolation
  - Prevent the fear of dying alone.
    - Make your presence known by answering call lights in a timely manner and making frequent contact.
    - Keep the client informed of procedure and assessment times.
    - Allow family members to stay overnight.
    - Determine where the client is most comfortable, such as in a room close to the nurses' station.
- Support for the Grieving Family
  - Suggest that family members plan visits to promote the client's rest.
  - Ensure that the family receives appropriate information as the treatment plan changes.
  - Provide privacy so family members have the opportunity to communicate and express feelings among themselves without including the client.
  - Determine family members' desire to provide physical care while maintaining awareness of possible caregiver fatigue. Provide instruction as necessary.
  - Educate the family about physical changes to expect as the client moves closer to death.

POSTMORTEM CARE

- Nurses are responsible for following federal and state laws regarding requests for organ or tissue donation, obtaining permission for autopsy, ensuring the certification and appropriate documentation of the death, and providing postmortem (after-death) care.

> **M** View Video: Postmortem Care

- After postmortem care is completed, the client's family becomes the nurse's primary focus.

Nursing Interventions

- Care of the Body
  - Provide care with respect and compassion while attending to the desires of the client and family per their cultural, religious, and social practices.
  - Recognize that the provider certifies death by pronouncing the time and documenting therapies used, and actions taken prior to the death.
  - Preparing the body for viewing
    - Maintain privacy.
    - Remove all tubes (unless organs are to be donated or this is a medical examiner's case).
    - Remove all personal belongings to be given to the family.
    - Cleanse and align the body with a pillow under the head, arms outside the sheet and blanket, dentures in place, and eyes closed.
    - Apply fresh linens and a gown.

- Brush/comb the client's hair; replace any hairpieces.
- Remove excess supplies, equipment, and soiled linens from the room.
- Dim the lights and minimize noise to provide a calm environment.
  - ○ Viewing considerations
    - Ask the family whether they would like to visit with the body, honoring any decision.
    - Clarify where the client's personal belongings should go – with the body or to a designated person.
    - Adhere to the same procedures when the client is an infant, with the following exceptions:
      - □ Swaddle the infant's body in a clean blanket.
      - □ Transport the infant in the nurse's arms or in an infant carrier based on facility protocol.
      - □ Offer mementos of the infant (identification bracelets, footprints, the cord clamp, a lock of hair, photos).
  - ○ Postviewing
    - Apply identification tags according to facility policy.
    - Complete documentation.
    - Remain aware of visitor and staff sensibilities during transport.
- Organ/Tissue Donation
  - ○ Recognize that requests for tissue and organ donations must be made by specially trained personnel.
  - ○ Provide support and education to family members as decisions are being made. Use private areas for any family discussions concerning donation.
  - ○ Be sensitive to cultural and religious influences.
  - ○ Maintain ventilatory and cardiovascular support for vital organ retrieval.
- Autopsy Considerations
  - ○ The provider typically approaches the family about performing an autopsy.
  - ○ The nurse's role is to answer the family members' questions and support their choices.
  - ○ Autopsies can be conducted to advance scientific knowledge regarding disease processes, which can lead to the development of new therapies.
  - ○ The law may require an autopsy to be performed if the death is due to homicide, suicide, or accidental death, or if death occurs within 24 hr of hospital admission.
  - ○ Most facilities require that all tubes remain in place for an autopsy.
- Documentation and completion of forms following federal and state laws typically includes the following:
  - ○ Who pronounced the death and at what time
  - ○ Consideration of and preparation for organ donation
  - ○ Description of any tubes or lines left in or on the body
  - ○ Disposition of personal articles
  - ○ Who was notified, and any decisions made
  - ○ The location of identification tags
  - ○ The time the body left the facility and the destination

- Care of Nurses Who are Grieving
  - Caring long term for clients can create personal attachments for nurses.
  - Nurses can use coping strategies:
    - Going to the client's funeral.
    - Communicating in writing to the family.
    - Attending debriefing sessions with colleagues.
    - Using stress management techniques.
    - Talking with a professional counselor.

APPLICATION EXERCISES

1. A nurse is caring for a client who has terminal lung cancer. The nurse observes the client's family assisting with all ADLs. Which of the following rationales for self-care should the nurse communicate to the family?

    A. Allowing the client to function independently will strengthen her muscles and promote healing.

    B. The client needs to be given privacy at times for self-reflecting and organizing her life.

    C. The client's sense of loss can be lessened through retaining control of certain areas of her life.

    D. Performing ADLs is required prior to discharge from an acute care facility.

2. A nurse is caring for a client who has stage 4 lung cancer and is 3 days postoperative following a wedge resection. The client states, "I told myself that I would go through with the surgery and quit smoking, if I could just live long enough to attend my daughter's wedding." Based on Kübler-Ross' Five Stages of Grief, which stage is the client experiencing?

    A. Anger

    B. Denial

    C. Bargaining

    D. Acceptance

3. A nurse is consoling the partner of a client who just expired after a long battle with liver cancer. The partner is displaying grief and states, "I hate him for leaving me." Which of the following statements by the nurse successfully facilitate mourning for the grieving partner? (Select all that apply.)

    _____ A. "Would you like me to contact the chaplain to come speak with you?"

    _____ B. "You will feel better soon. You have been expecting this for a while now."

    _____ C. "Let's talk about your children and how they are going to react."

    _____ D. "You know, it is quite normal to feel anger toward your husband at this time."

    _____ E. "Tell me more about how you are feeling."

4. A nurse is caring for a client who has a terminal illness. Death is expected within 24 hr. The client's family is at the bedside and asks the nurse what are anticipated clinical findings at this time. Which of the following is an appropriate response by the nurse?

    A. Regular breathing patterns

    B. Warm extremities

    C. Increased urine output

    D. Decreased muscle tone

5. A nurse is assisting a newly licensed nurse with postmortem care of a client. The family wishes to view the body. Which of the following statements by the newly licensed nurse indicate an understanding of the procedure? (Select all that apply.)

_____ A. "I will remove the dentures from the body."

_____ B. "I will make sure the body is lying completely flat."

_____ C. "I will apply fresh linens and place a clean gown on the body."

_____ D. "I will remove all equipment from the bedside."

_____ E. "I will dim the lights in the room."

6. A nurse educator is teaching a module on palliative care to a group of newly licensed nurses. Use the ATI Active Learning Template: Basic Concept to complete this item. Under Nursing Interventions, list five physical care interventions and five psychological care interventions appropriate for the care of a dying client.

APPLICATION EXERCISES KEY

1.   A. INCORRECT: The strengthening of muscles is not a priority of palliative care.

   B. INCORRECT: Privacy for periods of self-reflection can be achieved at times apart from performance of ADLs.

   C. **CORRECT:** Allowing the client as much control as possible maintains dignity and self-esteem.

   D. INCORRECT: Performance of ADLs is not a criterion for discharge from an acute care facility.

   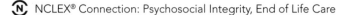 NCLEX® Connection: Psychosocial Integrity, End of Life Care

2.   A. INCORRECT: This client statement does not display anger.

   B. INCORRECT: The client is not denying the severity of the diagnosis and prognosis.

   C. **CORRECT:** The client is displaying bargaining by attempting to negotiate more time to live to see his daughter get married.

   D. INCORRECT: Although the client may have accepted his diagnosis and prognosis, this client statement does not convey coming to terms with the situation.

   NCLEX® Connection: Psychosocial Integrity, End of Life Care

3.   A. **CORRECT:** Asking the client whether she would like spiritual support at this time is an acceptable nursing intervention to facilitate mourning.

   B. INCORRECT: Giving false reassurance and offering assumptions are not recommended to facilitate mourning.

   C. INCORRECT: Changing the subject and bringing the focus away from the grieving individual are not recommended to facilitate mourning.

   D. **CORRECT:** Educating the client's partner on the grieving process and expected emotions is recommended at this time.

   E. **CORRECT:** Encouraging the open communication of feelings by using therapeutic communication is recommended to facilitate mourning.

   NCLEX® Connection: Psychosocial Integrity, Therapeutic Communication

4. A. INCORRECT: Labored breathing and irregular patterns are indicative of imminent death.

    B. INCORRECT: Cool extremities would be indicative of imminent death.

    C. INCORRECT: Decreased urine output would be indicative of imminent death.

    D. **CORRECT:** Muscle relaxation is an expected finding when a client is approaching death.

    Ⓝ NCLEX® Connection: Psychosocial Integrity, End of Life Care

5. A. INCORRECT: Dentures should be inserted so that the face looks as natural as possible.

    B. INCORRECT: The body should not be completely flat. One pillow is placed under the head and shoulders to prevent discoloration of the face.

    C. **CORRECT:** The body and the environment should be as clean as possible. This includes washing soiled areas of the body and applying fresh linens and a clean gown.

    D. **CORRECT:** The environment should be as clutter-free as possible. All equipment and supplies should be removed from the bedside.

    E. **CORRECT:** Dimming the lights helps to provide a calm environment for the family.

    Ⓝ NCLEX® Connection: Basic Care and Comfort, Personal Hygiene

6. *Using the ATI Active Learning Template: Basic Concept*

- Nursing Interventions
  - Physical Care
    - Give priority to controlling clinical findings.
    - Administer medications that manage pain, air hunger, and anxiety.
    - Perform ongoing assessment to determine the effectiveness of treatment and the need for modifications of the treatment plan, such as lower or higher doses of medications.
    - Manage adverse effects of medications.
    - Reposition the client to maintain airway patency and comfort.
    - Maintain the integrity of skin and mucous membranes.
    - Provide an environment that promotes dignity and self-esteem.
      - Remove products of elimination as soon as possible to maintain a clean and odor-free environment.
      - Offer comfortable clothing.
    - Provide careful grooming for hair, nails, and skin.
    - Encourage family members to bring in comforting possessions to make the client feel at home.
    - If appropriate, encourage the use of relaxation techniques, such as guided imagery and music.
    - Promote decision-making in food selection, activities, and health care to give the client as much control as possible.
    - Encourage the client to perform ADLs as able and willing to do so.
  - Psychosocial Care
    - Use an interprofessional approach.
    - Provide care to the client and family.
    - Use volunteers when appropriate to provide nonmedical care.
    - Use therapeutic communication to develop and maintain a nurse-client relationship.
    - Facilitate the understanding of information regarding disease progression and treatment choices.
    - Facilitate communication between the client, the family, and the provider.
    - Encourage the client to participate in religious practices that bring comfort and strength, if appropriate.
    - Assist the client in clarifying personal values in order to facilitate effective decision-making.
    - Encourage the client to use coping mechanisms that have worked in the past.
    - Be sensitive to comments made in the presence of clients who are unconscious because hearing is the last sensation lost.

(N) NCLEX® Connection: Basic Care and Comfort, Non-Pharmacological Comfort Interventions

UNIT 4	Physiological Integrity
SECTION:	BASIC CARE AND COMFORT

› Hygiene
› Rest and Sleep
› Nutrition and Oral Hydration
› Mobility and Immobility
› Pain Management
› Complementary and Alternative Therapies
› Bowel Elimination
› Urinary Elimination
› Sensory Perception

NCLEX® CONNECTIONS

When reviewing the chapters in this unit, keep in mind the relevant sections of the NCLEX® outline, in particular:

Client Needs: Basic Care and Comfort

› Relevant topics/tasks include:
  » Assistive Devices
    › Assess the client's use of assistive devices.
  » Elimination
    › Provide skin care to clients who are incontinent.
  » Mobility/Immobility
    › Apply knowledge of nursing procedures and psychomotor skills when providing care to clients with immobility.
  » Nutrition and Oral Hydration
    › Calculate the client's intake and output.
  » Personal Hygiene
    › Assess the client for personal hygiene habits/routine.
  » Rest and Sleep
    › Schedule client care activities to promote adequate rest.

chapter 37

Overview

- Personal hygiene needs vary with clients' health status, social and cultural practices, and the daily routines they follow at home. For most clients, personal hygiene includes:
  - Bathing
  - Oral care
  - Nail and foot care
  - Perineal care
  - Hair care
  - Shaving (especially for men)
- Because personal hygiene has a profound impact on overall health, comfort, and well-being, it is an integral component of individualized nursing care plans.
- When clients become ill, have surgery, or are injured and are unable to manage their own personal hygiene needs, it becomes the nurse's responsibility to meet those needs.
- Before beginning any personal care delivery, it is important to evaluate each client's ability to participate in personal hygiene. Encourage clients to participate in any way they can.

Hygiene Care

- Bathing
  - Bathe clients to cleanse the body, relax it, and enhance healing.
  - Perform a skin assessment and wound care at this time.
  - Bathe clients whose health problems have exhausted them or limited their mobility.
    - Give a complete bath to clients who can tolerate it and whose hygiene needs warrant it.
    - Partial baths are useful when clients cannot tolerate a complete bath, they need particular cleansing of odorous or uncomfortable areas, or they can perform part of the bath independently.
- Proper oral hygiene helps decrease the risk of infection for clients living in long-term care facilities, especially from the transmission of pathogens that can cause pneumonia.
- Foot care prevents skin breakdown, pain, and infection. Foot care is extremely important for clients who have diabetes mellitus, and a qualified professional must perform it.
- Perineal care helps maintain skin integrity, relieve discomfort, and prevent transmission of micro-organisms (catheter care).

- Cultural and Social Practices
  - Clients vary in their hygiene preferences and practices. These include bathing routines, oral care, grooming preferences, and health beliefs. Culture also plays an important role, because some cultures have unique hygiene practices. Be sure to be respectful and observant of each client's specific cultural needs.
  - Socioeconomic status may affect clients' hygiene status. If a client is homeless, alter the discharge instructions and follow-up care accordingly.
  - Respect each client's dignity. Many clients are dealing with a loss of control when others must provide their hygiene care. Reassuring clients and allowing them to have as much control as possible may help.
- Safety
  - Before starting any care, understand how to complete each task to avoid injuring the client. This includes knowing the equipment and what the proper techniques are for each hygiene procedure.
  - Never leave clients in a position where injury could occur during routine hygiene care. For example, avoid leaving a client who is at risk for aspiration alone with oral hygiene supplies.
- Special Considerations for Older Adult Clients
  - Older adults' skin is drier and thinner and may not tolerate as much bathing as younger adults' skin.
  - Older adults have higher incidences of infection and periodontal disease because of the weakening of the periodontal membrane.
  - Dentures must fit correctly, or they can cause digestive issues, pain, and discomfort. Dentures are a client's personal property. Never leave them on a meal tray or in a place where they could be damaged or lost.
  - Dry mouth is common in older adults due to decreased saliva production and medications this population commonly uses (antihypertensives, diuretics, anti-inflammatory agents, antidepressants).
  - Poor nutritional status is often due to dental problems, socioeconomic status, or a limited ability to prepare healthful foods.

Assessment/Data Collection

- Inspect the skin for color, hydration, texture, turgor, and any lesions or other impaired integrity.
- Check the condition of the gums and teeth for dryness or inflammation of the oral mucosa. Does the client report any pain?
- Assess the skin surfaces including the feet and nails, and note the shape and size of each foot, any lesions, and areas of dryness or inflammation. Significant alterations may indicate neuropathy and/or vascular insufficiency. Are all pulses palpable and equal bilaterally?
- Identify hygiene preferences to understand how clients perform hygiene at home and what additional education and care to provide.
- Assess for safety issues (altered positioning, decreased mobility) and the ability to participate in self-care.

Nursing Interventions

- To give a bed bath:
  - ○ Collect equipment, provide for privacy, and explain the procedure.
  - ○ Apply gloves.
  - ○ Lock the wheels on the bed.
  - ○ Place a bath blanket over the client and remove the gown.
  - ○ Obtain bath water.
  - ○ Wash the face first. Allow the client to perform this task if able.
  - ○ Perform the bath systematically by starting with the upper body and continuing on to the lower extremities. Keep cleaned areas covered with a blanket or towel. Change water as indicated, using fresh water to perform perineal care.
    - ▪ Perineal Care
      - □ It is important to maintain skin integrity to relieve discomfort and prevent transmission of infection (catheter care).
      - □ Principles of perineal care include:
        - ▸ Providing privacy.
        - ▸ Maintaining a professional demeanor.
        - ▸ Removing any fecal material from the skin.
        - ▸ Cleansing the perineal area from front to back.
        - ▸ Drying thoroughly.
        - ▸ Retracting the foreskin of male clients to wash the tip of the penis, then replacing the foreskin.
    - ▪ Foot Care
      - □ It is important to prevent any infection or pain that may interfere with gait. This care is extremely important for clients who have diabetes mellitus, and a qualified professional must perform it.
      - □ Instruct clients at risk for injury to:
        - ▸ Inspect the feet daily, paying special attention to the area between the toes.
        - ▸ Use lukewarm water and dry the feet thoroughly.
        - ▸ Apply moisturizer to the feet but avoid applying it between the toes.
        - ▸ Avoid over-the-counter products that contain alcohol or other strong chemicals.
        - ▸ Wear clean cotton socks daily.
        - ▸ Check shoes for any objects, rough seams, or edges that may cause injury.
        - ▸ Cut the nails straight across and use an emery board to file nail edges.
        - ▸ Avoid self-treating corns or calluses.
        - ▸ Buy and wear comfortable shoes that do not restrict circulation.
        - ▸ Do not apply heat unless prescribed.
        - ▸ Contact the provider if any signs of infection or inflammation appear.

- ○ Apply lotion and powder (if neither is contraindicated), and a clean gown.

- ○ Document skin assessment, type of bath, and the client's response.

- ○ To change linens on an occupied bed:

    - Roll the bottom linens up in the bottom sheet or mattress pad under the client who is turned on his side, facing the opposite direction.

    - Apply clean bottom linens to the bed, and extend them to the middle of the bed with the remainder of the linen fan folded underneath the client.

    - Have the client roll over the linens and face the opposite direction, then remove the used linens and apply the clean linens.

    - Apply the upper sheet and blanket.

    - To remove the pillowcase, insert one hand into the opening, grab the pillow, and turn the pillowcase inside out.

    - Apply the clean pillowcase by grasping the center of the closed end, turning the case inside out, fitting the pillow into the corner of the case, and pulling the case until it is right side out over the pillow.

- Oral Hygiene

    - ○ Clients who have fragile oral mucosa require gentle brushing and flossing.

    - ○ Have suction apparatus ready at the bedside when providing oral hygiene to clients who are unconscious to help prevent aspiration. Position them side-lying with the head turned toward you in either a semi-Fowler's position, or with the head of the bed flat. This will allow fluid and oral secretions to collect in the dependent side of the mouth and drain out.

    - ○ Perform denture care for clients who are unable to do so themselves.

        - Remove the dentures with a gloved hand, pulling down and out at the front of the upper denture, and lifting up and out at the front of the lower denture.

        - Place the dentures in a denture cup, an emesis basin, or on a washcloth in the sink.

        - Brush them with a soft brush and denture cleaner.

        - Rinse them in tepid water.

        - Store the dentures in a denture cup with water to keep them moist, or help the client reinsert the dentures.

- Nail Care

    - ○ Observe the size, shape, and condition of the nails and nail beds.

    - ○ Check for cracking, clubbing, and fungus.

    - ○ Before cutting any client's nails, check the facility's/agency's policy; some require a prescription from the provider, while others allow only a podiatrist or other qualified professional to cut some or all clients' nails.

    - ○ Foot and nail care will vary from the standard when you care for a client who has diabetes mellitus. Do not soak the feet due to the risk of infection and do not cut the nails. Instead, file them using a nail file. Do not apply lotion between the fingers or toes since the moisture can cause skin irritation and breakdown.

- Hair Care
  - Caring for the hair and scalp is important for clients' appearance and sense of well-being, and is an essential component of personal hygiene.
  - Brush or comb the hair daily to remove tangles, massage the scalp, stimulate circulation to the scalp, and distribute natural oils along the shaft of the hair. Use a soft-bristled brush to prevent injury or trauma to the scalp and a wide-toothed comb or hair pick to comb through tightly curled hair.
  - For clients who cannot shower but can sit in a chair and lean back, shampoo the hair at the sink. For clients on bed rest, use a plastic shampoo trough. Dry or no-rinse shampoos and shampoo caps are also options for clients on bed rest.
  - Start shampooing the hair at the hairline and work toward the neck. To wash the hair on the back of the head, gently lift the head with one hand and shampoo with the other.
  - Place a folded or rolled towel behind the neck to pad the edge of the sink. Then rinse, comb, and dry the hair.
- Shaving
  - Safety is important. Clients prone to bleeding or receiving anticoagulants should use an electric razor.
  - Apply soap or shaving cream to warm, moist skin.
  - Move the razor over the skin in the direction of hair growth using long strokes on large areas of the face and short strokes around the chin and lips.
  - Be sure to communicate with clients about personal shaving preferences.

APPLICATION EXERCISES

1. A nurse is admitting a client from a long-term care facility to an acute-care setting. An indwelling urinary catheter was inserted just prior to her transfer. Which of the following interventions will help prevent the development of a catheter-associated infection?

    A. Determining the client's ability to void independently

    B. Placing an absorbent pad under the client to protect the bed in case of incontinence

    C. Frequently cleaning the client's perineal area and caring for her catheter

    D. Giving the client a diet high in fluid and fiber to prevent constipation

2. A nurse is instructing a client who has diabetes mellitus about foot care. Which of the following guidelines should the nurse include? (Select all that apply.)

    _____ A. Inspect the feet daily.

    _____ B. Use moisturizing lotions on the feet.

    _____ C. Wash the feet with warm water and let them air dry.

    _____ D. Use over-the-counter products to treat abrasions.

    _____ E. Check shoes for any foreign objects.

3. A client develops dyspnea and feels tired after completing her morning care. Which of the following should the nurse include in the client's plan of care for the next day?

    A. Plan for several rest periods during morning care.

    B. Do not offer any morning care.

    C. Perform all of the client's care as quickly as possible.

    D. Ask a family member to come in to give the client a bath.

4. A nurse is beginning a complete bed bath for a client. After removing the client's gown and placing a bath blanket over him, which of the following areas should the nurse wash first?

    A. Face

    B. Feet

    C. Chest

    D. Arms

5. A nurse is preparing to perform denture care for a client who prefers to keep the dentures in a cup while he is resting. Which of the following is an appropriate action for caring for the dentures?

A. Soak the dentures in a cup of cleansing solution.

B. Brush the dentures with a toothbrush and denture cleaner.

C. Rinse the dentures with hot water after cleaning them.

D. Place the dentures in a clean, dry storage container after cleaning them.

6. A nurse is about to perform perineal care for a client whose ability to assist with care is limited. Use the ATI Active Learning Template: Nursing Skill to complete this item. Under Nursing Actions, list the steps the nurse should take to perform this procedure.

APPLICATION EXERCISES KEY

1. A. INCORRECT: Determining the client's ability to void independently might eliminate the need for the catheter, but it will not prevent infection while she has the catheter.

    B. INCORRECT: Placing an absorbent pad under the client might increase the risk of infection by creating a warm, moist environment from perspiration or stool around the catheter.

    C. **CORRECT:** Most catheter-associated infections develop in the urinary tract, and regular cleaning of the perineal area along with catheter care reduces the number of micro-organisms.

    D. INCORRECT: Giving the client a diet high in fiber will help prevent constipation, but it will not reduce the risk of infection.

     NCLEX® Connection: Reduction of Risk Potential, Potential for Complications of Diagnostic Tests/Treatments/Procedures

2. A. **CORRECT:** Clients who have diabetes mellitus are at increased risk for infection and diminished sensitivity in the feet, so they should inspect them daily.

    B. **CORRECT:** The client should use moisturizing lotions (but not between the toes) to help keep the skin smooth and supple.

    C. INCORRECT: The client should wash the feet with lukewarm water and should dry them thoroughly.

    D. INCORRECT: Over-the-counter products often contain harmful chemicals that can cause skin impairment.

    E. **CORRECT:** Decreased sensation can impair the client's ability to feel loose objects (such as pebbles or sand) or rough areas of the inside of the shoe, and these can cause injury.

     NCLEX® Connection: Reduction of Risk Potential, Potential for Alterations in Body Systems

3. A. **CORRECT:** Planning for several rest periods during morning care will help prevent fatigue and continue to foster independence.

    B. INCORRECT: Fatigue and dyspnea do not eliminate the need for morning care.

    C. INCORRECT: Performing all of the client's care quickly might affect the client's self-esteem and reduce his independence.

    D. INCORRECT: Having a family member bathe the client reduces his self-esteem and independence.

     NCLEX® Connection: Basic Care and Comfort, Rest and Sleep

4.   A.   **CORRECT:** The greatest risk to a client during bathing is the transmission of pathogens from one area of the body to another. Thus, the nurse should begin with the cleanest area of the body and proceed to the least clean area. The face is generally the cleanest area, and washing it first follows a systematic head-to-toe approach to client care.

    B.   INCORRECT: Among these options, the nurse should wash the feet last.

    C.   INCORRECT: Among these options, there are two other options that are higher priorities.

    D.   INCORRECT: Among these options, there is another option that is a higher priority.

 NCLEX® Connection: Safety and Infection Control, Standard Precautions/Transmission-Based Precautions/Surgical Asepsis

5.   A.   INCORRECT: Soaking dentures in a commercial cleaning solution can help remove staining, but it is not enough to clean them adequately.

    B.   **CORRECT:** Brushing the dentures thoroughly with a toothbrush and denture cleaner removes debris that accumulates on and between the teeth.

    C.   INCORRECT: Using hot water to rinse dentures can damage some denture materials. The nurse should use tepid water to rinse dentures.

    D.   INCORRECT: Dentures should be moist when not in use to prevent warping and to facilitate insertion. The nurse should store them in water in a denture cup with the client's identification on the cup.

 NCLEX® Connection: Basic Care and Comfort, Assistive Devices

6. *Using the ATI Active Learning Template: Nursing Skill*
   - Nursing Actions
     - Provide privacy.
     - Maintain a professional demeanor.
     - Remove any fecal material from the skin.
     - Cleanse the perineal area from front to back.
     - Dry skin thoroughly.
     - Retract the foreskin of male clients to wash the tip of the penis then replace the foreskin.

 NCLEX® Connection: Safety and Infection Control, Standard Precautions/Transmission-Based Precautions/Surgical Asepsis

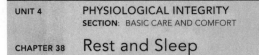

chapter 38

Overview

- Adequate amounts of sleep and rest promote health. Too little sleep leads to an inability to concentrate, poor judgment, moodiness, and an increased risk for accidents.
- Chronic sleep loss can increase the risk of obesity, depression, hypertension, diabetes mellitus, heart attack, and stroke.

Sleep Cycle

- The sleep cycle consists of nonrapid eye movement (NREM) sleep and rapid eye movement (REM) sleep. Typically, after Stage 1 of NREM sleep, people cycle four to six times through the other stages of sleep. With each cycle, the length of time in REM sleep increases. NREM sleep accounts for 75% to 80% of sleep time.

STAGE	CHARACTERISTICS	
Stage 1 NREM	› Very light sleep › Only a few minutes long › Vital signs and metabolism beginning to diminish	› Awakens easily › Feels relaxed and drowsy
Stage 2 NREM	› Deeper sleep › 10 to 20 min in length › Vital signs and metabolism continuing to diminish	› Requires slightly more stimulation to awaken › Increased relaxation
Stage 3 NREM	› Deep sleep › 15 to 30 min in length › Vital signs continuing to decrease	› Difficult to awaken › Relaxation with little movement
Stage 4 NREM	› Called delta sleep › Deepest sleep › 15 to 30 min in length › Vital signs low › Very difficult to awaken	› Physiologic rest and restoration › Enuresis, sleepwalking, sleeptalking possible › Repair and renewal of tissue
REM	› Vivid dreaming › About 90 min after falling asleep › Longer with each sleep cycle › Average length 20 min	› Varying vital signs › Very difficult to awaken › Cognitive restoration

- Sleep Duration
  - Sleep averages vary with the developmental stage, with infants and toddlers averaging 14 to 16 hr/day. This declines gradually throughout childhood, with adolescents averaging 9 to 10 hr/day and adults 7 to 9 hr/day.
- Common Sleep Disorders
  - Insomnia, the most common sleep disorder, is the inability to get an adequate amount of sleep and to feel rested. It might mean difficulty falling asleep, difficulty staying asleep, awakening too early, or not getting refreshing sleep. Acute insomnia lasts a few days and may be due to personal stressors. Chronic insomnia lasts a month or more. Some people have intermittent insomnia, sleeping well for a few days and then having insomnia for a few days. Women and older adults are more prone to insomnia.
  - Sleep apnea is more than five breathing cessations lasting longer than 10 seconds per hour during sleep, resulting in decreased arterial oxygen saturation levels. Sleep apnea can be a single disorder or a mixture of the following:
    - Central – central nervous system dysfunction that fails to trigger breathing during sleep.
    - Obstructive – structures in the mouth and throat occlude the upper airway.
  - Narcolepsy – sudden attacks of sleep during waking hours. It often happens at inappropriate times and increases the risk for injury.

Assessment/Data Collection

- Ask about sleep patterns, history, and any recent changes.
- Ask about sleep problems (type, symptoms, timing, seriousness, related factors, aftereffects).
- Use a linear scale or visual with "best sleep" on one end and "worst sleep" on the opposite end and ask for a sleep rating on a 0 to 10 scale.
- Check for common factors that interfere with sleep:
  - Illness – may require more sleep or disrupt sleep, such as nocturia.
  - Current life events (traveling more, change in work hours).
  - Emotional stress or mental illness (anxiety, fear).
  - Diet (caffeine consumption, heavy meals before bedtime).
  - Exercise – promotes sleep if at least 2 hr before bedtime; otherwise, it can disrupt sleep.
  - Sleep environment too light, the wrong temperature, or too noisy (children, pets, loud noise, snoring partner).
  - Medications – may induce sleep but interfere with restorative sleep; others cause insomnia (bronchodilators, antihypertensives).

Nursing Interventions

- Help clients establish and follow a bedtime routine.
- Limit waking clients during the night.
- Help with personal hygiene needs or a back rub prior to sleep to increase comfort.
- Instruct clients to:
  - Exercise regularly at least 2 hr before bedtime.
  - Arrange the sleep environment for comfort.
  - Limit alcohol, caffeine, and nicotine at least 4 hr before bedtime.
  - Limit fluids 2 to 4 hr before bedtime.
  - Engage in muscle relaxation if anxious or stressed.
- Instruct clients with narcolepsy to:
  - Exercise regularly.
  - Eat small meals that are high in protein.
  - Avoid activities that increase sleepiness (sitting too long, warm environments, drinking alcohol).
  - Avoid activities that would cause injury should the client fall asleep (driving, heights).
  - Take naps when drowsy or when narcoleptic events are likely.
  - Take stimulants the provider prescribes.
- Consider continuous positive airway pressure (CPAP) devices for clients who have sleep apnea.
- Consult the provider about trying sleep-promoting, over-the-counter products (melatonin, valerian, chamomile).
- As a last resort, suggest that the provider prescribe a pharmacological agent. Medications of choice for insomnia are benzodiazepine-like medications, which include the sedative-hypnotics zolpidem (Ambien), eszopiclone (Lunesta), and zaleplon (Sonata).

APPLICATION EXERCISES

1. A nurse in a provider's office is caring for a client who states that, for the past week, she has felt tired during the day and cannot sleep at night. Which of the following questions should the nurse ask when collecting data about the client's difficulty sleeping? (Select all that apply.)

_____ A. Does your lack of sleep interfere with your ability to function during the day?

_____ B. Do you feel confused in the late afternoon?

_____ C. Do you drink coffee, tea, or other caffeinated drinks? If so, how many cups per day?

_____ D. Has anyone ever told you that you seem to stop breathing for a few seconds while you are asleep?

_____ E. Tell me about any personal stress you are experiencing.

2. A nurse is talking with a client about ways to help him sleep and rest. Which of the following recommendations should the nurse give to the client to promote sleep and rest? (Select all that apply.)

_____ A. Practice muscle relaxation techniques.

_____ B. Exercise each morning.

_____ C. Take an afternoon nap.

_____ D. Alter the sleep environment for comfort.

_____ E. Limit fluid intake at least 2 hr before bedtime.

3. A nurse is caring for an older adult client who has been following the facility's routine and bathing in the morning. However, at home, she always takes a warm bath just before bedtime. Now she is having difficulty sleeping at night. Which of the following actions should the nurse take first?

A. Rub her back for 15 min before bedtime.

B. Offer her warm milk and crackers at 2100.

C. Allow her to take a bath in the evening.

D. Ask the provider for a sleeping medication.

4. A nurse is preparing a presentation at a local community center about sleep hygiene. When explaining rapid eye movement (REM) sleep, which of the following characteristics should the nurse include? (Select all that apply.)

_____ A. REM sleep provides cognitive restoration.

_____ B. REM sleep lasts about 90 min.

_____ C. It is difficult to awaken a person in REM sleep.

_____ D. Sleepwalking occurs during REM sleep.

_____ E. Vivid dreams are common during REM sleep.

5. A nurse is instructing a client who has a new diagnosis of narcolepsy about measures that might help with self-management. Which of the following client statements indicates understanding of the instructions?

A. "I'll add plenty of carbohydrates to my meals."

B. "I'll take a short nap whenever I feel a little sleepy."

C. "I'll make sure I stay warm when I am at my desk at work."

D. "It's okay to drink alcohol as long as I limit it to one drink per day."

6. A nurse on a medical unit is collecting data from a client who reports a persistent inability to sleep. Use the ATI Active Learning Template: Basic Concept to complete this item. Include the following:

A. Underlying Principles: List at least three common factors that might be interfering with the client's sleep.

B. Nursing Interventions: List at least three strategies the nurse can implement to help the client sleep while in the hospital.

APPLICATION EXERCISES KEY

1. A. **CORRECT:** Daytime sleepiness, which can interfere with functioning, is common during the day when people cannot sleep at night.

    B. INCORRECT: Chronic sleep deprivation or lack of rapid eye movement sleep can cause confusion, but sleep difficulties for 1 week should not result in confusion.

    C. **CORRECT:** Caffeinated drinks act as a stimulant and can interfere with sleep.

    D. **CORRECT:** Periods of apnea warrant a prompt referral for diagnostic sleep studies.

    E. **CORRECT:** Emotional stress is the most common cause of short-term sleep problems.

    Ⓝ NCLEX® Connection: Basic Care and Comfort, Rest and Sleep

2. A. **CORRECT:** Relaxation techniques, especially muscle relaxation, can help promote sleep and rest.

    B. **CORRECT:** Following an exercise routine regularly, at least 2 hr before bedtime, can help promote rest and sleep.

    C. INCORRECT: Napping during the day can keep some people from getting the sleep they need during their usual sleeping hours.

    D. **CORRECT:** For example, rather than trying to sleep with a restless pet at the foot of the bed, move the pet to another sleep area.

    E. **CORRECT:** Limiting fluids for a few hours before bedtime helps minimize getting up to urinate.

    Ⓝ NCLEX® Connection: Basic Care and Comfort, Rest and Sleep

3. A. INCORRECT: Rubbing the client's back might help promote sleep, but there is another option the nurse should try first.

    B. INCORRECT: Offering the client warm milk and crackers might help promote sleep, but there is another option the nurse should try first.

    C. **CORRECT:** When providing nursing care, the nurse should first use the least restrictive intervention. Of these options, allowing the client to follow her usual bedtime routine represents the least change, so it is the first intervention to try.

    D. INCORRECT: Asking for a prescription for sleep medication might help, but there is another option the nurse should try first.

    Ⓝ NCLEX® Connection: Basic Care and Comfort, Rest and Sleep

4. A. **CORRECT:** Cognitive and brain tissue restoration occur during REM sleep.

    B. INCORRECT: REM sleep lasts an average of 20 min. It typically begins about 90 min after falling asleep.

    C. **CORRECT:** In this stage, awakening is difficult. Awakening is relatively easy in stages 1 and 2 of non-REM sleep.

    D. INCORRECT: Sleepwalking and sleeptalking tend to occur during Stage 4 non-REM sleep.

    E. **CORRECT:** Dreaming does occur in other stages, but it is less vivid and possibly less colorful.

    Ⓝ NCLEX® Connection: Physiological Adaptations, Pathophysiology

5. A. INCORRECT: Clients who have narcolepsy should eat light, high-protein meals.

    B. **CORRECT:** Clients who have narcolepsy should take short naps to reduce feelings of drowsiness.

    C. INCORRECT: Clients who have narcolepsy should avoid sitting for prolonged periods in warm environments.

    D. INCORRECT: Clients who have narcolepsy should avoid ingesting any substance that could increase drowsiness, such as alcohol.

    Ⓝ NCLEX® Connection: Basic Care and Comfort, Rest and Sleep

6. *Using the ATI Active Learning Template: Basic Concept*

    A. Underlying Principles
      - Illness
      - Current life events (travel, change in work hours)
      - Emotional stress or mental illness (anxiety, fear)
      - Caffeine consumption
      - Heavy meals before bedtime
      - Exercise within 2 hr of bedtime
      - A sleep environment that is noisy, too light, or the wrong temperature
      - Medications that cause insomnia

    B. Nursing Interventions
      - Help the client establish and follow a bedtime routine.
      - Limit waking client during the night.
      - Assist with personal hygiene needs.
      - Offer a back rub.
      - Request a prescription for a sleep medication from the provider.

    Ⓝ NCLEX® Connection: Basic Care and Comfort, Rest and Sleep

chapter 39

Overview

- Nutrients provide energy for cellular metabolism and for repair, organ function, growth, and physical activity. Water, the most basic of all nutrients, is crucial for all body fluid and cellular functions.

- The proper balance of nutrients and fluid along with consideration of energy intake and requirements is essential for ensuring proper nutritional status. Early recognition and treatment of clients who are malnourished or at risk can have a positive influence on client outcomes.

- A nutritional assessment helps identify areas to modify, either through adding or avoiding specific nutrients or by increasing or decreasing caloric intake.

- When planning a nutritional or hydration intervention, it is important to consider beliefs and culture, the environment, and the presentation of the food, as well as any illnesses or allergies clients might have.

Basic Nutrients the Body Requires

- Carbohydrates provide most of the body's energy and fiber. Each gram produces 4 kcal. Sources include whole grain breads, baked potatoes, and brown rice.

- Fats provide energy and vitamins. No more than 30% of caloric intake should be from this source. Each gram produces 9 kcal. Sources include olive oil, salmon, and egg yolks.

- Proteins contribute to the growth and repair of body tissues. Each gram produces 4 kcal. Sources include ground beef, whole milk, and poultry.

- Vitamins are necessary for metabolism. The fat-soluble vitamins are A, D, E, and K. The water-soluble vitamins include C and B complex (eight vitamins).

- Minerals complete essential biochemical reactions in the body (calcium, potassium, sodium, iron).

- Water replaces fluids lost through perspiration, elimination, and respiration.

Factors Affecting Nutrition and Metabolism

Q
PCC

- Religious and cultural practices may guide food preparation and choices.

- Financial issues may prevent clients from buying foods that are high in protein, vitamins, and minerals.

- Appetite decreases with illness, medications, pain, depression, and unpleasant environmental stimuli.

- Negative experiences with certain foods or familiarity with foods clients like help determine preferences.

Q
S

- Disease/illness can affect the functional ability to prepare and eat food.

- Medications can alter taste and appetite and can interfere with the absorption of certain nutrients.

- Age affects nutritional requirements.

AGE GROUP	CONSIDERATIONS

Infants (Birth to 1 year)	› High energy requirements.
	› Breast milk (preferred) or formula to provide:
	  » 108 kcal/kg of weight the first 6 months.
	  » 98 kcal/kg of weight the second 6 months.
	› Solid food starting after 6 months of age.
	› No cow's milk or honey for the first year.

Toddlers (12 months to 3 years) and preschoolers (3 to 6 years)	› Toddlers and preschoolers need fewer calories per kg of weight than infants. › Toddlers and preschoolers need increased protein from sources other than milk. › Calcium and phosphorus are important for bone health.
School-age children (6 to 12 years)	› School-age children need supervision to consume adequate protein and vitamins C and A. › School-age children tend to eat foods high in carbohydrates, fats, and salt.
Adolescents (12 to 20 years)	› Metabolic demands are high and require more energy. › Protein, calcium, iron, iodine, folic acid, and vitamin B needs are high. › One fourth of dietary intake comes from snacks. › Increased water consumption is important for active adolescents.
Young adults (20 to 35 years) and middle adults (35 to 65 years)	› There is a decreased need for most nutrients (except during pregnancy). › Calcium and iron are essential minerals for women. › Good oral health is important.
Older adults (over 65 years)	› A slower metabolic rate requires fewer calories. › Thirst sensations diminish. › Older adults need the same amount of most vitamins and minerals as younger adults. › Calcium may be necessary and is important for both men and women. › Many older adults require carbohydrates that provide fiber and bulk to enhance gastrointestinal function.

- Eating Disorders
  - Anorexia nervosa
    - Body weight less than 85% of ideal
    - Fear of being fat
    - Feeling fat
    - With female clients, no menses for at least 3 consecutive months
  - Bulimia nervosa – a cycle of binge eating followed by purging (vomiting, using diuretics or laxatives, exercise, fasting)
    - Lack of control during binges
    - Average at least two binges per week for at least 3 months
  - Obesity
    - Dividing weight (in kg) by height (in m²) determines body mass index (BMI).
    - A BMI of 25 is the upper boundary of healthy weight. Adults who have a BMI above 30 are obese.

Assessment/Data Collection

- Dietary history should include the following:
  - Number of meals per day
  - Fluid intake
  - Food preferences, amounts
  - Food preparation, purchasing practices, access to food
  - History of indigestion, heartburn, gas
  - Allergies
  - Taste
  - Chewing and swallowing
  - Appetite
  - Elimination patterns
  - Medication use
  - Activity levels
  - Religious, cultural food restrictions
- Clinical Measures
  - Height, weight to calculate BMI and ideal body weight (IBW)
  - Laboratory values of cholesterol, triglycerides, hemoglobin, electrolytes, albumin, nitrogen levels
- Intake and Output (I&O)
  - Record I&O.
  - Monitor I&O for clients who have fluid or electrolyte imbalances.
  - Weigh clients each day at the same time, after voiding, and while wearing the same type of clothes.
  - If using bed scales, use the same amount of linen each day, and reset the scale to zero if possible.

- Subjective and objective data indicating poor nutrition:
  - Nausea, vomiting, diarrhea, constipation
  - Flaccid muscles
  - Mental status changes
  - Loss of appetite
  - Change in bowel pattern
  - Spleen, liver enlargement
  - Dry, brittle hair
  - Loss of subcutaneous fat
  - Dry, scaly skin
  - Inflammation, bleeding of gums
  - Poor dental health
  - Dry, dull eyes
  - Enlarged thyroid
  - Prominent protrusions over bony areas
  - Weakness
  - Change in weight
  - Poor posture

Nursing Interventions

- Assist in advancing the diet as appropriate.
- Instruct clients about the appropriate diet regimen.
- Provide interventions to promote appetite (good oral hygiene, favorite foods, minimal environmental odors).
- Educate clients about medications that may affect nutritional intake.
- Assist clients with feeding to promote optimal independence.
- Assist with preventing aspiration.
  - Position in Fowler's position or in a chair.
  - Support the upper back, neck, and head.
  - Have clients tuck their chin when swallowing to help propel food down the esophagus.
  - Observe for aspiration and pocketing of food in the cheeks or other areas of the mouth.
  - Observe for signs of dysphagia, such as coughing, choking, gagging, and drooling of food.
  - Keep clients in semi-Fowler's position for at least 1 hr after meals.
  - Provide oral hygiene after meals and snacks.

- Provide therapeutic diets.
  - Clear liquid – liquids that leave little residue (clear fruit juices, gelatin, broth)
  - Full liquid – clear liquids plus liquid dairy products, all juice, pureed vegetables
  - Pureed – clear and full liquids plus pureed meats, fruits, scrambled eggs
  - Mechanical soft – clear and full liquids plus diced or ground foods
  - Soft/low-residue – foods that are low in fiber and easy to digest
  - High-fiber (whole grains, raw and dried fruits)
  - Low sodium – no added salt or 1 to 2 g of sodium
  - Low cholesterol – no more than 300 mg/day of dietary cholesterol
  - Diabetic – balanced intake of protein, fats, and carbohydrates of about 1,800 calories
  - Dysphagia – pureed food and thickened liquids
  - Regular – no restrictions
- Administer and monitor enteral feedings via nasogastric, gastrostomy, or jejunostomy tubes.
- Administer and monitor parenteral nutrition to clients who are unable to use their gastrointestinal tract to acquire nutrients.
  - Parenteral nutrients include lipids, electrolytes, minerals, vitamins, dextrose, and amino acids.
- Maintain fluid balance by:
  - Administering IV fluids.
  - Restricting oral fluid intake.
    - Remove the water pitcher from the bedside.
    - Inform the dietary staff of the amount of fluid to serve with each meal tray.
    - Inform the staff of each shift of the amount of fluid clients may have in addition to what they receive with each meal tray.
    - Record all oral intake, and inform the family of the restriction.
  - Encouraging oral intake of fluids.
    - Provide fresh drinking water.
    - Ask about beverage preferences.

APPLICATION EXERCISES

1. A nurse is caring for a client who is at high risk for aspiration. Which of the following is an appropriate nursing intervention?

    A. Give the client thin liquids.

    B. Instruct the client to tuck her chin when swallowing.

    C. Have the client use a straw.

    D. Encourage the client to lie down and rest after meals.

2. A nurse is preparing a presentation about basic nutrients for a group of high school athletes. She should explain that which of the following is the body's priority energy source?

    A. Fat

    B. Protein

    C. Glycogen

    D. Carbohydrates

3. A nurse is caring for a client who is on a low-residue diet. The nurse should expect to see which of the following foods on the client's meal tray?

    A. Cooked barley

    B. Pureed broccoli

    C. Vanilla custard

    D. Lentil soup

4. A nurse is caring for a client who weighs 80 kg (176 lb) and is 1.6 m (5 ft 3 in) tall. Calculate her body mass index (BMI) and determine whether this client is obese based on her BMI.

5. A nurse in a senior center is counseling a group of older adults about their nutritional needs and considerations. Which of the following information should the nurse include? (Select all that apply.)

_____ A. Older adults are more prone to dehydration than younger adults are.

_____ B. Older adults need the same amount of most vitamins and minerals as younger adults do.

_____ C. Many older men and women need calcium supplementation.

_____ D. Older adults need more calories than they did when they were younger.

_____ E. Older adults should consume a diet low in carbohydrates.

6. A nurse is preparing a presentation in a community center on eating disorders that affect adolescents and young adults. Use the ATI Active Learning Template: Basic Concept to complete this item. Under Related Content, list two common eating disorders and their characteristics.

APPLICATION EXERCISES KEY

1. A. INCORRECT: Thin liquids increase the client's risk for aspiration.

    B. **CORRECT:** Tucking the chin when swallowing allows food to pass down the esophagus more easily.

    C. INCORRECT: Using a straw increases the client's risk for aspiration.

    D. INCORRECT: Sitting for an hour after meals helps prevent gastroesophageal reflux and possible aspiration of stomach contents after a meal.

     NCLEX® Connection: Reduction of Risk Potential, Potential for Complications of Diagnostic Tests/Treatments/Procedures

2. A. INCORRECT: Although the body gets about half of its energy supply from fat, it is an inefficient means of obtaining energy. It produces end products the body has to excrete, and it requires energy from another source to burn the fat.

    B. INCORRECT: Protein can supply energy, but it has other very essential and specific functions that only it can perform. So it is not the body's priority energy source.

    C. INCORRECT: Glycogen, which the body stores in the liver, is a backup source of energy, not a primary or priority source.

    D. **CORRECT:** Carbohydrates are the body's priority energy source; providing energy for cells is their primary function. They provide glucose, which burns completely and efficiently without end products to excrete, and carbohydrates are a ready source of energy, and spare proteins from depletion.

    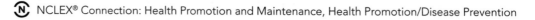 NCLEX® Connection: Health Promotion and Maintenance, Health Promotion/Disease Prevention

3. A. INCORRECT: Whole grains, such as barley and oats, are high in fiber and thus inappropriate components of a low-residue diet.

    B. INCORRECT: Raw and gas-producing vegetables, such as the cabbage in coleslaw, are high in fiber and thus inappropriate components of a low-residue diet.

    C. **CORRECT:** A low-residue diet consists of foods that are low in fiber and easy to digest. Dairy products and eggs, such as custard and yogurt, are appropriate for a low-residue diet.

    D. INCORRECT: Legumes, such as lentils and black beans, are high in fiber and thus inappropriate components of a low-residue diet.

    NCLEX® Connection: Basic Care and Comfort, Nutrition and Oral Hydration

4. BMI = weight (kg) ÷ height (m²). BMI = 80 ÷ 1.62² = 80 ÷ 2.56 = 31.25 = 31. A BMI above 30 identifies obesity, so this client is obese.

    N NCLEX® Connection: Basic Care and Comfort, Nutrition and Oral Hydration

5. A. **CORRECT:** Sensations of thirst diminish with age, leaving older adults more prone to dehydration.

    B. **CORRECT:** These requirements do not change from middle adulthood to older adulthood.

    C. **CORRECT:** They may ingest insufficient calcium in the diet and may need supplements to help prevent bone demineralization (osteoporosis).

    D. INCORRECT: They have a slower metabolic rate, so they require less energy (unless they are very active), and therefore need fewer calories.

    E. INCORRECT: Many older adults need more carbohydrates for the fiber and bulk they contain. They should, however, reduce their intake of fats and of "empty" calories, such as pastries and soda pop.

    N NCLEX® Connection: Basic Care and Comfort, Nutrition and Oral Hydration

6. *Using the ATI Active Learning Template: Basic Concept*
    - Related Content
      - Anorexia Nervosa
        - Body weight less than 85% of ideal
        - Fears being fat
        - Feeling fat
        - For females, no menses for at least 3 consecutive months
      - Bulimia Nervosa
        - Cycle of binge eating followed by purging (vomiting, using diuretics or laxatives, exercise, fasting)
        - Lack of control during binges
        - Average of at least two binges per week for at least 3 months

    N NCLEX® Connection: Health Promotion and Maintenance, Health Promotion/Disease Prevention

chapter 40

Overview

- Mobility is freedom and independence in purposeful movement. Mobility refers to adapting to and having self-awareness of the environment. Functional musculoskeletal and nervous systems are essential for mobility.

- Immobility is the inability to move freely and independently at will. The risk of complications increases with the degree of immobility and the length of time of immobilization.

- Cutaneous stimulation in the form of cold and heat applications helps relieve pain and promote healing.

- Promoting venous return is another key component of reducing the complications of immobility.

Mobility and Immobility

- Immobility may be the following:
  - Temporary, such as following knee arthroplasty
  - Permanent, such as paraplegia
  - Sudden onset, such as a fractured arm and leg following a motor-vehicle crash
  - Slow onset, such as multiple sclerosis
- The principles of body mechanics are based on alignment, balance, gravity, and friction.
- Movement depends on an intact skeletal system, skeletal muscles, and nervous system.
- Assessment focuses on mobility, range of motion (ROM), gait, exercise status, activity tolerance, and body alignment while standing, sitting, and lying.
- Factors affecting mobility include the following:
  - Alterations in muscles
  - Injury to the musculoskeletal system
  - Poor posture
  - Impaired central nervous system
  - Health status and age

- Changes that occur in body systems include the following:

BODY SYSTEM CHANGES	
Integumentary	
› Increased pressure on skin, which is aggravated by metabolic changes	› Decreased circulation to tissue causing ischemia, which can lead to pressure ulcers
Respiratory	
› Decreased respiratory movement resulting in decreased oxygenation and carbon dioxide exchange	› Stasis of secretions and decreased and weakened respiratory muscles, resulting in atelectasis and hypostatic pneumonia
	› Decreased cough response
Cardiovascular	
› Orthostatic hypotension	› Decreased cardiac output leading to poor cardiac effectiveness, which results in increased cardiac workload
› Less fluid volume in the circulatory system	
› Stasis of blood in the legs	› Increased oxygenation requirement
› Diminished autonomic response	› Increased risk of thrombus development
Metabolic	
› Altered endocrine system	› Decreased protein resulting in loss of muscle
› Decreased basal metabolic rate	› Loss of weight
› Changes in protein, carbohydrate, and fat metabolism	› Alterations in calcium, fluid, and electrolytes
	› Resorption of calcium from bones
› Decreased appetite with altered nutritional intake	› Decreased urinary elimination of calcium resulting in hypercalcemia
› Negative nitrogen balance	
Elimination	
› Genitourinary	› Gastrointestinal
» Urinary stasis	» Decreased peristalsis
» Change in calcium metabolism with hypercalcemia resulting in renal calculi	› Decreased fluid intake
	› Constipation, then fecal impaction, then diarrhea
» Decreased fluid intake, poor perineal care, and indwelling urinary catheters resulting in urinary tract infections	
Musculoskeletal	
› Decreased muscle endurance, strength, and mass	› Altered calcium metabolism
› Impaired balance	› Osteoporosis
› Atrophy of muscles	› Contractures
› Decreased stability	› Foot drop
	› Altered joint mobility

BODY SYSTEM CHANGES

Neurological/Psychosocial

› Changes in emotional status – depression, alteration in self-concept, and anxiety

› Behavioral changes – withdrawal, altered sleep/wake pattern, hostility, inappropriate laughter, and passivity

› Altered sensory perception

› Ineffective coping

Developmental

› Infants, toddlers, and preschoolers

» Slower progression in gross motor skills and intellectual and musculoskeletal development

» Body aligned with line of gravity, resulting in unbalanced posture

› Adolescents

» Imbalanced growth spurt possibly altered with immobility

» Delayed development of independence

» Social isolation

› Adults

» Alterations in every physiological system

» Alterations in family and social systems

» Alterations in job identity

› Older adults

» Alterations in balance resulting in a major risk for falls and injuries

» Steady loss of bone mass resulting in weakened bones

» Decreased coordination

» Slower walk with smaller steps

» Alterations in functional status

» Increased dependence on staff and family

Assessment/Data Collection and Patient-Centered Care

ASSESSMENT	NURSING INTERVENTIONS
Integumentary – Maintain intact skin.	
› Observe the skin for breakdown, warmth, and change in color. Look for pallor or redness in fair-skinned clients, and purple or blue discoloration in dark-skinned clients. › Observe bony prominences. › Check skin turgor. › Use a pressure ulcer risk scale such as Norton or Braden. › Assess at least every 2 hr. › Observe for urinary or bowel incontinence.	› Identify clients at risk for pressure ulcer development. › Position using corrective devices such as pillows, foot boots, trochanter rolls, and wedge pillows. › Turn every 1 to 2 hr, and use devices for support or per protocol. › Teach clients who can move independently to turn at least every 15 min. › Provide clients who are sitting in a chair with a device to decrease pressure. › Limit sitting in a chair to less than 2 hr. Instruct clients to shift their weight every 15 min. › Use a therapeutic bed or mattress for clients in bed for an extended time. › Monitor nutritional intake. › Provide skin and perineal care.

ASSESSMENT	NURSING INTERVENTIONS
Respiratory – Maintain airway patency, achieve optimal lung expansion and gas exchange, and mobilize airway secretions.	

› Complete every 2 hr:
  » Observe chest wall movement for symmetry.
  » Auscultate breath sounds.
  » Observe for productive cough, and note the color, amount, and consistency of secretions.
	› Reposition every 1 to 2 hr.
	› Instruct clients to turn, cough, and breathe deeply every 1 to 2 hr while awake.
	› Instruct clients to yawn every hr while awake.
	› Instruct clients to use an incentive spirometer while awake.
	› Remove abdominal binders every 2 hr and replace correctly.
	› Use chest physiotherapy.
	› Auscultate the lungs to determine the effectiveness of chest physiotherapy or other respiratory therapy.
	› Instruct clients to consume at least 2,000 mL of fluid per day, unless intake is restricted.
	› Monitor the ability to expectorate secretions.
	› Use suction if unable to expectorate secretions.

Cardiovascular – Maintain cardiovascular function, increase activity tolerance, and prevent thrombus formation.	
› Measure orthostatic blood pressure and pulse (lying to sitting to standing), and assess for vertigo. › Palpate the apical and peripheral pulses. › Auscultate the heart at the apex for S_3 (an early sign of heart failure). Older adult clients may not adapt well to immobility. › Palpate for edema in the sacrum, legs, and feet. › Palpate the skin for warmth in peripheral areas to include the nose, ear lobes, hands, and feet. › Assess for deep-vein thrombosis by observing the calves for redness and palpating for warmth and tenderness. › Measure the circumference of both calves and thighs and compare in size.	› Increase activity as soon as possible by dangling feet on side of bed or transferring to a chair. › Instruct clients to perform isometric exercises to increase activity tolerance. › Change position as often as possible. › Instruct clients to avoid the Valsalva maneuver. › Give a stool softener to prevent straining. › Teach range of motion (ROM) exercises such as ankle pumps and knee flexion. › Instruct clients to avoid placing pillows under the knees or lower extremities, crossing the legs, wearing tight clothes around the waist or on the legs, sitting for long periods of time, and massaging the legs. › Use elastic stockings. › Use sequential compression devices (SCD) or intermittent pneumatic compression (IPC). › Increase fluid intake if no restrictions. › Give low-dose heparin prophylactically. › Contact the provider immediately if assessment data indicate venous thrombosis.

ASSESSMENT	NURSING INTERVENTIONS
Metabolic – Reduce skin injury and maintain metabolism.	
› Record anthropometric measurements of height, weight, and skinfold. › Assess I&O. › Assess food intake. › Review urinary and bowel elimination status. › Assess wound healing. › Auscultate bowel sounds. › Check skin turgor. › Review laboratory values for electrolytes, serum, total protein, and BUN.	› Provide a high-calorie and high-protein diet with vitamin B and C supplements. › Monitor and evaluate oral intake. For clients who cannot eat or drink, provide enteral or parenteral nutritional therapy.
Elimination – Maintain urinary and bowel elimination.	
› Assess I&O. › Assess the bladder for distention. › Observe urine for color, amount, clarity, and frequency. › Auscultate bowel sounds. › Observe feces for color, amount, frequency, and consistency.	› Maintain hydration (at least 2,000 mL/day unless fluid is restricted). › Instruct clients to consume a diet that includes fruits and vegetables and is high in fiber. › Give a stool softener. Consider laxatives only as a last resort. › Provide perineal care. › Teach bladder and bowel training. › Insert a straight or indwelling catheter to relieve or manage bladder distention. › Promote urination by pouring warm water over the perineal area.

ASSESSMENT	NURSING INTERVENTIONS
Musculoskeletal – Maintain or regain body alignment and stability, decrease skin and musculoskeletal system changes, achieve full or optimal ROM, and prevent contractures.	

› Assess ROM capability.
› Assess muscle tone and mass.
› Observe for contractures.
› Monitor gait.
› Monitor nutritional intake for calcium.
› Monitor use of assistive devices to assist with ADLs.
	› Make sure clients change position in bed at least every 2 hr and perform weight shifts in the wheelchair every 15 min.
	› Encourage active or provide passive ROM two or three times a day.
	› Instruct clients to perform ROM while bathing, eating, grooming, and dressing.
	› Monitor nutritional intake of calcium.
	› Develop an individualized program for each client. Older adult clients may require a program that addresses the aging process.
	› Cluster care to promote a proper sleep-wake cycle.
	› Request physical therapy for clients who have decreased mobility.
	› Use a continuous passive motion device.
	› Cane instructions
	  » Maintain two points of support on the ground at all times.
	  » Keep the cane on the stronger side of the body.
	  » Support body weight on both legs, move the cane forward 6 to 10 inches, then move the weaker leg forward toward the cane.
	  » Next, advance the stronger leg past the cane.
	› Crutch instructions
	  » Do not alter crutches after fitting.
	  » Follow the prescribed crutch gait.
	  » Support body weight at the hand grips with the elbows flexed at 30°.
	  » Position the crutches on the unaffected side when sitting or rising from a chair.

Psychosocial – Maintain an acceptable sleep/wake pattern, achieve socialization, and complete self-care independently.	
› Assess emotional status. › Assess mental status. › Assess behavior and decision-making skills. › Monitor mobility status. › Observe for unusual alterations in sleep/wake pattern. › Assess coping skills, especially for loss. › Monitor activities of daily living (ADLs). › Assess for family support and relationships. › Monitor social activities.	› Assist in using usual coping skills or in developing new coping skills. › Maintain orientation to time (clock and calendar with date), person (call by name and introduce self), and place (talk about treatments, therapy, and length of stay). › Develop a schedule of therapies, and place it on a calendar for clients. › Arrange for clients with limited mobility to be in a semiprivate room with an alert roommate. › Involve clients in daily care. › Provide stimuli such as books, television, newspapers, and radio. › Help clients maintain body image by performing or assisting with hygiene and grooming tasks such as shaving or applying makeup. › Have nurses and other staff interact on an informal social basis. › Recommend a referral for consultation (psychological, spiritual, or social worker) for clients who are not coping well.

ASSESSMENT	NURSING INTERVENTIONS
Developmental – Continue expected development and achieve physical and mental stimulation.	
› Infancy through school age » Gross motor skills, and intellectual and musculoskeletal development » Body alignment and posture » Developmental tasks specific to age	› Infancy through school age » Initiate events that stimulate physical and psychosocial systems. Increase mobility, and involve play therapists in age-appropriate activities. » Use measures to prevent falls. » Develop strategies for maintaining or enhancing the developmental process. » Teach families that their perception of immobility can affect progress and ability to cope. » Encourage parents to stay with children. » Incorporate children's involvement, if it is age-appropriate, in their treatments. » Place children in a room with others who are age-appropriate.
› Adolescents » Growth and development specific to age » Level of independence » Social activities	› Adolescents » Initiate care that facilitates independence. » Involve adolescents in decision-making for ADLs. » Provide stimuli to promote socialization (interaction with peers, use of adolescents' activity room).
› Adults » All physical systems » Family relationships » Social status » Meaning of career/job	› Adults » Provide care that promotes activity in all physical systems. » Discuss with families the importance of interaction with clients. » Discuss social involvement. » Discuss the meaning of career/job.
› Older adults » Balance » Coordination » Gait » Functional status » Level of independence » Social isolation	› Older adults » Plan care with clients and families to increase independence with ADLs and decision-making skills. » Teach the staff to facilitate clients' independence in all activities. » Provide stimuli such as a clock, newspaper, calendar, and weather status. » Encourage families to visit to maintain socialization. » Plan for staff to spend some time talking and listening to clients.

Application of Heat and Cold

THERAPEUTIC EFFECTS OF HEAT AND COLD APPLICATIONS	
Heat	Cold
› Increases blood flow	› Decreases inflammation
› Increases tissue metabolism	› Prevents swelling
› Relaxes muscles	› Reduces bleeding
› Eases joint stiffness and pain	› Reduces fever
	› Diminishes muscle spasms
	› Decreases pain by decreasing the velocity of nerve conduction

- For clients at risk for injury from heat/cold applications:
  - Use extreme caution with clients who are very young, fair-skinned, and older because they have fragile skin.
  - Clients who are immobile may not be able to move away from the application if it becomes uncomfortable; they are at risk for skin injuries.
  - Clients who have impaired sensory perception may not feel pain or burning.
  - Avoid extremely long applications of either heat or cold because they will result in a reaction opposite to the intended response.
  - Heat
    - Monitor bony prominences carefully because they are more sensitive to heat applications.
    - Avoid the use of heat applications over metal devices (pacemakers, prosthetic joints) to prevent deep tissue burns.
    - Do not apply heat to the abdomen of a client who is pregnant to prevent harm to the fetus.
    - Do not place a heat application under a client who is immobile because this may increase the risk of burns.
  - Cold application is inappropriate for clients who have cold intolerance, vascular insufficiency, and disorders aggravated by cold, such as Raynaud's phenomenon.
  - Make sure the provider has written a prescription that includes the following:
    - Location
    - Duration and frequency
    - Specific type (moist or dry)
    - Temperature to use

Patient-Centered Care

- Heat application supplies include the following:
  - Moist
    - Hot compresses – towel, bath thermometer, hot water, plastic covering, hot pack or aquathermia pad (with distilled water), tape
    - Hot soaks – water, bath thermometer, basin, waterproof pads
    - Sitz baths – sitz bath (disposable or built-in), bath thermometer, bath blanket, towels
  - Dry
    - Hot pack (disposable or reusable) or an aquathermia pad with distilled water, and a pillowcase
    - Warming blanket
- Cold application supplies include the following:
  - Moist
    - Cold water
    - Cold pack
  - Dry
    - Ice bag, ice collar, ice glove, or a cold pack
    - Cooling blanket
- Apply to the area.
- Make sure the call light is within reach, and instruct clients to report any discomfort.
- Assess the site every 5 to 10 min to check for:
  - Redness or pallor
  - Pain or burning
  - Numbness
  - Shivering (with cold applications)
  - Blisters
  - Decreased sensation
  - Cyanosis (with cold applications)
- Discontinue the application if any of the above occur, or remove the application at the predetermined time (usually 15 to 20 min).
- Document
  - Location, type, and length of the application
  - Condition of the skin before and after the application
  - Clients' tolerance of the application

PROMOTING VENOUS RETURN

- Elastic (antiembolic) stockings or thromboembolic device (TED) hose help maintain external pressure on the muscles of the lower extremities and promote blood return to the heart.

- Sequential compression devices (SCDs) and intermittent pneumatic compression (IPC) have plastic or fabric sleeves that wrap around the leg and secure with hook-and-loop closures. The sleeves are then attached to an electric pump that alternately inflates and deflates the sleeve around the leg. These machines are set to cycle, typically a 10- to 15-second inflation and a 45- to 60-second deflation.

- Positioning techniques reduce compression of leg veins.

- ROM exercises cause skeletal muscle contractions, which promote blood return. Specific exercises that help prevent thrombophlebitis include ankle pumps, foot circles, and knee flexion.

- TED hose, SCDs, and IPC require a prescription.

- Clients who are immobile should perform leg exercises, increase their fluid intake, and change positions frequently.

- When suspecting poor venous return or possible thrombus, notify the provider and do not apply pressure to a thrombus to avoid dislodging it.

Patient-Centered Care

- TED hose
  - Equipment
    - Tape measure
    - TED hose
  - Procedure
    - Perform hand hygiene.
    - Assess skin and circulation in the legs.
    - Measure the calf and/or thigh circumference and the length of the leg to select the correct size stocking.
    - Turn the stockings inside to the heel.
    - Put the stocking on the foot.
    - Pull the remainder of the stocking over the heel and up the leg.
    - Smooth any creases or wrinkles.
    - Remove the stockings and reapply them at least twice a day.
    - Make sure the stockings are not too tight over the toes.
    - Keep the stockings clean and dry. Clients who are postoperative or have special needs may need a second pair of hose.
    - Document the application and removal of the stockings.

- SCDs and IPC
  - Equipment
    - Tape measure
    - Sequential stockings
    - Stockinette
  - Procedure
    - Perform hand hygiene.
    - Assess circulation and skin prior to application.
    - Measure around the largest part of the thigh to determine the stocking size.
    - Place the stockinette on first.
    - Apply the sleeves.
    - Attach the sleeves to the inflator.
    - Turn on the device.
    - Monitor circulation and skin after application.
    - Document the application and removal of the stockings.
- Positioning techniques to reduce compression of leg veins
  - Procedure – Instruct clients to avoid the following:
    - Crossing legs
    - Sitting for long periods
    - Wearing restrictive clothing on the lower extremities
    - Putting pillows behind the knees
    - Massaging legs
- ROM exercises hourly while awake.
  - Procedure – Instruct clients to perform the following:
    - Ankle pumps – Point the toes toward the head and then away from the head.
    - Foot circles – Rotate the feet in circles at the ankles.
    - Knee flexion – Flex and extend the legs at the knees.

Complications

- Thrombophlebitis/deep-vein thrombosis is an inflammation of a vein (usually in the lower extremities) that results in clot formation.
  - Clinical manifestations are pain, edema, warmth, and erythema at the site.
  - Nursing Actions
    - Notify the provider immediately.
    - Position the client in bed with the leg elevated.
    - Avoid any pressure at the site of the inflammation.
    - Anticipate giving anticoagulants.
- A pulmonary embolism is a potentially life-threatening occlusion of blood flow to one or more of the pulmonary arteries by a clot. The clot or embolus often originates in the venous system of the lower extremities.
  - Clinical manifestations are shortness of breath, chest pain, hemoptysis (coughing up blood), decreased blood pressure, and rapid pulse.
  - Nursing actions
    - Prepare to give thrombolytics or anticoagulants.

APPLICATION EXERCISES

1. A nurse is caring for a client who has been sitting in a chair for 3 hr. Which of the following problems is the client at risk for developing?

    A. Stasis of secretions

    B. Muscle atrophy

    C. Pressure ulcer

    D. Fecal impaction

2. A nurse is caring for a client who is on bed rest. Which of the following interventions should the nurse implement to maintain the patency of the client's airway?

    A. Encourage isometric exercises.

    B. Suction every 8 hr.

    C. Give low-dose heparin.

    D. Promote incentive spirometer use.

3. A nurse is caring for a client who is postoperative. Which of the following nursing interventions reduce the risk of thrombus development? (Select all that apply.)

    _____ A. Instruct the client not to use the Valsalva maneuver.

    _____ B. Apply elastic stockings.

    _____ C. Review laboratory values for total protein level.

    _____ D. Place pillows under the client's knees and lower extremities.

    _____ E. Assist the client to change position often.

4. A nurse is instructing a client who is postoperative about the sequential compression device the provider has prescribed. Which of the following client statements should indicate to the nurse that the client understands the teaching?

    A. "This device will keep me from getting sores on my skin."

    B. "This thing will keep the blood pumping through my leg."

    C. "With this thing on, my leg muscles won't get weak."

    D. "This device is going to keep my joints in good shape."

5. To promote the safe use of a cane for a client who is recovering from a minor musculoskeletal injury of the left lower extremity, which of the following instructions should the nurse provide? (Select all that apply.)

_____ A. Hold the cane on the right side.

_____ B. Keep two points of support on the floor.

_____ C. Place the cane 15 inches in front of the feet before advancing.

_____ D. After advancing the cane, move the weaker leg forward.

_____ E. Advance the stronger leg so that it aligns evenly with the cane.

6. A nurse is reviewing the effects of immobility on the various body systems with a group of nursing students. Use the ATI Active Learning Template: Basic Concept to complete this item. Under Related Content, list at least two effects of immobility on the cardiovascular system and at least two on the respiratory system.

APPLICATION EXERCISES KEY

1. A. INCORRECT: Sitting up in a chair will help prevent stasis of secretions.

    B. INCORRECT: Muscle atrophy is a complication for a client on prolonged bed rest, not for one who is sitting in a chair.

    C. **CORRECT:** Unrelieved pressure over a bony prominence for too long increases the risk for skin breakdown.

    D. INCORRECT: Fecal impaction is a complication for a client on prolonged bed rest, not for one who is sitting in a chair.

     NCLEX® Connection: Basic Care and Comfort, Mobility/Immobility

2. A. INCORRECT: Performing isometric exercises strengthens skeletal muscles.

    B. INCORRECT: The nurse should not suction the client's airway routinely.

    C. INCORRECT: Low-dose heparin helps prevent thrombus formation.

    D. **CORRECT:** Using an incentive spirometer helps keep the airways open and prevents atelectasis.

     NCLEX® Connection: Basic Care and Comfort, Mobility/Immobility

3. A. INCORRECT: The Valsalva maneuver increases the workload of the heart, but it does not affect peripheral circulation.

    B. **CORRECT:** Elastic stockings promote venous return and prevent thrombus formation.

    C. INCORRECT: A review of the client's total protein level is important for evaluating his ability to heal and prevent skin breakdown.

    D. INCORRECT: Placing pillows under the knees and lower extremities further impairs circulation of the lower extremities.

    E. **CORRECT:** Frequent position changes prevent venous stasis.

     NCLEX® Connection: Basic Care and Comfort, Mobility/Immobility

4.   A. INCORRECT: A sequential pressure device is a temporary intervention that remains in use only until the client is ambulatory. The device is not in place long enough to cause pressure ulcers.

    B. **CORRECT:** Sequential pressure devices promote venous return in the deep veins of the legs and thus help prevent thrombus formation.

    C. INCORRECT: Continuous passive motion machines, not sequential pressure devices, provide some muscle movement that may assist in preserving some muscle strength.

    D. INCORRECT: Continuous passive motion machines, not sequential pressure devices, exercise the knee joint after arthroplasty.

     NCLEX® Connection: Basic Care and Comfort, Mobility/Immobility

5.   A. **CORRECT:** The client should hold the cane on the uninjured side to provide support for the injured left leg.

    B. **CORRECT:** The client should keep two points of support on the ground at all times for stability.

    C. INCORRECT: The client should place the cane 6 to 10 inches in front of her feet before advancing.

    D. **CORRECT:** The client should advance the weaker leg first, followed by the stronger leg.

    E. INCORRECT: The client should advance the stronger leg past the cane.

     NCLEX® Connection: Basic Care and Comfort, Mobility/Immobility

6.   *Using the ATI Active Learning Template: Basic Concept*
- Related Content
  - ○ Cardiovascular system
    - Orthostatic hypotension
    - Less fluid volume in the circulatory system
    - Stasis of blood in the legs
    - Diminished autonomic response
    - Decreased cardiac output leading to poor cardiac effectiveness, which results in increased cardiac workload
    - Increased oxygenation requirement
    - Increased risk of thrombus development
  - ○ Respiratory system
    - Decreased respiratory movement resulting in decreased oxygenation and carbon dioxide exchange
    - Stasis of secretions and decreased and weakened respiratory muscles, resulting in atelectasis and hypostatic pneumonia
    - Decreased cough response

     NCLEX® Connection: Basic Care and Comfort, Mobility/Immobility

chapter 41

Overview

- Effective pain management includes the use of pharmacological and nonpharmacological pain management therapies. Invasive therapies such as nerve ablation may be appropriate for intractable cancer-related pain.

- Clients have a right to adequate assessment and management of pain. Nurses are accountable for the assessment of pain. The nurse's role is that of an advocate and educator for effective pain management.

- Nurses have a priority responsibility for the continual assessment of the client's pain level and to provide individualized interventions. They should assess the effectiveness of the interventions 30 to 60 min after implementation.

- Assessment challenges may occur with clients who are cognitively impaired or on a ventilator.

- Undertreatment of pain is a serious health care problem. Consequences of undertreatment of pain include physiological and psychological components.

  ○ Acute/chronic pain can cause anxiety, fear, and depression.

  ○ Poorly managed acute pain may lead to chronic pain syndrome.

Physiology of Pain

- Transduction is the conversion of painful stimuli to an electrical impulse through peripheral nerve fibers (nociceptors).

- Transmission occurs as the electrical impulse travels along the nerve fibers, where neurotransmitters regulate it.

- The pain threshold is the point at which a person feels pain.

- Pain tolerance is the amount of pain a person is willing to bear.

SUBSTANCES THAT INCREASE PAIN TRANSMISSION AND CAUSE AN INFLAMMATORY RESPONSE		SUBSTANCES THAT DECREASE PAIN TRANSMISSION AND PRODUCE ANALGESIA
› Substance P	› Bradykinin	› Serotonin
› Prostaglandins	› Histamine	› Endorphins

- Perception or awareness of pain occurs in various areas of the brain, with influences from thought and emotional processes.

- Modulation occurs in the spinal cord, causing muscles to contract reflexively, moving the body away from painful stimuli.

Pain Categories

ACUTE PAIN

› Acute pain is protective, temporary, usually self-limiting, and resolves with tissue healing.

› Physiological responses (sympathetic nervous system) are fight-or-flight responses (tachycardia, hypertension, anxiety, diaphoresis, muscle tension).

› Behavioral responses include grimacing, moaning, flinching, and guarding.

› Interventions include treatment of the underlying problem.

CHRONIC PAIN

› Chronic pain is not protective. It is ongoing or recurs frequently, lasting longer than 6 months and persisting beyond tissue healing.

› Physiological responses do not usually alter vital signs, but clients may have depression, fatigue, and a decreased level of functioning.

› Psychosocial implications may lead to disability.

› Chronic pain may not have a known cause, and it may not respond to interventions.

› Management aims at symptomatic relief.

› Chronic pain can be malignant or nonmalignant.

NOCICEPTIVE PAIN

› Nociceptive pain arises from damage to or inflammation of tissue, which is a noxious stimulus that triggers the pain receptors called nociceptors and causes pain.

› It is usually throbbing, aching, and localized.

› This pain typically responds to opioids and nonopioid medications.

› Types of nociceptive pain include:

» Somatic – in bones, joints, muscles, skin, or connective tissues.

» Visceral – in internal organs such as the stomach or intestines. It can cause referred pain in other body locations separate from the stimulus.

» Cutaneous – in the skin or subcutaneous tissue.

NEUROPATHIC PAIN

› Neuropathic pain arises from abnormal or damaged pain nerves.

› It includes phantom limb pain, pain below the level of a spinal cord injury, and diabetic neuropathy.

› Neuropathic pain is usually intense, shooting, burning, or described as "pins and needles."

› This pain typically responds to adjuvant medications (antidepressants, antispasmodic agents, skeletal muscle relaxants).

- Risk factors for undertreatment of pain include the following:
  ○ Cultural and societal attitudes
  ○ Lack of knowledge
  ○ Fear of addiction
  ○ Exaggerated fear of respiratory depression

- Populations at risk for undertreatment of pain include the following:
  - Infants
  - Children
  - Older adults
  - Clients who have substance use disorder
- Causes of acute and chronic pain include the following:
  - Trauma
  - Surgery
  - Cancer (tumor invasion, nerve compression, bone metastases, associated infections, immobility)
  - Arthritis
  - Fibromyalgia
  - Neuropathy
  - Diagnostic or treatment procedures (injection, intubation, radiation)
- Factors that affect the pain experience include the following:
  - Age
    - Infants cannot verbalize or understand their pain.
    - Older adult clients may have multiple pathologies that cause pain and limit function.
  - Fatigue, which can increase sensitivity to pain.
  - Genetic sensitivity, which can increase or decrease pain tolerance.
  - Cognitive function.
    - Clients who are cognitively impaired may not be able to report pain or report it accurately.
  - Prior experiences, which can increase or decrease sensitivity depending on whether clients obtained adequate relief.
  - Anxiety and fear, which can increase sensitivity to pain.
  - Support systems that are present and can decrease sensitivity to pain.
  - Culture, which may influence how clients express pain or the meaning they give to pain.

Assessment/Data Collection

- According to noted pain experts Margo McCaffery and Chris Pasero, pain is whatever the person experiencing it says it is, and it exists whenever the person says it does. The client's report of pain is the most reliable diagnostic measure of pain. Self-report using standardized pain scales is useful for clients over the age of 7 years. Specialized pain scales are available for use with younger children.
- Assess and document pain (the fifth vital sign) frequently.
- Use a symptom analysis to obtain subjective data.

DESCRIPTION	QUESTIONS
› Use anatomical terminology and landmarks to describe location.	› Ask, "Where is your pain? Does it radiate anywhere else?" Ask clients to point to the location.
› Quality refers to how the pain feels: sharp, dull, aching, burning, stabbing, pounding, throbbing, shooting, gnawing, tender, heavy, tight, tiring, exhausting, sickening, terrifying, torturing, nagging, annoying, intense, or unbearable.	› Ask, "What does the pain feel like?" Give more than two choices ("Is the pain throbbing, burning, or stabbing?").
› Intensity, strength, and severity are "measures" of the pain. Use visual analog scales (description scale, number rating scale) to measure pain, monitor pain, and evaluate the effectiveness of interventions.	› Ask the following questions: » "How much pain do you have now?" » "What is the worst/best the pain has been?" » "Rate your pain on a scale of 0 to 10."
› Timing – onset, duration, frequency	› Ask the following questions: » "When did it start?" » "How long does it last?" » "How often does it occur?" » "Is it constant or intermittent?"
› Setting – how the pain affects daily life or how activities of daily living (ADLs) affect the pain	› Ask the following questions: » "Where are you when the symptoms occur?" » "What are you doing when the symptoms occur?" » "How does the pain affect your sleep?" » "How does the pain affect your ability to work and do your job?"
› Document associated symptoms (fatigue, depression, nausea, anxiety).	› Ask, "What other symptoms do you have when you are feeling pain?"
› Aggravating/relieving factors	› Ask the following questions: » "What makes the pain better?" » "What makes the pain worse?" » "Are you currently taking any prescription, herbal, or over-the-counter medications?"

 View Video: Pain Assessment

- Objective Data
  - ○ Behaviors complement self-report and assist in pain assessment of nonverbal clients.
    - ▪ Facial expressions (grimacing, wrinkled forehead), body movements (restlessness, pacing, guarding)
    - ▪ Moaning, crying
    - ▪ Decreased attention span
- Blood pressure, pulse, and respiratory rate increase temporarily with acute pain. Eventually, increases in vital signs will stabilize despite the persistence of pain. Therefore, physiologic indicators may not be an accurate measure of pain over time.

Nonpharmacological Pain Management

- Cutaneous (skin) stimulation – transcutaneous electrical nerve stimulation (TENS), heat, cold, therapeutic touch, and massage
  - ○ Interruption of pain pathways
  - ○ Cold for inflammation
  - ○ Heat to increase blood flow and to reduce stiffness
- Distraction
  - ○ Includes ambulation, deep breathing, visitors, television, and music
- Relaxation
  - ○ Includes meditation, yoga, and progressive muscle relaxation
- Imagery
  - ○ Focusing on a pleasant thought to divert focus
  - ○ Requires an ability to concentrate
- Acupuncture – vibration or electrical stimulation via tiny needles inserted into the skin and subcutaneous tissues at specific points
- Reduction of pain stimuli in the environment
- Elevation of edematous extremities to promote venous return and decrease swelling

Pharmacological Interventions

- Analgesics are the mainstay for relieving pain. The three classes of analgesics are nonopioids, opioids, and adjuvants.
- Nonopioid analgesics (acetaminophen, nonsteroidal anti-inflammatory drugs [NSAIDs], including salicylates) are appropriate for treating mild to moderate pain.
  - ○ Be aware of the hepatotoxic effects of acetaminophen. Clients who have a healthy liver should take no more than 4 g/day. Make sure clients are aware of opioids that contain acetaminophen, such as hydrocodone bitartrate 5 mg/acetaminophen 500 mg (Vicodin).
  - ○ Monitor for salicylism (tinnitus, vertigo, decreased hearing acuity).
  - ○ Prevent gastric upset by administering the medication with food or antacids.
  - ○ Monitor for bleeding with long-term NSAID use.

- Opioid analgesics, such as morphine sulfate, fentanyl (Sublimaze), and codeine, are appropriate for treating moderate to severe pain (postoperative pain, myocardial infarction pain, cancer pain).

  - Managing acute severe pain with short-term (24 to 48 hr) around-the-clock administration of opioids is preferable to following a PRN schedule.

  - The parenteral route is best for immediate, short-term relief of acute pain. The oral route is better for chronic, nonfluctuating pain.

  - Consistent timing and dosing of opioid administration provide consistent pain control.

  - It is essential to monitor and intervene for adverse effects of opioid use.

    - Constipation – Use a preventative approach (monitoring of bowel movements, fluids, fiber intake, exercise, stool softeners, stimulant laxatives, enemas).

    - Orthostatic hypotension – Advise clients to sit or lie down if symptoms of light-headedness or dizziness occur. Instruct clients to avoid sudden changes in position by slowly moving from a lying to a sitting or standing position. Provide assistance with ambulation.

    - Urinary retention – Monitor I&O, assess for distention, administer bethanechol (Urecholine), and catheterize.

    - Nausea/vomiting – Administer antiemetics, advise clients to lie still and move slowly, and eliminate odors.

    - Sedation – Monitor level of consciousness and take safety precautions. Sedation usually precedes respiratory depression.

    - Respiratory depression – Monitor respiratory rate prior to and following administration of opioids (especially for clients who are opioid-naïve). Initial treatment of respiratory depression and sedation is generally a reduction in opioid dose. If necessary, slowly administer diluted naloxone (Narcan) to reverse opioid effects.

- Adjuvant analgesics enhance the effects of nonopioids, help alleviate other symptoms that aggravate pain (depression, seizures, inflammation), and are useful for treating neuropathic pain.

  - Adjuvant medications include:

    - Anticonvulsants: carbamazepine (Tegretol)

    - Antianxiety agents: diazepam (Valium)

    - Tricyclic antidepressants: amitriptyline (Elavil)

    - Antihistamine: hydroxyzine (Vistaril)

    - Glucocorticoids: dexamethasone (Decadron)

    - Antiemetics: ondansetron (Zofran)

- Patient-controlled analgesia (PCA) is a medication delivery system that allows clients to self-administer safe doses of opioids.

  - Small, frequent dosing ensures consistent plasma levels.

  - Clients have less lag time between identified need and delivery of medication, which increases their sense of control and may decrease the amount of medication they need.

  - Morphine and hydromorphone (Dilaudid) are typical opioids for PCA delivery.

  - Clients should let the nurse know if using the pump does not control the pain.

  - To prevent inadvertent overdosing, the client is the only person who should push the PCA button.

- Other strategies for effective pain management include the following:

  - Taking a proactive approach by giving analgesics before pain becomes too severe. It takes less medication to prevent pain than to treat pain.

  - Instructing clients to report developing or recurrent pain and not wait until pain is severe (for PRN pain medication).

  - Explaining misconceptions about pain.

  - Helping clients reduce fear and anxiety.

  - Creating a treatment plan that includes both nonpharmacological and pharmacological pain-relief measures.

- Strategies specific for relieving chronic pain include the above interventions, plus:

  - Administering long-acting or controlled-release opioid analgesics (including the transdermal route).

  - Administering analgesics around the clock rather than PRN.

Complications and Nursing Implications

- Undertreatment of pain is a serious complication and may lead to increased anxiety with acute pain and depression with chronic pain. Assess clients for pain frequently, and intervene as appropriate.

- Sedation, respiratory depression, and coma can occur as a result of overdosing. Sedation always precedes respiratory depression.

  - Identify high-risk clients (older adult clients, clients who are opioid-naïve).

  - Carefully titrate doses while closely monitoring respiratory status.

  - Stop the opioid and give the antagonist naloxone (Narcan) if respiratory rate is below 8/min and shallow, or the client is difficult to arouse.

  - Identify the cause of sedation.

  - Use a sedation scale in addition to a pain rating scale to assess pain, especially when administering opioids.

APPLICATION EXERCISES

1. A nurse is assessing the pain level of a client who has come to the emergency department reporting severe abdominal pain. The nurse asks the client whether he has nausea and has been vomiting. The nurse is assessing which of the following?

    A. Presence of associated symptoms

    B. Location of the pain

    C. Pain quality

    D. Aggravating and relieving factors

2. A nurse is assessing a client who is reporting pain despite analgesia. The nurse can best assess the intensity of the client's pain by

    A. asking what precipitates the pain.

    B. questioning the client about the location of the pain.

    C. offering the client a pain scale to measure his pain.

    D. using open-ended questions to identify the sensation.

3. A nurse is obtaining a history from a client who has pain. The nurse's guiding principle throughout this process should be that

    A. some clients exaggerate their level of pain.

    B. pain must have an identifiable source to justify the use of opioids.

    C. objective data are essential in assessing pain.

    D. pain is whatever the client says it is.

4. A nurse is caring for a client who is receiving morphine via a patient-controlled analgesia (PCA) infusion device after abdominal surgery. Which of the following statements indicates that the client knows how to use the device?

    A. "I'll wait to use the device until it's absolutely necessary."

    B. "I'll be careful about pushing the button so I don't get an overdose."

    C. "I should tell the nurse if the pain doesn't stop after I use this device."

    D. "I will ask my son to push the dose button when I am sleeping."

5. A nurse is monitoring a client who is receiving opioid analgesia for adverse effects of the medication. Which of the following effects should the nurse anticipate? (Select all that apply.)

_____ A. Urinary incontinence

_____ B. Diarrhea

_____ C. Bradypnea

_____ D. Orthostatic hypotension

_____ E. Nausea

6. A nurse on a medical-surgical unit is reviewing with a group of nursing students the various types of pain the clients on the unit have. Use the ATI Active Learning Template: Basic Concept to complete this item. Include under Underlying Principles: list the four different types of pain, their definitions, and characteristics.

APPLICATION EXERCISES KEY

1. A. **CORRECT:** Nausea and vomiting are common symptoms clients have when they are in pain.

    B. INCORRECT: The location of the pain is where the client feels the pain.

    C. INCORRECT: Pain quality is what the pain feels like, such as throbbing and dull.

    D. INCORRECT: Aggravating and relieving factors are what might make the pain better or worse.

    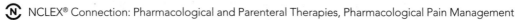 NCLEX® Connection: Pharmacological and Parenteral Therapies, Pharmacological Pain Management

2. A. INCORRECT: Assessment of pain triggers will provide valuable information to help select pain-control interventions, but it does not provide information about the intensity of pain.

    B. INCORRECT: Identification of the location of the client's pain provides valuable information to help select pain-control interventions, but it does not provide information about the intensity of pain.

    C. **CORRECT:** A pain scale can help the client measure the amount of pain he has and its intensity.

    D. INCORRECT: Asking open-ended questions is important in pain assessment, but it does not provide for consistent quantification of pain intensity.

    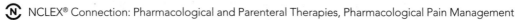 NCLEX® Connection: Pharmacological and Parenteral Therapies, Pharmacological Pain Management

3. A. INCORRECT: A misconception about pain is that clients exaggerate their pain level.

    B. INCORRECT: Clients can have pain without being able to identify the source.

    C. INCORRECT: Objective data are not always present when clients have pain.

    D. **CORRECT:** Pain is a subjective experience, and the client is the best source of information about it.

    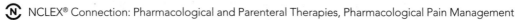 NCLEX® Connection: Pharmacological and Parenteral Therapies, Pharmacological Pain Management

4. A. INCORRECT: The client may use the device when he begins to feel pain. It will help prevent unnecessary worsening of the pain and more doses of analgesia to relieve it.

    B. INCORRECT: A feature of PCA devices is the timing control or lockout mechanism, which enforces a preset minimum interval between medication doses. This safety feature is one means of preventing an overdose because the client cannot self-administer another dose of medication until that time interval has passed.

    C. **CORRECT:** PCA is a method of delivering pain medication through an electronic infusion device that allows the client to self-administer pain medication on an as-needed basis. If the client is not achieving adequate pain control, he should let the nurse know so that she can initiate a reevaluation of the client's pain management plan.

    D. INCORRECT: The client is the only one who should operate the PCA pump. In situations where the client is not able to do so, the provider may authorize a nurse or a family member to operate the pump.

    Ⓝ NCLEX® Connection: Pharmacological and Parenteral Therapies, Pharmacological Pain Management

5. A. INCORRECT: Urinary retention, not urinary incontinence, is a common adverse effect of opioid analgesia.

    B. INCORRECT: Constipation, not diarrhea, is a common adverse effect of opioid analgesia.

    C. **CORRECT:** Respiratory depression, which causes respiratory rates to drop to dangerously low levels, is a common adverse effect of opioid analgesia.

    D. **CORRECT:** Dizziness or light-headedness when changing positions is a common adverse effect of opioid analgesia.

    E. **CORRECT:** Nausea and vomiting are common adverse effects of opioid analgesia.

    Ⓝ NCLEX® Connection: Pharmacological and Parenteral Therapies, Pharmacological Pain Management

6. *Using the ATI Active Learning Template: Basic Concept*
   - Underlying Principles
     - Acute Pain
       - Definition: protective, temporary, usually self-limiting, resolves with tissue healing
       - Physiological responses: tachycardia, hypertension, anxiety, diaphoresis, muscle tension
       - Behavioral responses: grimacing, moaning, flinching, guarding
     - Chronic Pain
       - Definition: not protective; ongoing or recurs frequently, lasts longer than 6 months, persists beyond tissue healing, can be malignant or nonmalignant
       - Physiological responses: no change in vital signs, depression, fatigue, decreased level of functioning, disability
     - Nociceptive Pain
       - Definition: arises from damage to or inflammation of tissue, which is a noxious stimulus that triggers the pain receptors called nociceptors and causes pain, and is usually throbbing, aching, localized; pain typically responds to opioids and nonopioid medications
       - Types of nociceptive pain:
         - Somatic – in bones, joints, muscles, skin, or connective tissues
         - Visceral – in internal organs such as the stomach or intestines, can cause referred pain
         - Cutaneous – in skin or subcutaneous tissue
     - Neuropathic Pain
       - Definition: arises from abnormal or damaged pain nerves (phantom limb pain, pain below the level of a spinal cord injury, diabetic neuropathy), usually intense, shooting, burning, or "pins and needles"
       - Physiological responses to adjuvant medications (antidepressants, antispasmodic agents, skeletal muscle relaxants).

Ⓝ NCLEX® Connection: Pharmacological and Parenteral Therapies, Pharmacological Pain Management

chapter **42**

Overview

- In combination with allopathic therapies (conventional Western medicine), complementary and alternative therapies comprise integrative health care, which focuses on optimal health of the whole person. Another term for these therapies is complementary and alternative medicine (CAM).

- Alternative therapies are unconventional treatment approaches.

- Complementary therapies are unconventional treatment approaches used in addition to or to enhance conventional medical care.

- Many health care entities are developing programs of integrative medicine or integrative therapies to provide clients with conventional and unconventional health care choices, particularly for chronic health problems.

- An important prerequisite for implementing complementary or alternative therapies is the client's acceptance of and involvement in the therapeutic intervention.

- Categories of CAM include the following:

  ○ Alternative medical philosophy (traditional Chinese medicine, acupuncture, homeopathy)

  ○ Biological and botanical therapies (diets, vitamins, minerals, herbal preparations)

  ○ Body manipulation (massage, touch, chiropractic therapy)

  ○ Mind-body therapies (biofeedback, art therapy, meditation, yoga, psychotherapy, tai chi)

  ○ Energy therapies (Reiki, therapeutic touch)

Nursing and CAM

- Nurses should do the following:
  - Understand the varieties of therapies available.
  - Be receptive to learning about clients' alternative health beliefs and practices (home remedies, cultural practices, vitamin use, modification of prescriptions).
  - Identify clients' needs for complementary or alternative therapies.
  - Incorporate complementary or alternative therapies into clients' care plans.
- Specialized licensed or certified practitioners may provide complementary or alternative therapies. These include:

THERAPY	CHARACTERISTICS
Acupuncture/pressure	› Needles or pressure along meridians to alter body function or produce analgesia
Homeopathic medicine	› Administering doses of substances (remedies) that would produce symptoms of the disease state in a well person to ill clients to bring about healing
Naturopathic medicine	› Diet, exercise, environment, and herbal remedies to promote natural healing
Chiropractic medicine	› Spinal manipulation for healing
Massage therapy	› Stretching and loosening muscles and connective tissue for relaxation and circulation
Biofeedback	› Using technology to increase awareness of various neurological body responses to minimize extremes
Therapeutic touch	› Using hands to help bring energy fields into balance

- Nursing interventions can provide some aspects of complementary alternative therapies, including the following:

THERAPY	CHARACTERISTICS
Guided imagery/ visualization therapy	› Encourages healing and relaxation of the body by having the mind focus on images
Healing intention	› Techniques that use caring, compassion, and empathy in the context of prayer to facilitate healing
Breath work	› Various breathing patterns to reduce stress and increase relaxation
Humor	› A coping mechanism to reduce tension and improve mood
Meditation	› A technique to calm the mind and body
Simple touch	› Communicates presence, appreciation, and acceptance
Music therapy	› Type of relaxation therapy that provides distraction from pain; earphones improve concentration
Therapeutic communication	› Allows clients to verbalize and become aware of emotions and fears in a safe, nonjudgmental environment

APPLICATION EXERCISES

1. A nurse admits a client for abdominal surgery. The client's initial vital signs are temperature 37° C (98.6° F), pulse 98/min, respirations 20/min, and blood pressure 148/88 mm Hg. The client states, "I am really worried. This is the first surgery I have ever had." Which of the following is an appropriate use of a complementary alternative intervention?

    A. Offer information and ask the client if he is interested in trying a relaxation technique.

    B. Call the provider and get permission to use relaxation techniques with the client.

    C. Provide the client with reassurance and information about the procedure.

    D. Give the client a therapeutic back massage and tell him to try to relax.

2. A nurse is caring for a client who reports back pain and tells the nurse that a friend has recommended a chiropractor. She asks the nurse what a chiropractor does to relieve back pain. Which of the following responses by the nurse is correct?

    A. "Chiropractors use their hands to manipulate the spine to treat back pain."

    B. "Chiropractors insert needles or put pressure along meridians in the back."

    C. "Chiropractors use herbal remedies to treat back pain."

    D. "Chiropractors use their hands to balance the energy fields in the back."

3. A nurse is reviewing complementary and alternative therapies with a group of nursing students. The nurse should classify which of the following as mind-body therapies? (Select all that apply.)

    _____ A. Art therapy

    _____ B. Acupressure

    _____ C. Yoga

    _____ D. Therapeutic touch

    _____ E. Biofeedback

4. A nurse is coaching a group of nursing students in learning to use complementary and alternative therapies they can incorporate into their practice without the need for specialized licensing or certification. Which of the following should the nurse encourage the students to use? (Select all that apply.)

_____ A. Guided imagery

_____ B. Massage therapy

_____ C. Meditation

_____ D. Music therapy

_____ E. Therapeutic touch

5. A nurse is planning to use healing intention with a client who is recovering from a lengthy illness. Which of the following is the priority action the nurse should take before attempting this particular mind-body intervention?

A. Ask the client's permission.

B. Explain to the client that this therapy involves prayer.

C. Request that the client participate actively.

D. Encourage the client to relax for this therapy.

6. A nursing instructor is reviewing the various categories of complementary and alternative therapies with a group of nursing students. Use the ATI Active Learning Template: Basic Concept to complete this item. Under Related Content, list at least four different types of therapies with examples of each.

APPLICATION EXERCISES KEY

1. A. **CORRECT:** Providing information will help the client make an informed decision.

    B. INCORRECT: The nurse does not need a provider's prescription for relaxation therapy.

    C. INCORRECT: Providing reassurance may negate the client's fear. Providing more information without validating this as a need may increase his anxiety.

    D. INCORRECT: The nurse should not give any therapy without informing the client and obtaining his consent. Telling him to relax does not acknowledge the impact of his anxiety.

    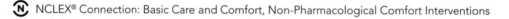 NCLEX® Connection: Basic Care and Comfort, Non-Pharmacological Comfort Interventions

2. A. **CORRECT:** Chiropractors use their hands to manipulate the spine.

    B. INCORRECT: Acupuncture involves needles or pressure.

    C. INCORRECT: Naturopathic medicine uses herbal remedies.

    D. INCORRECT: Therapeutic touch practitioners use their hands to balance energy fields.

    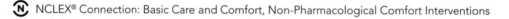 NCLEX® Connection: Management of Care, Concepts of Management

3. A. **CORRECT:** Mind-body therapies use the emotional connections between thinking (mind) and functioning (body) to promote health.

    B. INCORRECT: Acupressure is a body-based therapy because it focuses specifically on body structures and systems.

    C. **CORRECT:** Mind-body therapies use the emotional connections between thinking (mind) and functioning (body) to promote health.

    D. INCORRECT: Therapeutic touch is an energy therapy, not a mind-body therapy.

    E. **CORRECT:** Mind-body therapies use the emotional connections between thinking (mind) and functioning (body) to promote health.

    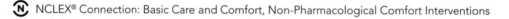 NCLEX® Connection: Basic Care and Comfort, Non-Pharmacological Comfort Interventions

4.   A. **CORRECT:** Nurses need to understand the general principles of using guided imagery with clients, but they do not need certification or licensure for this therapy.

   B. INCORRECT: Massage therapists undergo extensive training as well as certification and/or licensure.

   C. **CORRECT:** Nurses need to understand the general principles of using meditation with clients, but they do not need certification or licensure for this therapy.

   D. **CORRECT:** Nurses need to talk with clients to determine their preferences related to music and the effects different types of music have on them, but they do not require special training to do so.

   E. INCORRECT: Therapeutic touch requires specific training to perform this energy therapy effectively.

   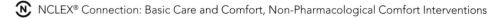 NCLEX® Connection: Basic Care and Comfort, Non-Pharmacological Comfort Interventions

5.   A. INCORRECT: Before beginning any therapy, the nurse must obtain the client's permission. However, this is not the nurse's highest priority with the use of healing intention.

   B. **CORRECT:** The first action the nurse should take using the nursing process is to assess or collect data from the client. Because people may have personal, cultural, or religious sensitivities or aversions to religious practices such as prayer, the nurse must first determine that the client is comfortable with a therapy that involves prayer.

   C. INCORRECT: The success of any complementary therapy depends on the client's active participation. However, this is not the nurse's highest priority with the use of healing intention.

   D. INCORRECT: Before beginning any complementary therapy, the nurse should use strategies such as controlled breathing to encourage the client to relax. However, this is not the nurse's highest priority with the use of healing intention.

   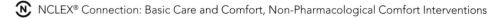 NCLEX® Connection: Basic Care and Comfort, Non-Pharmacological Comfort Interventions

6.   *Using the ATI Active Learning Template: Basic Concept*
   • Related Content
      ○ Alternative medical philosophy: traditional Chinese medicine, acupuncture, homeopathy
      ○ Biological and botanical therapies: diets, vitamins, minerals, herbal preparations
      ○ Body manipulation: massage, touch, chiropractic therapy
      ○ Mind-body therapies: biofeedback, art therapy, meditation, yoga, psychotherapy, tai chi
      ○ Energy therapies: Reiki, therapeutic touch

   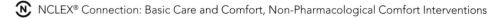 NCLEX® Connection: Basic Care and Comfort, Non-Pharmacological Comfort Interventions

chapter 43

Overview

- Interventions such as surgery, immobility, medications, and therapeutic diets can affect bowel elimination.

- Constipation is having bowel movements that are infrequent, hard or dry, and difficult to pass.

- Diarrhea is an increased number of loose, liquid stools.

- There are objective ways to assess for the presence of constipation or diarrhea, but individual bowel patterns vary greatly.

- Various disease processes necessitate the creation of bowel diversions to allow fecal elimination to continue.

- Stool specimens are collected both for screening and for diagnostic tests, such as for the detection of occult blood, bacteria, or parasites.

Bowel Elimination Needs and Specimen Collection

- Collect stool specimens for serial fecal occult blood (guaiac) testing three times from three different defecations. Stool samples should come from fresh stools that are not contaminated with water or urine.

- Bowel diversions through ostomies are temporary or permanent openings (stomas) in the abdominal wall to allow fecal matter to pass.

- End stomas are a result of colorectal cancer or some types of bowel disease. Colostomies end in the colon, and ileostomies end in the ileum.

- Loop colostomies help resolve a medical emergency and are temporary.

- Double-barrel colostomies consist of two abdominal stomas – one proximal and one distal.

FACTORS AFFECTING BOWEL ELIMINATION	
Age	› Infants: » Breast milk stools – watery and yellow brown » Formula stools – pasty and brown › Toddlers: bowel control at 2 to 3 years old › Older adults: decreased peristalsis, relaxation of sphincters
Diet	› Fiber requirement: 25 to 30 g/day › Lactose intolerance: difficulty digesting milk products
Fluids	› Fluid requirement: 2,000 to 3,000 mL/day from fluid and food sources
Physical activity	› Stimulates intestinal activity
Psychosocial factors	› Emotional distress increasing peristalsis and exacerbating chronic conditions (colitis, Crohn's disease, ulcers, irritable bowel syndrome) › Depression decreases peristalsis and can lead to constipation.
Personal habits	› Use of public toilets, false perception of the need for "one-a-day" bowel movements, lack of privacy when hospitalized
Positioning	› Normal: squatting › Immobilized client: difficulty defecating
Pain	› Normal defecation is painless. Discomfort leads to suppression of the urge to defecate. › Opioid use contributing to constipation
Pregnancy	› Growing fetus compromising intestinal space › Slower peristalsis › Straining increasing the risk of hemorrhoids
Surgery and anesthesia	› Temporary slowing of intestinal activity › Paralytic ileus – rationale for auscultating bowel sounds before advancing diet
Medications	› Laxatives – to soften stool › Cathartics – to promote peristalsis › Laxative abuse leading to diarrhea and dehydration

- Diagnostic Tests
  - Visualization of the bowel
    - Colonoscopy – the provider visualizes and may collect tissue for biopsy or remove polyps from the colon and sometimes a portion of the lower small bowel.
    - Sigmoidoscopy – the provider visualizes and may collect tissue for biopsy or remove polyps from the sigmoid colon and rectum.
  - Preparation
    - Protocols vary with the provider and the facility, but generally include clear liquids only and a bowel cleanser.
    - Clients receive moderate (conscious) sedation and may not drive home afterwards.

Patient-Centered Care

PROMOTING HEALTHY BOWEL ELIMINATION	
Equipment	

› Bedpans
  » Fracture pan – for supine clients and clients in body casts or leg casts
  » Regular pan – for seated clients
› Beside commode
› Toilet
	› Adequate fiber in the diet
	› Adequate fluid intake – minimum of 1,500 mL/day of water and/or juices
	› Adequate activity – walking 15 to 20 min/day if mobile and exercises in bed or chair (pelvic tilt, single leg lifts, lower trunk rotation)

Procedure	
› Encourage the client to set aside time to defecate – sometimes after a meal works best. › If not contraindicated or restricted, encourage the client to drink plenty of fluids and to consume a diet high in fiber to prevent constipation. › Wear gloves when addressing toileting needs. › Provide privacy. › Assist the client to a sitting position whether using a regular bedpan, commode, or toilet. › For clients using a fracture pan, raise the head of the bed to 30°.	› If the client cannot lift his hips to get the bedpan under him, roll him onto one side, position the bedpan over his buttocks, and roll the client back onto the bedpan. › Encourage the client to decrease stress when sitting or rising by using an elevated toilet seat or a footstool. › Never leave a client lying flat on a regular bedpan. › After the client defecates, provide skin care to the perianal area.

 View Video: Bowel Elimination

SPECIMEN COLLECTION

Equipment

- › Appropriate specimen container
- › Soap/cleansing solution or wipe
- › Gloves
- › Specimen label
- › Fecal occult blood test cards
- › Wooden applicator or tongue depressor
- › Developer solution
- › Stool collection container (bedside commode, bedpan, receptacle in toilet)

Procedure

- › Fecal occult blood testing (guaiac test)
  - » Explain the procedure to the client.
  - » Ask the client to collect a specimen in the toilet receptacle, bedpan, or bedside commode.
  - » Apply gloves, and, with a wooden applicator, place small amounts of stool on the windows of the test card or as directed.
  - » Follow the facility's procedures for handling.
    - › Apply a label to the cards and send them to the laboratory for processing.
    - › Or, if for point-of-care testing, place a couple of drops of developer on the opposite side of the card. A blue color is positive for blood.
  - » Remove the gloves and perform hand hygiene.

- › Stool for culture, parasites, and ova
  - » Explain the procedure to the client.
  - » Ask the client to collect the specimen in the toilet receptacle, bedside commode, or bedpan.
  - » Put on gloves.
  - » Use a wooden tongue depressor to transfer the stool to a specimen container.
  - » Label the container with the client's identifying information.
  - » Remove the gloves.
  - » Perform hand hygiene.
  - » Transport the specimen to the laboratory.

CLEANSING ENEMA

The height of the bag above the rectum determines the depth of cleansing.

Equipment

- › Gloves
- › Lubricant
- › Absorbent, waterproof pads
- › Bedpan, beside commode, or toilet
- › IV pole
- › Enema bag with tubing or prepackaged enema
- › Solutions and additives – vary with the type of enema
  - » Tap water or hypotonic solution
    - › Stimulates evacuation
    - › Never repeated due to potential water toxicity
  - » Soapsuds
    - › Pure castile soap in tap water or normal saline
    - › Acts as an irritant to promote bowel peristalsis

- » Normal saline
  - › Safest due to equal osmotic pressure
  - › Volume stimulates peristalsis
- » Low-volume hypertonic
  - › Good for clients who cannot tolerate high-volume enemas
  - › Fleet® – a commercially prepared hypertonic enema
- » Oil retention – lubricates the rectum and colon for easier passage of stool
- » Medicated enemas – contains medications to retain

Procedure

- › Perform hand hygiene.
- › Prepare and warm the enema solution.
- › Pour the solution into the enema bag, allowing it to fill the tubing, and then close the clamp.
- › Explain the procedure to the client.
- › Provide privacy.
- › Provide quick access to a commode or bedpan.
- › Place absorbent pads under the client to protect the bed linens.
- › Position the client on the left side with the right leg flexed forward.
- › Put on gloves.
- › Lubricate the rectal tube or nozzle.
- › Slowly insert the rectal tube 7.5 to 10 cm (3 to 4 in). For a child, insert the tube 5 to 7.5 cm (2 to 3 in).
- › With the bag level with the client's hip, open the clamp.
- › Raise the bag 30 to 45 cm (12 to 18 in) above the anus, depending on the level of cleansing.

- › Slow the flow of solution by lowering the container if the client reports cramping, or if fluid leaks around the tube at the anus.
- › If using a prepackaged solution, insert the lubricated tip into the rectum and squeeze the container to instill all of the solution.
- › Ask the client to retain the solution for the prescribed amount of time, or until the client is no longer able to retain it.
- › Discard the enema bag and tubing.
- › Assist the client to the appropriate position to defecate.
- › Remove the gloves.
- › Perform hand hygiene.
- › For clients who have little or no sphincter control, administer the enema on a bedpan.
- › Document the results and the client's tolerance of the procedure.

OSTOMY CARE	
Equipment	
› Pouch system (skin barrier and pouch)	› Towel
› Pouch closure clamp	› Warm water
› Barrier pastes (optional)	› Scissors
› Gloves	› Pen
› Washcloths	
Procedure	
› If a wound ostomy continence nurse is not available, educate the client about stoma care.	› Apply paste if necessary.
› Perform hand hygiene.	› Measure and draw where to cut the skin barrier, allowing only the stoma to appear through the opening.
› Put on gloves.	› Cut the opening in the skin barrier.
› Remove the pouch from the stoma.	› If necessary, apply barrier pastes to creases.
› Inspect the stoma. It should appear moist, shiny, and pink. The peristomal area should be intact, and the skin should appear healthy.	› Apply the skin barrier and pouch.
› Use mild soap and water to cleanse the skin, then dry it gently and completely. Moisturizing soaps can interfere with adherence of the pouch.	› Fold the bottom of the pouch and place the closure clamp on the pouch.
	› Dispose of the used pouch. Remove the gloves and perform hand hygiene.

Complications

- Constipation
    - Bowel pattern of difficult and infrequent evacuation of hard, dry feces.
    - May be the result of improper diet, decreased fluid intake, lack of exercise, or side effects of medications.
    - Increase fiber and water consumption before treating constipation with laxatives.
    - Give bulk-forming products before stool softeners, stimulants, or suppositories to promote bowel elimination.
    - Enemas are a last resort for stimulating defecation.
- Impaction
    - Stool that is wedged into the rectum with diarrhea fluid leaking around the impacted stool.
    - Use a gloved, lubricated finger for digital removal of stool.
    - Loosen the stool around the edges and then remove it in small pieces, allowing the client to rest as necessary.
    - When evacuating the rectum, be careful to avoid stimulating the vagus nerve.
- Diarrhea
    - Frequent, liquid stools caused by various disorders.
    - Help determine and treat the cause.
    - Administer medications to slow peristalsis.
    - Provide perineal care after each stool and apply a moisture barrier.
    - Clients and caregivers should perform hand hygiene frequently.

- Fecal Incontinence
  - Inability to control defecation, often caused by diarrhea.
  - Assess for causes, such as medications, infections, or impaction.
  - Provide perineal care after each stool and apply a moisture barrier.
- Flatulence
  - Distention of the bowel from gas accumulation (may cause cramping or a feeling of fullness)
    - Assess for abdominal distention and the ability to pass gas through the anus.
    - Encourage ambulation to promote the passage of flatus.
    - Notify the provider if the problem continues.
- Hemorrhoids
  - Engorged, dilated blood vessels in the rectal wall from difficult defecation, pregnancy, liver disease, and heart failure.
    - Hemorrhoids may be itchy, painful, and bloody after defecation.
    - Use moist wipes for cleansing the perianal area.
    - Apply ointments or creams.

CONSTIPATION AND DIARRHEA

- For healthy clients, constipation and diarrhea are not serious. But for older adult clients and clients with pre-existing health problems, constipation and diarrhea can be serious.
- Causes of constipation include:
  - Frequent use of laxatives.
  - Advanced age.
  - Inadequate fluid intake.
  - Inadequate fiber intake.
  - Immobilization due to injury.
  - A sedentary lifestyle.
- Causes of diarrhea include:
  - Viral gastroenteritis.
  - Bacterial gastroenteritis.
  - Overuse of laxatives.
  - Antibiotic therapy.
  - Inflammatory bowel disease.
  - Irritable bowel syndrome.
  - Foodborne pathogens.

FUNDAMENTALS FOR NURSING

Assessment/Data Collection

- Monitor for constipation.
  - Abdominal bloating
  - Abdominal cramping
  - Straining at defecation

- Monitor for diarrhea.
  - Dehydration (postural hypotension, dizziness when changing positions)
  - Frequent loose stools
  - Abdominal cramping
- Collect assessment data.
  - Perform a physical examination of the abdomen (bowel sounds, tenderness) daily.
  - Assess for fluid deficit.
  - Assess skin integrity around the anal area.
  - Collect a detailed history of diet, exercise, and bowel habits.
- Perform specimen collection and diagnostic testing.
  - Fecal occult blood test – obtain a fecal sample using medical asepsis while wearing disposable gloves. Some foods (red meat, fish, poultry, raw vegetables) and medications can cause false positive results. Bleeding can be a sign of cancer, which can be a contributing factor for constipation.
  - Digital rectal examination for impaction – position on the left side with the knees flexed. The examiner inserts a gloved, lubricated index finger gently into the rectum. During.the procedure, monitor vital signs and response.
  - Specimens for stool cultures – obtain using medical asepsis while wearing disposable gloves. Label the specimen and promptly send it to the laboratory. Intestinal bacteria can cause diarrhea.

Patient-Centered Care

- Closely monitor fluid status. Record of intake and output.
- Monitor for dehydration.
- Closely monitor elimination pattern.
- Observe and document the character of bowel movements.
- Carefully check for blood or pus. For diarrhea, measure the volume of the stools.
- Administer laxatives and/or enemas.
- Encourage fluids (especially water), fiber, and exercise.
- After diarrhea stops, suggest eating yogurt to help re-establish an intestinal balance of beneficial bacteria.

Complications

- Complications of constipation include:
  - Fecal impaction.
  - Hemorrhoids, rectal fissures.
  - Bradycardia, hypotension, syncope associated with the Valsalva maneuver (occurs with straining/ bearing down).
  - Interventions
    - Monitor for constipation. Instruct clients not to strain to have bowel movements. Encourage measures to treat and prevent constipation.
    - Remove fecal impactions. Administering a glycerin or bisacodyl (Dulcolax) suppository might help.
- Complications of diarrhea include:
  - Dehydration and fluid and electrolyte disturbances (metabolic acidosis from excessive loss of bicarbonate).
  - Skin breakdown around the anal area.
  - Interventions
    - Replace losses.
    - Provide care and treatment for any skin breakdown.

Meeting the Needs of Older Adults

- Older adult clients are more susceptible to developing constipation as bowel tone decreases with age, and they are more at risk for developing fecal impaction.
- Adequate fluid and fiber intake and exercise are very important.
- Older adult clients are less able to compensate for fluid lost due to diarrhea.

APPLICATION EXERCISES

1. A nurse is caring for a client who will perform fecal occult blood testing at home. Which of the following information should the nurse include when explaining the procedure to the client?

    A. Eating more protein is optimal prior to testing.

    B. One stool specimen is sufficient for testing.

    C. A red color change indicates a positive test.

    D. The specimen cannot be contaminated with urine.

2. A nurse is talking with a client who reports constipation. When the nurse discusses dietary changes that can help prevent constipation, which of the following foods should the nurse recommend?

    A. Macaroni and cheese

    B. Fresh fruit and whole wheat toast

    C. Rice pudding and ripe bananas

    D. Roast chicken and white rice

3. A nurse is caring for a client who has had diarrhea for the past 4 days. When assessing the client, the nurse should expect which of the following findings? (Select all that apply.)

    _____ A. Bradycardia

    _____ B. Hypotension

    _____ C. Fever

    _____ D. Poor skin turgor

    _____ E. Peripheral edema

4. A nurse is preparing to administer a cleansing enema to an adult client in preparation for a diagnostic procedure. Which of the following are appropriate steps for the nurse to take? (Select all that apply.)

    _____ A. Warm the enema solution prior to instillation.

    _____ B. Position the client on the left side with the right leg flexed forward.

    _____ C. Lubricate the rectal tube or nozzle.

    _____ D. Slowly insert the rectal tube about 2 inches.

    _____ E. Hang the enema container 24 inches above the client's anus.

5. While a nurse is administering a cleansing enema, the client reports abdominal cramping. Which of the following is the appropriate intervention?

   A. Have the client hold his breath briefly.

   B. Discontinue the fluid instillation.

   C. Remind the client that cramping is common at this time.

   D. Lower the enema fluid container.

6. A nurse is explaining to a group of nursing students the various factors that alter bowel elimination patterns. Use the ATI Active Learning Template: Basic Concept to complete this item. Under Underlying Principles, list at least eight factors that affect bowel elimination, along with a brief example or description of each.

APPLICATION EXERCISES KEY

1. A. INCORRECT: Some proteins such as red meat, fish, and poultry can alter the test results.

    B. INCORRECT: Three specimens from three different bowel movements are required.

    C. INCORRECT: A blue color indicates blood in the stool.

    D. **CORRECT:** For fecal occult blood testing at home, the stool specimens cannot be contaminated with water or urine.

    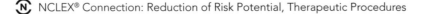 NCLEX® Connection: Reduction of Risk Potential, Therapeutic Procedures

2. A. INCORRECT: Macaroni and cheese is a low-residue option that could actually worsen constipation.

    B. **CORRECT:** A high-fiber diet promotes normal bowel elimination. The choice of fruit and toast is the highest fiber option.

    C. INCORRECT: Rice pudding and ripe bananas are low-residue options that could actually worsen constipation.

    D. INCORRECT: Roast chicken and white rice are low-residue options that could actually worsen constipation.

    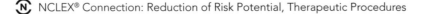 NCLEX® Connection: Basic Care and Comfort, Elimination

3. A. INCORRECT: Prolonged diarrhea is more likely to cause tachycardia than bradycardia

    B. **CORRECT:** Prolonged diarrhea leads to dehydration, which causes a decrease in blood pressure.

    C. **CORRECT:** Prolonged diarrhea leads to dehydration, which causes fever.

    D. **CORRECT:** Prolonged diarrhea leads to dehydration, which causes poor skin turgor.

    E. INCORRECT: Peripheral edema results from a fluid overload. Prolonged diarrhea is more likely to cause a fluid deficit.

    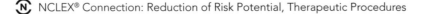 NCLEX® Connection: Physiological Adaptations, Illness Management

4.   A. **CORRECT:** The nurse should warm the enema solution because cold fluid can cause abdominal cramping and hot fluid can injure the intestinal mucosa.

    B. **CORRECT:** This position allows a downward flow of solution by gravity along the natural anatomical curve of the sigmoid colon.

    C. **CORRECT:** Lubrication prevents trauma or irritation to the rectal mucosa.

    D. INCORRECT: This is an appropriate length of insertion for a child. For an adult client, the nurse should insert the tube 3 to 4 inches.

    E. INCORRECT: The height of the fluid container affects the speed of instillation. The maximum recommended height is 18 inches. Hanging the container higher than that can cause rapid instillation and possibly painful distention of the colon.

    ⓝ NCLEX® Connection: Reduction of Risk Potential, Diagnostic Tests

5.   A. INCORRECT: Taking slow, deep breaths is more therapeutic for easing discomfort than holding the breath.

    B. INCORRECT: The nurse should stop the instillation if the client's abdomen becomes rigid and distended or if the nurse notes bleeding from the rectum.

    C. INCORRECT: This intervention is nontherapeutic as it implies that the client must tolerate the discomfort and that the nurse cannot or will not do anything to ease it.

    D. **CORRECT:** To relieve the client's discomfort, the nurse should slow the rate of instillation by reducing the height of the enema solution container.

    ⓝ NCLEX® Connection: Reduction of Risk Potential, Potential for Complications of Diagnostic Tests/ Treatments/Procedures

6. *Using the ATI Active Learning Template: Basic Concept*
    - Underlying Principles
        - Age
            - Infants
                - Breast milk stools – watery and yellow brown
                - Formula stools – pasty and brown
            - Toddlers: bowel control at 2 to 3 years old
            - Older adults: decreased peristalsis, relaxation of sphincters
        - Diet
            - Fiber requirement: 25 to 30 g/day
            - Lactose intolerance: difficulty digesting milk products
        - Fluids: Fluid requirement: 2,000 to 3,000 mL/day from fluid and food sources
        - Physical activity: Stimulates intestinal activity
        - Psychosocial factors
            - Emotional distress increasing peristalsis and exacerbating chronic conditions (colitis, Crohn's disease, ulcers, irritable bowel syndrome)
            - Depression decreasing peristalsis
        - Personal habits: Use of public toilets, false perception of the need for "one-a-day" bowel movements, lack of privacy when hospitalized
        - Positioning
            - Normal: squatting
            - Immobilized client: difficulty defecating
        - Pain
            - Discomfort leading to suppression of the urge to defecate
            - Opioid use contributing to constipation
        - Pregnancy
            - Growing fetus compromising intestinal space
            - Slower peristalsis
            - Straining increasing the risk of hemorrhoids
        - Surgery and anesthesia
            - Temporary slowing of intestinal activity
            - Paralytic ileus
        - Medications
            - Laxatives – to soften stool, abuse leading to diarrhea
            - Cathartics – to promote peristalsis
        - Ⓝ NCLEX® Connection: Physiological Adaptations, Pathophysiology

chapter 44

Overview

- Urinary elimination is a precise system of filtration, reabsorption, and excretion. These processes help maintain fluid and electrolyte balance while filtering and excreting water-soluble wastes.

- The primary organs involved in urinary elimination are the kidneys, with the nephrons performing most of the functions of filtration and elimination. Most adults produce between 1,500 and 2,000 mL of urine per day.

- Once filtered, the urine passes through the ureters into the bladder, the storage reservoir for urine. Once an adequate amount of urine collects in the bladder (150 to 200 mL), it sends a signal to the brain to indicate the need to urinate. The person then relaxes the internal and external sphincters located at the bottom of the bladder and the urethra. Urine passes from the bladder through the urethra where it exits the body.

- Interventions such as surgery, immobility, medications, and therapeutic diets may affect urinary elimination.

Urinary Diversions

- Urinary diversions – temporary or permanent, a stoma for the drainage of urine

  - Ureterostomy – one or both ureters to the abdominal surface

  - Nephrostomy – a tube from the renal pelvis to the abdominal surface

  - Pouched systems for urine diversions are similar to those for bowel diversions with similar body image concerns.

- Surgeons create urinary diversions for clients who have cancer of the bladder or injury to the bladder.

Factors Affecting Normal Urinary Elimination

- Age

  - Full bladder control by 4 to 5 years of age

  - Enlargement of the prostate after 40 years of age leading to urinary frequency, hesitancy, retention, incontinence, and urinary tract infections (UTIs).

  - Childbirth and gravity weaken the pelvic floor, putting clients at risk for prolapse of the bladder, leading to stress incontinence, which clients can manage with pelvic floor (Kegel) exercises.

Ⓖ
- ○ Older adult clients
  - ▪ Fewer nephrons
  - ▪ Loss of muscle tone of the bladder – frequency occurs
  - ▪ Inefficient emptying of the bladder – residual urine increasing the risk of UTIs
  - ▪ Increase in nocturia
- • Pregnancy
  - ○ A growing fetus compromises bladder space and compresses the bladder.
  - ○ There is a 30% to 50% increase in circulatory volume, which increases renal workload and output.
  - ○ The hormone relaxin causes relaxation of the sphincter.
- • Diet
  - ○ An increase in sodium leads to decreased urination.
  - ○ Caffeine and alcohol intake lead to increased urination.
- • Poor abdominal and pelvic muscle tone
- • Acute and chronic disorders
- • Spinal cord injury
- • Immobility
  - ○ Incontinence is not associated with aging. It is a result of neurological or mobility impairments.
- • Psychosocial factors
  - ○ Emotional stress and anxiety
  - ○ Having to use public toilets, lack of privacy when hospitalized
  - ○ Not having enough time to urinate (predetermined bathroom breaks in elementary schools)
- • Pain
  - ○ Suppression of the urge to urinate when there is pain in the urinary tract
  - ○ Obstruction in the ureter leading to renal colic
  - ○ Arthritis or painful joints causing immobility, which leads to delayed urination
- • Surgical procedures
  - ○ Alterations in glomerular filtration rate from anesthesia/opioid analgesics, resulting in decreased urine output
  - ○ Lower abdominal surgery creating obstructing edema and inflammation
- • Medications
  - ○ Diuretics preventing reabsorption of water
  - ○ Antihistamines and anticholinergics causing urinary retention
  - ○ Medications changing urine color
    - ▪ Phenazopyridine (Pyridium) – orange
    - ▪ Amitriptyline – green/blue
    - ▪ Levodopa (Dopar) – brown/black
  - ○ Chemotherapy creating a toxic environment for the kidneys

Diagnostic Tests

- Bedside sonography/bladder scanner – Portable ultrasound scanner noninvasively measures bladder volume to measure residual volume after voiding.

- Kidneys/ureters/bladder (KUB) – X-ray to determine size, shape, and position of these structures.

- Intravenous pyelogram (IVP) – Injecting contrast media (iodine) allows for viewing of ducts, renal pelvis, ureters, bladder, and urethra. Determine whether the client has an allergy to shellfish.

- Renal scan – View of renal blood flow and anatomy of the kidneys – no contrast.

- Renal ultrasound – View of gross renal structures.

- Cystoscopy – Uses an endoscope to visualize the bladder and urethra.

- Urodynamic testing – Tests bladder muscle function by filling the bladder with CO_2 or 0.9% sodium chloride and comparing pressure readings with the client's reported sensations.

Nursing Interventions

PROMOTING HEALTHY URINARY ELIMINATION
Equipment
› Urinal for men
› Toilet, bedpan, or commode
» Fracture pan – for supine clients and clients in body or leg casts
» Regular pan – for seated clients
Procedure
› Have the client sit when possible.
› Provide for privacy needs with adequate time for urinating (generally, at least 30 min).

I&O
Equipment
› Hard plastic urometer on indwelling catheter drainage bag is a reliable measuring tool.
› Graduated cylinders, urinal, or toilet receptacle
Procedure
› Measure output from a bedpan, commode, or collection bag into a graduated container.
› Use a receptacle to measure urine voided into the toilet.
› Use markings on the side of the urinal to measure urine.
› Less than 30 mL/hr for more than 2 hr is a cause for concern.

BLADDER RETRAINING FOR THE TREATMENT OF URGE INCONTINENCE
Equipment
› Clock
Procedure
› Use timed voidings to increase intervals between voidings/decrease voiding frequency.
› Perform pelvic floor (Kegel) exercises.
› Perform relaxation techniques.
› Offer undergarments while the client is retraining.
› Teach the client not to ignore the urge to void.
› Provide positive reinforcement as the client maintains continence.
› Eliminate or decrease caffeine drinks.
› Take diuretics in the morning.

- Specimen Collection
  - Equipment
    - Appropriate specimen container
      - Nonsterile for urinalysis
      - Sterile for clean-catch midstream and specimens obtained from a catheter
    - Soap/cleansing solution or towel
    - Gloves (for contact with any body fluids)
    - Specimen label
    - Urine collection container (catheter, urinal, receptacle in toilet, commode)

PROCEDURE	NURSING INTERVENTION
Urinalysis – random nonsterile specimen	› Explain the procedure. › Label the container with the client's identifying information, and follow facility policy for transport and sending specimen to the laboratory.
Clean-catch midstream (CCMS) for culture and sensitivity (C&S)	› Teach the technique for obtaining the specimen. › After thorough cleansing of the urethral meatus, the client "catches" the urine sample midstream.
Catheter urine specimen for C&S	› This requires obtaining a sterile specimen from a straight or indwelling catheter using surgical asepsis (sterile technique).
Timed urine specimens	› Collect for 24 hr or other prescribed duration. › Discard the first voiding. › Collect all other voidings following facility policy on appropriate refrigerated storage, labeling, and transport of the specimen.

- Straight or Indwelling Catheter Insertion
  - Equipment
    - Correct size and type of catheter: usually 8 to 10 Fr for children, 14 to 16 Fr for women, and 16 to 18 Fr for men. (Use silicon or Teflon products for clients who have latex allergies.)
    - Catheterization kit – with sterile drainage bag for indwelling catheter insertion
    - Soap and water
    - Collection container for straight catheterization
  - Explain the procedure to the client, and provide for privacy.
    - Explain the procedure.
    - Use correct technique for insertion of indwelling catheter or straight catheterization.
- Closed Intermittent Irrigation
  - Use correct technique to perform closed intermittent irrigation.
- Routine Catheter Care
  - Equipment
    - Soap and water
    - Washcloth
    - Gloves
  - Procedure
    - Use soap and water at the insertion site.
    - Cleanse the catheter at least three times a day and after defecation.
    - Monitor the patency of the catheter.
      - If the client reports fullness in the bladder area, check for kinks in the tubing, and check for sediment in the tubing.
      - Make sure the catheter bag/system is at a level below the client's bladder to avoid reflux.
- Condom Catheter Application
  - Equipment
    - Gloves
    - Condom catheter
    - Elastic tape
    - Leg or standard collection bag
  - Procedure
    - Explain the procedure to the client.
    - Use correct technique for application of a condom catheter.

Complications and Nursing Implications

- Urinary tract infections (UTIs)
  - Most due to *Escherichia coli*
  - Factors that increase the risk of UTIs
    - Close proximity of the urethral meatus in women to the anus
    - Frequent sexual intercourse
    - Menopause decreasing estrogen levels and increasing susceptibility to UTIs
    - Uncircumcised males
    - Use of indwelling catheters
  - Nursing implications
    - Cleanse female clients from front to back.
    - Cleanse beneath the foreskin in males.
    - Provide catheter care regularly.

URINARY INCONTINENCE

Overview

- There are six major types of urinary incontinence:
  - Stress – The loss of small amounts of urine when laughing, sneezing, or lifting primarily due to weak pelvic muscles, urethra, or surrounding tissues.
  - Urge – The inability to stop urine flow long enough to reach the bathroom due to an overactive detrusor muscle with increased bladder pressure.
  - Overflow – Urinary retention from bladder overdistention and frequent loss of small amounts of urine due to obstruction of the urinary outlet or an impaired detrusor muscle.
  - Reflex – The involuntary loss of a moderate amount of urine usually without warning due to hyperreflexia of the detrusor muscle, usually from altered spinal cord activity.
  - Functional – The inability to get to the bathroom to urinate due to physical, cognitive, or social impairment.
  - Total – The unpredictable, involuntary loss of urine that does not generally respond to treatment.
- Urinary incontinence is a significant contributing factor to altered skin integrity and falls, especially in older adults.

Assessment

- Risk Factors
  - Female
  - History of multiple pregnancies and vaginal births, aging, chronic urinary retention, urinary bladder spasm, renal disease, chronic bladder infection (cystitis)
  - Neurological disorders: Parkinson's disease, cerebrovascular accident, spinal cord injury, multiple sclerosis
  - Medication therapy: Diuretics, opioids, anticholinergics, calcium channel blockers, sedative/hypnotics, adrenergic antagonists
  - Obesity
  - Confusion, dementia, immobility, depression
  - Physiological changes of aging
  - Decreased estrogen levels and decreased pelvic-muscle tone
  - Immobility, chronic degenerative diseases, dementia, diabetes mellitus, cerebrovascular accident
  - Urinary incontinence increases the risk for falls, fractures, pressure ulcers, and depression.
- Subjective Data
  - Loss of urine when laughing, coughing, sneezing
  - Enuresis (bed-wetting)
  - Bladder spasms
  - Urinary retention
  - Frequency, urgency, nocturia
- Objective Data
  - Laboratory Tests
    - Urinalysis and urine culture/sensitivity – to rule out urinary tract infection (presence of RBCs, WBCs, micro-organisms)
    - Serum creatinine and BUN – to assess renal function (elevated with renal dysfunction)
  - Diagnostic Procedures
    - Postvoid residual urine using a pelvis ultrasonographic scanner or postvoid catheterization – to rule out urinary retention (more than 100 mL retained urine post voiding)
    - Voiding cystourethrography (VCUG) – identifies the size, shape, support, and function of the urinary bladder, obstruction (prostate), postvoid residual urine
    - Urodynamic Testing
      - Cystourethroscopy – visualization of the inside of the bladder
      - Cystometrogram (CMG) – measures pressure inside the bladder while filling with urine
      - Uroflowmetry – measures rate and degree of bladder emptying
      - Urethral pressure profilometry (UPP) – compares urethral pressure to bladder pressure during certain activities (coughing, lifting)
    - Electromyography (EMG) – measures strength of pelvic muscle contractions
    - Ultrasound – detects bladder abnormalities and/or residual urine

Patient-Centered Care

- Nursing Care
  - Establish a toileting schedule.
  - Monitor fluid intake during the daytime, and decrease fluid intake prior to bedtime.
  - Remove or control barriers to toileting.
  - Apply and monitor electrical stimulation of the pelvic floor muscles.
  - Provide incontinence garments.
  - Apply an external or condom catheter to males.
  - Avoid the use of indwelling urinary catheters.
  - Provide incontinence care.
  - Teach the client
    - To keep an incontinence diary.
    - How to perform Kegel exercises. Tighten pelvic muscles for a count of 10, relax slowly for a count of 10, and repeat in sequences of 15 in the lying-down, sitting, and standing positions.
    - Bladder compression techniques (Credé, Valsalva, double-voiding, splinting) to help clients manage reflex incontinence.
    - To avoid caffeine and alcohol consumption because these produce diuresis and the urge to urinate.
    - The side effects of medications that may stimulate voiding.
    - Vaginal cone therapy to strengthen pelvic muscles (stress incontinence).
- Medications
  - Antibiotics
    - Gentamicin (Garamycin) and cephalexin (Keflex) for infection
    - Nursing Considerations
      - Administer medication with food to decrease gastrointestinal distress.
    - Client Education
      - Inform client that the antibiotic might change the urine's odor.
      - Instruct the client to report loose stools.
      - Encourage the client to complete the full course of therapy even if symptoms resolve.
  - Tricyclic antidepressants
    - Nortriptyline (Pamelor) has anticholinergic effects that help relieve urinary incontinence.
    - Nursing Considerations
      - Medication can cause dizziness.
      - Monitor blood pressure and signs of orthostatic hypotension.
      - Do not give if the client is taking an MAOI.
    - Client Education
      - Encourage the client to get up slowly.

- ○ Urinary antispasmodics or anticholinergic agents
  - ▪ Oxybutynin (Ditropan) and dicyclomine (Bentyl) decrease urgency and help alleviate pain from a neurogenic or overactive bladder.
  - ▪ Nursing Considerations
    - ▫ Ask the client about a history of glaucoma.
    - ▫ The medication increases intraocular pressure.
    - ▫ Monitor for dizziness and tachycardia.
    - ▫ Monitor for urinary retention.
  - ▪ Client Education
    - ▫ Instruct the client to report problems voiding or constipation.
    - ▫ Instruct the client to report palpitations.
    - ▫ Inform the client that dizziness and dry mouth are common with this medication.
- ○ Phenazopyridine (Pyridium)
  - ▪ This is a bladder analgesic that treats the symptoms of urinary tract infections.
  - ▪ Nursing Considerations
    - ▫ The medication will not treat infection but will help with bladder discomfort.
    - ▫ Monitor for a decrease in hemoglobin and hematocrit.
    - ▫ Hepatic disorders and renal insufficiency are contraindications.
  - ▪ Client Education
    - ▫ Encourage the client to take with food.
    - ▫ Inform the client that the medication turns urine orange in color.
    - ▫ Instruct the client to notify the provider immediately if skin becomes yellow-tinged.
- ○ Hormone replacement therapy
  - ▪ This is controversial, but it increases blood supply to the pelvis.
- • Therapeutic Procedures
  - ○ Bladder training program
    - ▪ Urinary bladder training increases the bladder's ability to hold urine and the client's ability to suppress urination.
    - ▪ Nursing Actions
      - ▫ The client should void at scheduled intervals.
      - ▫ Gradually increase voiding intervals if the client has no incontinence episodes for 3 days until client can achieve the optimal 4-hr interval.
    - ▪ Client Education
      - ▫ Remind the client to hold urine until the scheduled toileting time.
      - ▫ Encourage the client to keep track of voiding times.

- ○ Urinary habit training
  - ▪ Urinary habit training helps clients with limited cognitive ability to establish a predictable pattern of bladder emptying.
  - ▪ Nursing Actions
    - □ The client should void at scheduled intervals.
  - ▪ Client Education
    - □ Inform the client that voiding patterns determine the toileting schedules.
    - □ Encourage the client to follow a voiding schedule according to the pattern in which no incontinence occurs.
- ○ Intermittent urinary catheterization
  - ▪ Intermittent urinary catheterization is periodic catheterization to empty the bladder. It reduces the risk of infection from indwelling catheterization, which is a temporary intervention when the client is at risk for skin breakdown, or when other options have failed.
  - ▪ Nursing Actions
    - □ Adjust the frequency of catheterization to keep output at 300 mL or less.
    - □ Explain the procedure.
  - ▪ Client Education
    - □ Encourage the client to follow a voiding schedule according to the pattern in which no incontinence occurs.
- • Surgical Interventions
  - ○ Anterior vaginal repair, retropubic suspension, pubovaginal sling, insertion of an artificial sphincter
    - ▪ Catheters (suprapubic or urinary) are appropriate until the client has a postvoid residual of less than 50 mL. Traction (with tape) helps prevent movement of the bladder.
    - ▪ Surgeons insert suprapubic catheters into the abdomen above the pubic bone and in the bladder and suture the catheter in place. The care for the catheter tubing and drainage bag is the same as for an indwelling catheter.
    - ▪ Nursing Actions
      - □ Monitor output and for any signs of infection (color of urine, sediment, level of output).
      - □ Keep the catheter patent at all times.
      - □ Determine the client's ability to detect the urge to void.
    - ▪ Client Education
      - □ Teach proper skin care around the insertion site.
      - □ Teach proper care and emptying of the catheter bag.
  - ○ Periurethral collagen injections to bladder neck

- Care after Discharge

  - To alleviate stress incontinence, consult nutritional services for dietary modifications if the client is obese.

  - Consult home care services to provide intermittent catheter, portable commode, or stool riser. Suggest installing handrails to assist the client with bathroom needs.

  - Client Education

    - Instruct the client to drink at least 2 to 3 L of fluid daily.

    - Instruct the client to try to hold urine, and stay on schedule with bladder training.

    - Advise the client to drink cranberry juice to decrease the risk of infection.

    - Encourage the obese client to participate in a weight reduction program to improve stress incontinence.

    - Instruct the client to take medications to help with incontinence.

    - Educate the client regarding the proper use of an intermittent catheterization if necessary.

    - Encourage the client to express feelings regarding incontinence.

Complications

- Skin Breakdown (from chronic exposure to urine)
  - Nursing Actions
    - Keep the skin clean and dry.
    - Assess for signs of breakdown.
    - Apply protective barrier creams.
    - Implement bladder retraining program.
- Social Isolation
  - Nursing Actions
    - Assist with measures to conceal urinary leaking (perineal pad, external catheter, adult incontinence garments).
    - Offer emotional support.

APPLICATION EXERCISES

1. A nurse in a provider's office is assessing a client who reports losing control of urine whenever she coughs, laughs, or sneezes. The client relates a history of three vaginal births, but no serious accidents or illnesses. Which of the following interventions are appropriate for helping to control or eliminate the client's incontinence? (Select all that apply.)

_____ A. Limit total daily fluid intake.

_____ B. Decrease or avoid caffeine.

_____ C. Increase the intake of calcium supplements.

_____ D. Avoid the intake of alcohol.

_____ E. Use Credé maneuver.

2. A client who has an indwelling catheter reports a need to urinate. Which of the following interventions should the nurse perform?

A. Check to see whether the catheter is patent.

B. Reassure the client that it is not possible for her to urinate.

C. Recatheterize the bladder with a larger-gauge catheter.

D. Collect a urine specimen for analysis.

3. A provider prescribes a 24-hr urine collection for a client. Which of the following actions should the nurse take?

A. Discard the first voiding.

B. Keep all voidings in a container at room temperature.

C. Ask the client to urinate and pour the urine into a specimen container.

D. Ask the client to urinate into the toilet, stop midstream, and finish urinating into the specimen container.

4. A nurse is preparing to initiate a bladder training program for a client who has a voiding disorder. Which of the following actions should the nurse take? (Select all that apply.)

_____ A. Establish a schedule of voiding prior to meal times.

_____ B. Have the client record voiding times.

_____ C. Gradually increase the voiding intervals.

_____ D. Remind client to hold urine until next scheduled voiding time.

_____ E. Provide a sterile container for voiding.

5. A nurse educator on a medical unit is reviewing factors that increase the risk of urinary tract infections (UTIs) with a group of assistive personnel. Which of the following should be included in the review? (Select all that apply.)

_____ A. Having sexual intercourse on a frequent basis

_____ B. Lowering of testosterone levels

_____ C. Wiping from back to front

_____ D. The location of the urethra in relation to the anus

_____ E. Undergoing frequent catheterization

6. A nurse is teaching a group of nursing students about the various types of urinary incontinence. Use the ATI Active Learning Template: Systems Disorder to complete this item.

A. Description of Disorder/Disease Process: List at least four of the six types of urinary incontinence, along with a brief example or description of each.

B. Risk Factors: List at least 10 common risk factors for urinary incontinence.

APPLICATION EXERCISES KEY

1. A. INCORRECT: Because stress incontinence results from weak pelvic muscles and other structures, limiting fluids will not resolve the problem.

    B. **CORRECT:** Caffeine is a bladder irritant and can worsen stress incontinence.

    C. INCORRECT: Calcium has no effect on stress incontinence.

    D. **CORRECT:** Alcohol is a bladder irritant and can worsen stress incontinence.

    E. INCORRECT: The Credé maneuver helps manage reflex incontinence, not stress incontinence.

    Ⓝ NCLEX® Connection: Basic Care and Comfort, Elimination

2. A. **CORRECT:** A clogged or kinked catheter causes the bladder to fill and stimulates the need to urinate.

    B. INCORRECT: Reassuring the client that it is not possible to urinate is a nontherapeutic response because it dismisses the client's concern.

    C. INCORRECT: There are less invasive approaches the nurse can take before replacing the catheter.

    D. INCORRECT: Although it might become necessary to collect a urine specimen, there is a simpler approach the nurse can take to assess and possibly resolve the client's problem.

    Ⓝ NCLEX® Connection: Reduction of Risk Potential, Potential for Complications of Diagnostic Tests/ Treatments/Procedures

3. A. **CORRECT:** The nurse should discard the first voiding of the 24-hr urine specimen, and note the time.

    B. INCORRECT: The nurse should collect all voidings after that and keep them in a refrigerated container.

    C. INCORRECT: For a urinalysis, the nurse should ask the client to urinate and pour the urine into a specimen container.

    D. INCORRECT: For a culture, the nurse should ask the client to urinate first into the toilet, then stop midstream, and finish urinating in the specimen container.

    Ⓝ NCLEX® Connection: Reduction of Risk Potential, Diagnostic Tests

4. A. INCORRECT: Bladder training involves voiding at scheduled frequent intervals and gradually increasing these intervals to 4 hr. Meal times are not regular, and the intervals may be longer than every 4 hr.

    B. **CORRECT:** Asking the client to keep track of voiding times is an appropriate nursing action.

    C. **CORRECT:** Gradually increasing the voiding interval is an appropriate nursing action.

    D. **CORRECT:** The client should be reminded to hold urine until the next scheduled voiding time.

    E. INCORRECT: A sterile container is not used in a bladder training program.

     NCLEX® Connection: Reduction of Risk Potential, Potential for Complications of Diagnostic Tests/Treatments/Procedures

5. A. **CORRECT:** Having sexual intercourse on a frequent basis is a factor that increases the risk of UTIs in both males and females.

    B. INCORRECT: The decrease in estrogen levels during menopause increases a woman's susceptibility to UTIs.

    C. INCORRECT: Wiping from front to back decreases a woman's risk of UTIs.

    D. INCORRECT: The close proximity of the female urethra to the anus is a factor that increases the risk of UTIs.

    E. **CORRECT:** Undergoing frequent catheterization and the use of indwelling catheters are risk factors for UTIs.

    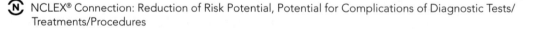 NCLEX® Connection: Reduction of Risk Potential, Potential for Complications of Diagnostic Tests/Treatments/Procedures

6. *Using the ATI Active Learning Template: Systems Disorder*

    A. Description of Disorder/Disease Process

    - Stress – Loss of small amounts of urine when laughing, sneezing, or lifting due to weak pelvic muscles or other structures

    - Urge – Inability to stop urine flow long enough to reach the bathroom due to an overactive detrusor muscle with increased bladder pressure

    - Overflow – Urinary retention from bladder overdistention and frequent loss of small amounts of urine due to obstruction of the urinary outlet or an impaired detrusor muscle

    - Reflex – Involuntary loss of a moderate amount of urine usually without warning due to hyperreflexia of the detrusor muscle, usually from altered spinal cord activity

    - Functional – Inability to get to the bathroom to urinate due to physical, cognitive, or social impairment

    - Total – Unpredictable, involuntary loss of urine; does not generally respond to treatment

    B. Risk Factors

    - Female

    - History of multiple pregnancies and vaginal births, aging, chronic urinary retention, urinary bladder spasm, renal disease, chronic bladder infection

    - Neurological disorders: Parkinson's disease, cerebrovascular accident, spinal cord injury, multiple sclerosis

    - Medications: diuretics, opioids, anticholinergics, calcium channel blockers, sedative/hypnotics, adrenergic antagonists

    - Obesity

    - Confusion, dementia, immobility, depression

    - Physiological changes of aging

    - Decreased estrogen levels, decreased pelvic-muscle tone

    - Immobility, chronic degenerative diseases, dementia, diabetes mellitus, stroke

    Ⓝ NCLEX® Connection: Physiological Adaptations, Pathophysiology

chapter 45

Overview

- Sensory perception is the ability to receive and interpret sensory impressions.
  - Consciousness
  - Arousal and awareness
  - Memory
  - Affect
  - Judgment
  - Awareness of reality
  - Language
- Sensory deficit is a change in reception and/or perception. Deficits can affect any of the senses. The body often will compensate for the deficit.
- Sensory deprivation is reduced sensory input either from the internal or the external environment. Sensory deprivation can be the result of illness, trauma, or isolation.
- Sensory overload is excessive, sustained, and unmanageable multisensory stimulation.

Contributing Factors

- Factors that contribute to loss of vision include presbyopia, cataracts, glaucoma, diabetic retinopathy, macular degeneration, infection, inflammation, injury, and brain tumor.
- Factors that contribute to conductive hearing loss include obstruction, tympanic membrane perforation, ear infections, and otosclerosis.
- Factors that contribute to sensorineural hearing loss include exposure to loud noises, ototoxic medications, aging, and acoustic neuroma.

Patient-Centered Care

- Nursing Care
  - Check for communication deficits and adjust care accordingly.
  - Collect equipment necessary to care for any assistive devices the client has (glasses, hearing aids).
  - Make every effort to communicate with clients who have sensoriperceptual losses because they tend to withdraw from interactions with others.

- Equipment
  - Assistive devices
  - Orientation tools (clocks, calendars)
  - Radio, television, CD/DVD player, digital audio player
  - Large-print materials
- Procedures
  - Keep clients safe and free from injury.
    - Make sure the call light is readily available.
    - Orient clients to the room.
    - Keep furniture clear from the path to the bathroom.
    - Keep personal items within reach.
    - Place the bed in its lowest position.
    - Make sure IV poles, drainage tubes, and bags are easy to maneuver.
  - Learn clients' preferred method of communication, and make accommodations.
  - For clients who are hearing impaired
    - Sit and face the client.
    - Avoid covering the mouth while speaking.
    - Encourage the use of hearing devices.
    - Speak slowly and clearly.
    - Do not shout.
    - Try lowering vocal pitch before increasing volume.
    - Use brief sentences with simple words.
    - Write down what clients do not understand.
    - Minimize background noise.
    - Ask for a sign language interpreter if necessary.
  - For clients who are visually impaired
    - Call clients by name before approaching to avoid startling them.
    - Identify yourself.
    - Stay within clients' visual field if they have a partial loss.
    - Give specific information about the location of items or areas of the building.
    - Explain interventions before touching clients.
    - Before leaving, inform clients of your departure.
    - Carefully appraise clients' clothing, and suggest changes if soiled or torn.
    - Make a radio, television, CD player, or digital audio player available.
    - Describe the arrangement of the food on the tray before leaving the room.

- For clients who have aphasia
  - Greet clients, and call them by name.
  - Speak clearly and slowly using short sentences.
  - Do not shout.
  - Pause between statements to allow time to understand.
  - Check for comprehension.
  - Ask questions that require simple answers.
  - Reinforce verbal with nonverbal communication (gestures, body language).
  - Allow plenty of time to respond.
  - Use methods speech therapists implement, such as a picture chart, to improve communication.
  - Acknowledge any frustration in communicating.
- For clients who are disoriented
  - Call clients by name, and identify yourself.
  - Maintain eye contact at eye level.
  - Use brief, simple sentences.
  - Ask only one question at a time.
  - Allow plenty of time for clients to respond.
  - Give directions one step at a time.
  - Avoid lengthy conversations.
  - Provide for adequate sleep and pain management.
- Encourage clients to verbalize feelings about sensoriperceptual loss.
- Orient clients to time, person, place, and situation.
  - Keep a clock in the room.
  - Post a calendar, or write the date where it is visible.
- Provide and/or use assistive devices.
- Provide care clients cannot perform (reading the menu, opening containers).
- Teamwork and Collaboration
  - Determine which assistive devices the client needs, and plan for their procurement.
  - Consult with rehabilitation therapists for restorative potential.
  - Refer clients to community-based support groups and organizations for additional resources.

Complications

- Risk for injury in the home environment
  - Teach ways to reduce hazards at home.
    - Visual
      - Remove throw rugs to prevent tripping hazards.
      - Keep walking pathways clear.
      - Ensure that stairways are well lit with secure handrails.
    - Auditory – Use flashing lights versus a warning sound from alarms.
    - Olfactory – Make sure smoke and carbon monoxide detectors are functioning to sense odors (burning food, natural gas).
    - Gustatory – Read dates on food packages to avoid contamination or spoilage.
    - Tactile – Protect and inspect body parts that lack sensation (burns, pressure ulcers, frostbite).
- Sensory deprivation and overload
  - Minimize overall stimuli and provide meaningful stimulation.
    - Minimize glare.
    - Manage pain effectively.
    - Allow for adequate sleep and rest periods.
    - Provide large-print materials or electronic players for audio books.
    - Amplify phones.
    - Season foods.
    - Reduce unpleasant odors.
    - Provide pleasant aromas.
    - Increase touch (if acceptable) with back rubs, hand holding, range-of-motion exercises, and hair care.
    - Organize care to minimize the activity surrounding the bed when possible.

REDUCED VISION

Overview

- Visual acuity of 20/200 or less with corrective lenses constitutes legal blindness.
- Reduced visual acuity can be unilateral (one eye) or bilateral (both eyes).

Health Promotion and Disease Prevention

- Advise clients to wear sunglasses while outside and protective eyewear while working in areas and at tasks with a risk for eye injury.
- Instruct clients to avoid rubbing eyes.
- Tell clients to get an eye examination regularly, especially after age 40.

Assessment

- Risk Factors

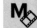

  - Age is the most significant risk factor for visual sensory alterations.
  - Presbyopia – age-related loss of the eye's ability to focus on close objects
  - Cataracts – opacity of lens
  - Glaucoma – loss of peripheral vision
  - Diabetic retinopathy – microaneurysms
  - Macular degeneration – loss of central vision
  - Eye infection, inflammation, or injury
  - Brain tumor
- Subjective Data
  - Frequent headaches
  - Frequent eye strain
  - Blurred vision
  - Poor judgment of depth
  - Diplopia – double vision
- Objective Data
  - Tendency to close or favor one eye
  - Poor hand-eye coordination
- Diagnostic Procedures
  - Ophthalmoscopy allows visualization of the back part of the eyeball (fundus), including the retina, optic disc, macula, and blood vessels.
  - Visual acuity tests include the Snellen and Rosenbaum eye charts.
  - Tonometry measures intraocular pressure (expected range: 10 to 21 mm Hg); elevated with glaucoma, especially angle-closure glaucoma.

> **M** View Image: Intraocular Pressure

  - Gonioscopy allows visualization of the iridocorneal angle or anterior chamber of the eyes.
  - Slit lamp allows visualization of the antérior portion of the eye, such as the cornea, anterior chamber, and the lens.

Patient-Centered Care

- Nursing Care
  - Nurses should monitor
    - Visual acuity using the Snellen and Rosenbaum eye charts – both measure distance vision.
      - The Snellen method has clients stand 20 ft away.
      - The Rosenbaum method has clients hold the chart 14 inches away from their eyes.
    - External and internal eye structures (ophthalmoscope)
    - Functional ability
  - Assess how clients adapt to the environment to maintain safety.
    - Increase the amount of light in a room.
    - Arrange the home to remove hazards, such as eliminating throw rugs.
    - Provide phones with large numbers and auto dial.
  - Provide the client with adaptive devices that accommodate for reduced vision.
    - Magnifying lens and large-print books and newspapers
    - Talking devices, such as clocks and watches
- Medications
  - Anticholinergics, such as atropine ophthalmic solution
    - Anticholinergics provide mydriasis (dilation of the pupil) and cycloplegia (ciliary paralysis) for examinations and surgery.
    - Client Education
      - Adverse effects include reduced accommodation, blurred vision, and photophobia. With systemic absorption, there could be anticholinergic effects (tachycardia, decreased secretions).
- Care After Discharge
  - Initiate referrals to social services, support groups, and reduced-vision resources.
  - Client Education
    - Wash hands before and after instilling eye medication.
    - Quit smoking.
    - Limit alcohol intake.
    - Keep blood pressure, blood glucose, and cholesterol under control.
    - Eat foods rich in antioxidants, such as green leafy vegetables.

Complications

- Risk for Injury
  - Reduced vision increases injury risk, especially for older adults.
  - Nursing Actions
    - Monitor for safety risks, such as the ability to drive safely, and intervene to reduce risks.

HEARING LOSS

Overview

- Hearing loss is difficulty in hearing or accurately interpreting speech and other sounds due to a problem in the middle or inner ear.
    - Conductive hearing loss is an alteration in the middle ear that blocks sound waves before they reach the inner ear.
    - Sensorineural hearing loss is an alteration in the inner ear that involves cranial nerve VIII or cochlear damage.

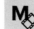 View Image: External, Middle, and Internal Ear

Health Promotion and Disease Prevention

- Advise clients to not place any objects in the ear, including cotton-tipped swabs.
- Tell clients to have an otologist remove any object lodged in the ear. Use a commercial ceruminolytic (ear drops that soften cerumen) for impactions, and follow with warm-water irrigation.
- Instruct clients to wear ear protection during exposure to high-intensity noise and risk for ear trauma.
- Tell clients to blow the nose gently and with both nostrils unobstructed.
- Advise clients when wearing headphones, keep the volume as low as possible.

Assessment

- Risk Factors
    - Risk for and degree of hearing loss advances with aging.
    - Use of ototoxic medications (aminoglycosides, monobactams).
    - Conductive hearing loss
        - History of middle ear infections
        - Older age (otosclerosis)
    - Sensorineural hearing loss
        - Prolonged exposure to loud noises
        - Ototoxic medications
        - Infectious processes
        - Age-related (presbycusis – decreased ability to hear high-pitched sounds)

- Subjective and Objective Data
  - Conductive hearing loss
    - Subjective
      - Hears better in a noisy environment
    - Objective
      - Speaks softly
      - Obstruction in external canal (packed cerumen)
      - Tympanic membrane findings (holes, scarring)
      - Rinne test that demonstrates that air conduction of sound is less than or equal to bone conduction (AC < or = to BC)
      - Weber test that lateralizes to the affected ear
  - Sensorineural hearing loss
    - Subjective
      - Tinnitus (ringing, roaring, humming in ears)
      - Dizziness
      - Hears poorly in a noisy environment
    - Objective
      - Speaks loudly
      - No otoscopic findings
      - Rinne test demonstrates expected response of air conduction is greater than bone conduction (AC > BC), but length of time is decreased for both.
      - Weber test lateralizes to unaffected ear
      - Diagnosis of acoustic neuroma (benign tumor cranial nerve VIII)

 View Video: Rinne and Weber Tests

  - Diagnostic Procedures
    - Audiometry
      - An audiogram identifies whether hearing loss is sensorineural and/or conductive.
      - Nursing Actions
        - Nurses use audiometry when screening for hearing loss in a school or older adult setting. The results will be more accurate in a quiet room.
        - Assess a client's ability to hear various frequencies (high vs. low pitch) at various decibels (soft vs. loud tones).
        - Have clients wear audiometer headphones and face away from the examiner.
        - Have clients indicate when they hear a tone and in which ear by raising their hand on the corresponding side. Comparing the responses on a graph with expected age and other norms yields information about the type and degree of hearing loss.

- Tympanogram
  - A tympanogram measures the mobility of the tympanic membrane and middle ear structures relative to sound to diagnose disorders of the middle ear.
- Otoscopy
  - An otoscope allows visualization of the external auditory canal, the tympanic membrane (TM), and malleus bone visible through the TM.

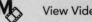 View Video: Otoscopic Examination

  - Nursing Actions
    - ▸ Perform an otoscopic examination when audiometry results indicate a possible impairment or for ear pain.
    - ▸ Select a speculum according to the size of the ear, then attach it and insert the otoscope into the external ear.
    - ▸ If the ear canal curves, pull up and back on the auricle of adults and down and back on the auricle of children younger than 3 years to straighten out the canal and enhance visualization.
    - ▸ The tympanic membrane should be pearly gray and intact. It should provide complete structural separation of the outer and middle ear structures.
    - ▸ The light reflex should be visible from the center of the TM anteriorly (5 o'clock right ear; 7 o'clock left ear).

M View Image: Light Reflex

    - ▸ With fluid or infection in the middle ear, the tympanic membrane will become inflamed and may bulge from the pressure of the exudate. This also will displace the light reflex, a significant finding.
    - ▸ Avoid touching the lining of the ear canal, which causes pain due to sensitivity.

Patient-Centered Care

- Nursing Care
  - Monitor functional ability.
  - Communication
    - Get the client's attention before speaking.
    - Stand or sit facing the client in a well-lit, quiet room without distractions.
    - Speak clearly and slowly without shouting and without hands or other objects covering the mouth.
    - Arrange for communication assistance (sign language interpreter, closed-captions, phone amplifiers, teletypewriter [TTY] capabilities).

- ○ Check the hearing of clients receiving ototoxic medications for more than 5 days. Reduced renal function that occurs with aging increases the risk for ototoxicity. Ototoxic medications include the following:

  - Multiple antibiotics – gentamicin (Garamycin), amikacin (Amikin), metronidazole (Flagyl)

  - Diuretics – furosemide (Lasix)

  - NSAIDs – aspirin, ibuprofen (Advil)

  - Chemotherapeutic agents – cisplatin (Abiplatin)

- Teamwork and Collaboration

  - ○ Refer clients with audiometry findings to an audiologist for more sensitive testing.

- Therapeutic Procedures

  - ○ Hearing aids

    - Hearing aids amplify sounds, but do not help clients interpret what they hear.

    - Amplification of sound in a loud environment can be distracting and disturbing.

  - ○ Nursing Actions

    - Use the lowest setting that allows hearing without feedback noise.

    - To clean the ear mold, use mild soap and water while keeping the hearing aid dry.

    - When the hearing aid is not in use, make sure to turn it off or remove the batteries to conserve battery power. Keep replacement batteries on hand.

- Surgical Interventions

  - ○ Tympanoplasty/myringoplasty – conductive hearing loss

    - Tympanoplasty is a surgical reconstruction of the middle ear structures; myringoplasty is an eardrum repair.

    - Nursing Actions

      - □ Place sterile ear packing postoperatively.

      - □ Position the client flat with the operative ear facing up for 12 hr.

    - Client Education

      - □ Tell the client to avoid air travel and forceful straining, coughing, or sneezing with the mouth closed.

      - □ Teach the client to cover the ear with a dressing to wash the hair and not to allow water to enter the ear.

      - □ Remind the client that hearing will be impaired while packing is in the ear.

APPLICATION EXERCISES

1. A nurse is caring for a client who recently had a cerebrovascular accident and has aphasia. Which of the following interventions should the nurse use to promote communication with this client? (Select all that apply.)

_____ A. Speak fast and loudly.

_____ B. Minimize background noise.

_____ C. Write down what the client does not understand.

_____ D. Allow plenty of time for the client to respond.

_____ E. Use brief sentences with simple words.

2. A nurse is caring for a client who had an amphetamine overdose and has sensory overload. Which of the following interventions should the nurse implement?

A. Immediately complete a thorough assessment.

B. Put the client in a room with a client who is hearing impaired.

C. Provide a private room, and limit stimulation.

D. Talk loudly to the client, and encourage ambulation.

3. A nurse is caring for a client who reports difficulty hearing. Which of the following assessment findings indicate a sensorineural hearing loss in the left ear? (Select all that apply.)

_____ A. Weber test showing lateralization to the right ear

_____ B. Light reflex at 10 o'clock in the left ear

_____ C. Signs of obstruction in the left ear canal

_____ D. Rinne test showing length of time is decreased for air and bone conduction

_____ E. Rinne test showing air conduction less than bone conduction in the left ear

4. A nurse is reviewing instructions with a client who is hearing impaired and has just started wearing hearing aids. Which of the following statements by the client indicates understanding of the instructions?

A. "I use a damp cloth to clean the outside part of my hearing aids."

B. "I clean the ear molds of my hearing aids with rubbing alcohol."

C. "I keep the volume of my hearing aids turned up so I can hear better."

D. "I take the batteries out of my hearing aids when I take them off at night."

5. A nurse is caring for a client who has several risk factors for hearing loss. As the nurse reviews the client's medication history, which of the following medications the client takes should alert the nurse to a further risk for ototoxicity? (Select all that apply.)

_____ A. Furosemide (Lasix)

_____ B. Ibuprofen (Advil)

_____ C. Cimetidine (Tagamet)

_____ D. Simvastatin (Zocor)

_____ E. Amiodarone (Cordarone)

6. A nurse is teaching a group of nursing students how to intervene for clients who have sensory impairment. Use the ATI Active Learning Template: Systems Disorder to complete this item. Under Management of Client Care, list at least six interventions for clients who are hearing impaired and at least six interventions for clients who are visually impaired.

APPLICATION EXERCISES KEY

1. A. **CORRECT:** The client is not hearing impaired, so speaking loudly will not promote communication.

    B. **CORRECT:** Minimizing background noise provides a calming environment.

    C. INCORRECT: Writing down what the client does not understand provides the same information in a format the client can understand, provided he is literate.

    D. INCORRECT: Allowing ample time for the client to respond helps enhance communication. Rushing ahead to the next question would be demeaning and could cause frustration.

    E. INCORRECT: Brief sentences with simple words are generally easy to understand.

    Ⓝ NCLEX® Connection: Psychosocial Integrity, Therapeutic Communication

2. A. INCORRECT: Immediately completing a thorough assessment might overwhelm the client at this time. Therefore, brief assessments during the course of the shift are better.

    B. INCORRECT: Rooming with a client who is hearing impaired would increase environmental stimuli.

    C. **CORRECT:** Minimizing stimuli helps clients who have sensory overload.

    D. INCORRECT: Talking loudly would increase environmental stimuli.

    Ⓝ NCLEX® Connection: Basic Care and Comfort, Assistive Devices

3. A. **CORRECT:** With sensorineural hearing loss, the Weber test demonstrates lateralization to the unaffected ear.

    B. INCORRECT: A light reflex at 10 o'clock in the left ear indicates that air or fluid has displaced the tympanic membrane, but it does not indicate sensorineural hearing loss.

    C. INCORRECT: Signs of obstruction in the ear canal indicate conductive, not sensorineural, hearing loss.

    D. **CORRECT:** With sensorineural hearing loss in the left ear, length of time is decreased for both air and bone conduction.

    E. INCORRECT: With sensorineural hearing loss in the left ear, air conduction is greater than bone conduction in the left ear.

    Ⓝ NCLEX® Connection: Safety and Infection Control, Accident/Error/Injury Prevention

4. A. INCORRECT: The client should keep the hearing aids completely dry at all times.

    B. INCORRECT: The client should clean the ear molds with mild soap and water.

    C. INCORRECT: To avoid feedback noise, the client should keep the volume on the lowest setting that allows her to hear.

    D. **CORRECT:** To conserve battery power, the client should turn off the hearing aids and remove the batteries when not in use.

     NCLEX® Connection: Psychosocial Integrity, Sensory/Perceptual Alterations

5. A. INCORRECT: Furosemide, a loop diuretic, can cause hearing loss as well as blurred vision.

    B. **CORRECT:** Ibuprofen, a nonsteroidal anti-inflammatory agent, can cause hearing loss as well as vision loss.

    C. **CORRECT:** Cimetidine, a medication that decreases gastric acid secretion, is unlikely to cause hearing loss.

    D. **CORRECT:** Simvastatin, a medication that helps lower cholesterol, is unlikely to cause hearing loss.

    E. **CORRECT:** Amiodarone, an antidysrhythmic medication, is more likely to cause blurred vision than hearing loss.

     NCLEX® Connection: Reduction of Risk Potential, System Specific Assessments

6. *Using the ATI Active Learning Template: Systems Disorder*

- Management of Client Care
  - ○ Hearing impairment
    - ▪ Sit and face the client.
    - ▪ Avoid covering the mouth while speaking.
    - ▪ Encourage the use of hearing devices.
    - ▪ Speak slowly and clearly.
    - ▪ Do not shout.
    - ▪ Try lowering vocal pitch before increasing volume.
    - ▪ Use brief sentences with simple words.
    - ▪ Write down what clients do not understand.
    - ▪ Minimize background noises.
    - ▪ Ask for a sign language interpreter if necessary.
  - ○ Vision impairment
    - ▪ Call clients by name before approaching to avoid startling them.
    - ▪ Identify yourself.
    - ▪ Stay within the clients' visual field if they have a partial loss.
    - ▪ Give specific information about the location of items or areas of the building.
    - ▪ Explain interventions before touching clients.
    - ▪ Before leaving, inform clients of your departure.
    - ▪ Carefully appraise clothing and suggest changes if soiled or torn.
    - ▪ Make a radio, television, compact disc (CD) player, or digital audio file player available.
    - ▪ Describe the arrangement of the food on the tray before leaving the room.

(N) NCLEX® Connection: Psychosocial Integrity, Sensory/Perceptual Alterations

UNIT 4   Physiological Integrity

SECTION: PHARMACOLOGICAL AND PARENTERAL THERAPIES

› Pharmacokinetics and Routes of Administration
› Safe Medication Administration and Error Reduction
› Dosage Calculation
› Intravenous Therapy
› Adverse Effects, Interactions, and Contraindications
› Individual Considerations of Medication Administration

NCLEX® CONNECTIONS

When reviewing the chapters in this unit, keep in mind the relevant sections of the NCLEX® outline, in particular:

Client Needs: Management of Care	Client Needs: Safety and Infection Control	Client Needs: Pharmacological and Parenteral Therapies

› Relevant topics/tasks include:
» Client Rights
  › Recognize the client's right to refuse treatment/procedures.
» Continuity of Care
  › Use approved abbreviations and standard terminology when documenting care.
	› Relevant topics/tasks include:
	» Error Prevention
	  › Ensure proper identification of the client when providing care.
		› Relevant topics/tasks include:
		» Dosage Calculation
		  › Perform calculations needed for medication administration.
		» Expected Actions/Outcomes
		  › Obtain information on prescribed medication for the client.
		» Medication Administration
		  › Prepare and administer medications, using the rights of medication administration.

chapter 46

Overview

- Pharmacokinetics refers to how medications travel through the body. Medications undergo a variety of biochemical processes that result in absorption, distribution, metabolism, and excretion.

Phases of Pharmacokinetics

- Absorption – The transmission of medications from the location of administration (gastrointestinal tract, muscle, skin, or subcutaneous tissue) to the bloodstream. The most common routes of administration are enteral (through the GI tract) and parenteral (by injection). Each of these routes will have a unique pattern of absorption.

  ○ The rate of medication absorption determines how soon the medication takes effect.

  ○ The amount of medication absorbed determines its intensity.

  ○ The route of administration affects the rate and amount of absorption.

ROUTES AND ABSORPTION	
BARRIERS TO ABSORPTION	**ABSORPTION PATTERN**
Oral	
› Medications must pass through the layer of epithelial cells that line the GI tract.	› Varies greatly due to: » Stability and solubility of the medication » Gastrointestinal pH and emptying time » Presence of food in the stomach or intestines » Other medications currently being administered » Forms of medications (enteric-coated pills, liquids)
Subcutaneous and intramuscular	

› The capillary wall has large spaces between cells. Therefore, there is no significant barrier.	› The rate of absorption is determined by:
	» Solubility of the medication in water.
	  › Highly soluble medications are absorbed in 10 to 30 min.
	  › Poorly soluble medications are absorbed slower.
	» Blood perfusion at the site of injection.
	  › Sites with high blood perfusion will have rapid absorption.
	  › Sites with low blood perfusion will have slow absorption.

Intravenous	
› No barriers	› Immediate – administered directly into the blood › Complete – all of it reaches the blood

- Distribution – The transportation of medications to sites of action by bodily fluids. Distribution may be influenced by:

  ○ Circulation: Conditions that inhibit blood flow or perfusion, such as peripheral vascular or cardiac disease, may delay medication distribution.

  ○ Permeability of the cell membrane: The medication must be able to pass through tissues and membranes in order to reach its target area. Medications that are lipid-soluble or have a transport system can cross the blood-brain barrier or the placenta.

  ○ Plasma protein binding: Medications compete for protein binding sites within the bloodstream, primarily albumin. The ability of a medication to bind to a protein can affect how much of the medication will leave and travel to target tissues. Two medications can compete for the same binding sites, resulting in toxicity.

- Metabolism (biotransformation) changes medications into less active forms or inactive forms by the action of enzymes. This occurs primarily in the liver, but also takes place in the kidneys, lungs, bowel, and blood.

  ○ Factors influencing the rate of medication metabolism

    ▪ Age – Infants have limited medication-metabolizing capacity. The aging process also can influence medication metabolism, but varies from individual to individual. In general, hepatic medication metabolism tends to decline with age.

    ▪ An increase in certain medication-metabolizing enzymes – This can cause a particular medication to be metabolized sooner, requiring an increase in dosage of that medication to maintain a therapeutic level. It can also cause an increase in the metabolism of other medications that are being used concurrently.

    ▪ First-pass effect – Some medications are inactivated on their first pass through the liver and must be given by a nonenteral route because of their high first-pass effect. These medications are usually given by routes such as SL or IV.

    ▪ Similar metabolic pathways – When two medications are metabolized by the same pathway, they can interfere with the metabolism of one or both of the medications. In this way, the rate of metabolism can be decreased for one or both of the medications leading to medication accumulation.

    ▪ Nutritional status – A malnourished client may be deficient in the factors that are necessary to produce specific medication-metabolizing enzymes. Consequently, medication metabolism may be impaired.

- Excretion – The elimination of medications from the body, primarily through the kidneys. Elimination also takes place through the liver, lungs, bowel, and exocrine glands. Kidney dysfunction may lead to an increase in duration and intensity of medication response.

Medication Responses

- Plasma medication levels can be regulated to control medication responses. Medication dosing attempts to maintain plasma levels between the minimum effective concentration (MEC) and the toxic concentration.

- A plasma medication level is in the therapeutic range when it is effective and not toxic. Therapeutic levels are well-established for many medications, and these levels can be used to monitor a client's response.

Therapeutic Index (TI)

- Medications with a high TI have a wide safety margin. Therefore, there is no need for routine serum medication level monitoring. Medications with a low TI should have serum medication levels monitored closely. Monitor peak levels based on the route of administration.

  ○ For example, an oral medication may have a peak of 1 to 3 hr after administration.

  ○ If the medication is given IV, the peak time might occur within 10 min.

  ○ Refer to a drug reference or a pharmacist for specific medication peak times.

  ○ For trough levels, blood is drawn immediately before the next medication dose, regardless of the route of administration.

Half-Life (t1/2)

- Refers to the period of time needed for the medication in the body to be reduced by 50%. May be affected by liver and kidney function. Usually takes four half-lives to achieve a steady state of serum concentration (medication intake = medication metabolism and excretion).

SHORT HALF-LIFE	LONG HALF-LIFE
› Medications leave the body quickly – 4 to 8 hr.	› Medications leave the body more slowly – more than 24 hr. Greater risk for medication accumulation and toxicity.
› Short-dosing interval or minimum effective concentration (MEC) will drop between doses.	› Medications are given at longer intervals without a loss of therapeutic effects. › Medications take a longer time to reach a steady state.

Pharmacodynamics (Mechanism of Action)

- Describes the interactions between medications and target cells, body systems, and organs to produce effects. These interactions result in functional changes that are considered the mechanism of action of the medication. Medications interact with cells in one of two ways.

  ○ Agonist – Medication that can mimic the receptor activity regulated by endogenous compounds. For example, morphine sulfate (Duramorph) is classified as an agonist because it activates the receptors that produce analgesia, sedation, constipation, and other effects.

  ○ Antagonist – Medication that can block normal receptor activity regulated by endogenous compounds or receptor activity caused by other medications. For example, losartan (Cozaar), an angiotensin II receptor blocker, is classified as an antagonist. Losartan works by blocking angiotensin II receptors on blood vessels, which prevents vasoconstriction.

  ○ Partial agonists – May act as an agonist/antagonist. Limited affinity to receptor site. For example, nalbuphine (Nubain) acts as an antagonist at mu receptors and an agonist at kappa receptors, causing analgesia at low doses, with minimal respiratory depression.

Routes of Administration

ROUTE OF ADMINISTRATION	NURSING IMPLICATIONS
Oral or enteral (tablets, capsules, liquids, suspensions, elixirs)	› Contraindications for oral medication administration include vomiting, decreased GI motility, absence of a gag reflex, difficulty swallowing, and a decreased level of consciousness. › Have the client in a seated position at a 90° angle to facilitate swallowing. › Administer irritating medications with small amounts of food. › Do not mix with large amounts of food or beverages in case the client is unable to consume the entire quantity. › Avoid administration with contraindicated foods or beverages such as grapefruit juice. › In general, administer oral medications on an empty stomach (30 min to 1 hr before meals, 2 hr after meals). › Follow the manufacturer's directions for crushing, cutting, and diluting medications. › Enteric-coated or time-release medications must be swallowed whole. › Use a liquid form of the medication to facilitate swallowing whenever possible.
Sublingual (under the tongue) and buccal (between the cheek and the gum)	› Instruct the client to have medication remain in place until absorbed. › The client should not eat or drink while the tablet is in place.
Liquids, suspensions, and elixirs	› Follow directions for dilution and shaking. › When administering the medication, the base of the meniscus (lowest fluid line) is at the level of the desired dose.
Transdermal – medication stored in a skin patch and absorbed through the skin producing systemic effects	› Instructions to the client should include: › Apply patches as provided to ensure proper dosing. › Wash the skin with soap and water, and dry it thoroughly before applying a new patch. › Place the patch on a hairless area of the skin and rotate sites to prevent skin irritation.
Topical	› Apply with a glove, tongue blade, or cotton-tipped applicator. › Never apply with a bare hand.

ROUTE OF ADMINISTRATION	NURSING IMPLICATIONS
Instillation (drops, ointments, sprays) – generally used for eyes, ears, and nose	› Eyes » Use medical aseptic technique when instilling medications in eyes. » Have the client sit upright or lie supine with the head tilted slightly and looking up at the ceiling. » Rest the dominant hand on the client's forehead, hold the dropper above the conjunctival sac about 1 to 2 cm, drop the medication into the center of the sac, and have the client close the eye gently. » Apply gentle pressure with the finger and a clean tissue on the nasolacrimal duct for 30 to 60 seconds to prevent systemic absorption of the medication. › Ears » Use medical aseptic technique when administering medications into the ears. » Have the client sit upright or maintain a side-lying position. » Straighten the ear canal by pulling the auricle upward and outward for adults or down and back for children. Hold the dropper 1 cm above the ear canal, instill medication, and then gently apply pressure with finger to tragus of ear unless contraindicated due to pain. » Do not press a cotton ball deep into the ear canal. If needed, gently place it into the outermost part of the ear canal. » Have the client remain in the side-lying position if possible for 2 to 3 min after installation of ear drops. › Nose » Use medical aseptic technique when administering medications into the nose. » Have the client supine with the head positioned to allow the medication to enter the appropriate nasal passage. » Use the dominant hand to instill drops, supporting the head with the nondominant hand. » Instruct the client to breathe through the mouth, stay in a supine position, and not to blow the nose for 5 min after drop insertion.

ROUTE OF ADMINISTRATION	NURSING IMPLICATIONS
Inhalation – administered through metered dose inhalers (MDI) or dry powder inhalers (DPI)	› For an MDI, instruct the client to: » Remove the cap from the inhaler mouthpiece. » Shake the inhaler five or six times. » Hold the inhaler with the mouthpiece at the bottom. » Hold the inhaler with the thumb near the mouthpiece and the index and middle fingers at the top. » Hold the inhaler about 2 to 4 cm (0.8 to 1.6 in) away from the front of the mouth or close the mouth around the mouthpiece of the inhaler with the opening pointing towards the back of the throat. » Take a deep breath and then exhale. » Tilt the head back slightly, press the inhaler, and, at the same time, begin a slow, deep breath. Continue to breathe slowly and deeply for 3 to 5 seconds to facilitate delivery to the air passages. » Hold the breath for 10 seconds to allow the medication to deposit in the airways. » Take the inhaler out of the mouth and slowly exhale through pursed lips. » Resume normal breathing. › A spacer may be used to keep the medication in the device longer thereby increasing the amount of medication delivered to the lungs and decreasing the amount of the medication in the oropharynx. › If a spacer is used: » Remove the covers from the mouthpieces of the inhaler and of the spacer. » Insert the MDI into the end of the spacer. » Shake the inhaler five or six times. » Exhale completely, then close the mouth around the spacer mouthpiece. Continue as with an MDI. › For a DPI: » Do not shake the device. » Take the cover off the mouthpiece. » Follow the directions of the manufacturer for preparing the medication, such as turning the wheel of the inhaler. » Exhale completely. » Place the mouthpiece between lips and take a deep breath through the mouth. » Hold the breath for 5 to 10 seconds » Take the inhaler out of the mouth and slowly exhale through pursed lips. » Resume normal breathing. › If more than one puff is prescribed, instruct the client to wait the length of time directed before administering the second puff. › Instruct the client to remove the canister and rinse the inhaler, cap, and spacer once a day with warm running water and dry it completely before using it again.

ROUTE OF ADMINISTRATION	NURSING IMPLICATIONS
Nasogastric and gastrostomy tubes	› Verify proper tube placement. › Use a syringe and allow the medication to flow in by gravity or push it in with the plunger of the syringe. › General guidelines » Liquid forms of medications must be used. » Sublingual medications should not be administered. » Do not crush specially prepared oral medications (extended/ time-release, fluid-filled, enteric-coated). » Each medication should be administered separately. » Do not mix medications with enteral feedings. » Completely dissolve crushed tablets and capsule contents in 15 to 30 mL of water prior to administration. › To prevent clogging, flush the tubing before and after each medication with 15 to 30 mL of water.
Suppositories	› Follow the manufacturer's directions for storage. › Wear gloves for the procedure. › Remove the foil wrapper, and lubricate the suppository if necessary. › Rectal suppositories » Position the client in the left lateral position. » Insert the suppository just beyond the internal sphincter. » Instruct the client to remain flat or in the left lateral position for at least 5 min after insertion to retain the suppository. Absorption times vary based on the medication. › Vaginal suppositories » Position the client supine with her knees bent, her feet flat on the bed and close to her hips (modified lithotomy position). » Vaginal suppositories can be inserted with an applicator. » Insert the suppository along the posterior wall of the vagina about 3 to 4 inches. » Instruct the client to remain supine for at least 5 min after insertion to retain the suppository.

ROUTE OF ADMINISTRATION	NURSING IMPLICATIONS
Parenteral	› General considerations for parenteral medications include: › The vastus lateralis site is usually the recommended site for infants 1 year and younger. › The ventrogluteal site is the preferred site for IM injections and is recommended for injecting volumes greater than 2 mL. › The deltoid site has a smaller muscle mass and only can accommodate up to 1 mL of fluid. › Use a needle size and length appropriate for the type of injection and the client's size. Syringe size should approximate the volume of medication. › Use a tuberculin syringe for solution volumes less than 0.5 mL. › Rotate injection sites to enhance medication absorption, and document each site used. › Do not use injection sites that are edematous, inflamed, or have moles, birthmarks, or scars. › If medication is given IV, immediately monitor the client for therapeutic and adverse effects. › Discard all sharps (broken ampule bottles, needle) in designated containers. Containers should be leak- and puncture-proof.
Intradermal	› Usually used for tuberculin testing or checking for medication/allergy sensitivities. › Use small amounts of solution (0.01 to 0.1 mL) in a tuberculin syringe with a fine-gauge needle (26- to 27-gauge) in lightly pigmented, thin-skinned, hairless sites (inner surface of the mid-forearm or scapular area of the back) at a 10° to 15° angle.
Subcutaneous	› Appropriate for small doses of nonirritating, water-soluble medications. Commonly used for insulin and heparin. › Use a 3/8- to 5/8-inch, 25- to 27-gauge needle or an insulin syringe of 28- to 31-gauge. Inject no more than 1.5 mL solution. For an average size client, pinch up the skin and inject at a 45 a to 90° angle. For an obese client, use a 90° angle. › Sites are selected for adequate fat-pad size (abdomen, upper hips, lateral upper arms, thighs).
Intramuscular	› Appropriate for irritating medications, solutions in oils, and aqueous suspensions. › Most common sites include ventrogluteal, deltoid, and vastus lateralis (pediatric). › Dorsogluteal is no longer used as a common injection site due to close proximity of the sciatic nerve. › Use a needle size 18- to 27-gauge (usually 22- to 25-gauge), 1- to 1.5-inch long, and inject at a 90° angle. Volume injected is usually 1 to 3 mL. If a greater amount is required, it should be divided into two syringes and two different sites should be used.

ROUTE OF ADMINISTRATION	NURSING IMPLICATIONS
Z-track	› Type of IM injection that prevents medication from leaking back into subcutaneous tissue. › It is often used for medications that cause visible and/or permanent skin stains, such as certain iron preparations.
Intravenous	› Appropriate for administration of medications, fluid, and blood products. › Vascular access devices can be for short-term use (catheters) or long-term use (infusion ports). Use 16-gauge for trauma clients, 18-gauge for surgical clients, and 22- to 24-gauge for children, older adults, medical clients, and stable postoperative clients. › Preferred sites are peripheral veins in the arm or hand. Ask the client which site he prefers. In neonates, veins of the head, lower legs, and feet may be used. After administration, immediately monitor for therapeutic and adverse effects.
Epidural	› Administration of intravenous opioid analgesia (morphine [Duramorph] or fentanyl [Sublimaze]). › The catheter is advanced through the needle that is inserted into the epidural space at the level of the fourth or fifth vertebrae. › Infusion pumps are necessary to administer medication.

- Advantages and Disadvantages of Different Routes

ADVANTAGES	DISADVANTAGES
Oral	
› Safe › Inexpensive › Easy and convenient	› Oral medications have a highly variable absorption. › Inactivation can occur by the GI tract or first-pass effect. › The client must be cooperative and conscious. › Contraindications include nausea and vomiting.
Subcutaneous and intramuscular (IM)	
› Use for poorly soluble medications. › This route is appropriate for administering medications that are absorbed slowly for an extended period of time (depot preparations).	› IM injections are associated with a higher cost. › IM injections are inconvenient. › There can be pain with the risk for local tissue damage and nerve damage. › There is a risk for infection at the injection site.
Intravenous (IV)	
› Onset is rapid, and absorption of the medication into the blood is immediate, which provides an immediate response. › This route allows control over the precise amount of medication administered. › This route allows for administration of large volumes of fluid. › Irritating medications can be given with free-flowing IV fluid.	› IV injections are associated with an even higher cost. › IV injections are more inconvenient. › Absorption of the medication into the blood is immediate. This can be potentially dangerous if the wrong dosage or the wrong medication is given. › There is an increased risk for infection or embolism with IV injections.

APPLICATION EXERCISES

1. A nurse is caring for a client who is 1 day postoperative following a total knee arthroplasty. The client states his pain level is 10 on a scale of 0 to 10. After reviewing the client's medication administration record, which of the following medications should the nurse administer?

    A. Meperidine (Demerol) 75 mg IM

    B. Fentanyl 50 mcg/hr transdermal patch

    C. Morphine 2 mg IV

    D. Oxycodone 10 mg PO

2. A nurse is teaching a client about taking multiple oral medications at home to include time-release capsules, liquid medications, enteric-coated pills, and narcotics. Which of the following statements by the client indicates an understanding of the teaching?

    A. "I can open the capsule with the beads in it and sprinkle them on my oatmeal."

    B. "If I am having difficulty swallowing, I will add the liquid medication to a batch of pudding."

    C. "The pills with the coating on them can be crushed."

    D. "I will eat two crackers with the pain pills."

3. A nurse is teaching a client how to administer medication through a jejunostomy tube. Which of the following instructions should the nurse include in the teaching?

    A. "Flush the tube before and after each medication."

    B. "Administer your medications with your enteral feeding."

    C. "Administer tablets through the tube slowly."

    D. "Mix all the crushed medications prior to dissolving in water."

4. A nurse educator is teaching a module on pharmacokinetics to a group of newly licensed nurses. Which of the following statements by a newly licensed nurse indicates an understanding of the first-pass effect?

    A. "Some medications block normal receptor activity regulated by endogenous compounds or receptor activity caused by other medications."

    B. "Some medications may have to be administered by a nonenteral route to avoid inactivation as they travel through the liver."

    C. "Some medications leave the body more slowly and therefore have a greater risk for medication accumulation and toxicity."

    D. "Some medications have a wide safety margin, so there is no need for routine serum medication level monitoring."

5. A nurse is teaching an adult client how to administer ear drops. Which of the following statements by the client indicates understanding of the proper technique?

    A. "I will straighten my ear canal by pulling my ear down and back."

    B. "I will gently apply pressure with my finger to the tragus of my ear after putting in the drops."

    C. "I will insert the nozzle of the ear drop bottle snug into my ear before squeezing the drops in."

    D. "After the drops are in, I will place a cotton ball all the way into my ear canal."

6. A nurse educator is teaching a module on biotransformation as a phase of pharmacokinetics during nursing orientation to a group of newly licensed nurses. Use the ATI Active Learning Template: Basic Concept to complete this item to include the following:

    A. Related Content: List four areas of the body where biotransformation takes place.

    B. Underlying Principles: List at least three factors that influence the rate of biotransformation.

APPLICATION EXERCISES KEY

1. A. INCORRECT: Although meperidine is used for pain control, the IM route of administration can allow for slow absorption delaying the onset of pain relief. The IM route also can cause additional pain from injection.

    B. INCORRECT: Although fentanyl is used for pain control, the transdermal route of administration can allow for slow absorption delaying the onset of pain relief.

    C. **CORRECT:** IV morphine is the best choice because the onset is rapid, and absorption of the medication into the blood is immediate, which provides an immediate response for a client who is reporting pain at a level of 10.

    D. INCORRECT: Although oxycodone is used for pain control, the oral route of administration of this medication can allow for onset of pain relief in 10 to 15 min, which can be a long time for a client who is reporting pain at a level of 10.

     NCLEX® Connection: Pharmacological and Parenteral Therapies, Pharmacological Pain Management

2. A. INCORRECT: Although this may assist a client with swallowing issues, enteric-coated or time-release medications should be swallowed whole.

    B. INCORRECT: Although it is recommended to add a liquid medication to food if the client is having difficulty swallowing, it is not recommended to mix the medication with large amounts of food or beverage in case the client is unable to consume the entire quantity.

    C. INCORRECT: Enteric-coated or time-release medications should be swallowed whole and cannot be crushed.

    D. **CORRECT:** It is recommended to administer irritating medications with small amounts of food. This will assist with prevention of nausea and vomiting so that the medication can be retained and take effect.

     NCLEX® Connection: Pharmacological and Parenteral Therapies, Pharmacological Pain Management

3. A. **CORRECT:** The client should flush the tubing before and after each medication with 15 to 30 mL of water to prevent clogging of the tube.

    B. INCORRECT: In order to maximize the therapeutic effect of a medication, it is recommended to never mix medications with enteral feeding. In addition, if the client does not receive the entire feeding he does not receive the entire medication. This can also delay the client receiving the medication.

    C. INCORRECT: The client should not administer tablets or undissolved medications through a jejunostomy tube because they may clog the tube.

    D. INCORRECT: The client should administer each medication separately.

    NCLEX® Connection: Pharmacological and Parenteral Therapies, Medication Administration

4. A. INCORRECT: This statement describes an antagonist medication, not the first pass-effect.

    B. **CORRECT:** Some medications are inactivated on their first pass through the liver and must be given by a nonenteral route to prevent this inactivation. These medications are usually given by routes such as sublingual or IV.

    C. INCORRECT: This statement describes a long half life, not the first-pass effect.

    D. INCORRECT: This statement describes a high therapeutic index, not the first-pass effect.

     NCLEX® Connection: Physiological Adaptations, Pathophysiology

5. A. INCORRECT: The adult client should straighten the ear canal by pulling the auricle upward and outward to open up the ear canal to allow the medication to reach the eardrum.

    B. **CORRECT:** The client should gently apply pressure with the finger to the tragus of the ear after administering the drops to help the drops go into the ear canal.

    C. INCORRECT: The client should never occlude the ear canal with the dropper when instilling ear drops because this can cause pressure that could injure the eardrum.

    D. INCORRECT: The client should not place a cotton ball past the outermost part of the ear canal because it could introduce bacteria to the inner or middle ear.

     NCLEX® Connection: Pharmacological and Parenteral Therapies, Medication Administration

6. *Using the ATI Active Learning Template: Basic Concept*

    A. Related Content
    - Biotransformation (metabolism) changes medications into less active forms or inactive forms by the action of enzymes. This occurs primarily in the liver, but also takes place in the kidneys, lungs, bowel, and blood.

    B. Underlying Principles
    - Age – Infants have limited medication-metabolizing capacity. The aging process also can influence medication metabolism, but varies from individual to individual. Hepatic medication metabolism tends to decline with age.

    - Increase in certain medication-metabolizing enzymes – This can cause a particular medication to be metabolized sooner, requiring an increase in dosage of that medication to maintain a therapeutic level. It also can cause an increase in the metabolism of other medications that are being used concurrently.

    - First-pass effect – Some medications are inactivated on their first pass through the liver and must be given by a nonenteral route because of their high first-pass effect. These medications usually are given by routes such as sublingual or IV.

    - Similar metabolic pathways – When two medications are metabolized by the same pathway, they can interfere with the metabolism of one or both of the medications. In this way, the rate of metabolism can be decreased for one or both of the medications leading to medication accumulation.

    - Nutritional status – A malnourished client may be deficient in the factors that are necessary to produce specific medication-metabolizing enzymes. Consequently, medication metabolism may be impaired.

    Ⓝ NCLEX® Connection: Physiological Adaptations, Pathophysiology

chapter 47

Overview

- The providers who are legally permitted to write prescriptions in the United States include physicians, advanced practice nurses, dentists, and physician assistants. These providers are responsible for:
  - Obtaining the client's medical history and physical examination.
  - Diagnosing.
  - Prescribing medications.
  - Monitoring the response to therapy.
  - Modifying medication prescriptions as necessary.
- Nurses are legally responsible for:
  - Having knowledge of federal, state (nurse practice acts), and local laws, and facility policies that govern the prescribing, dispensing, and administration of medications.
  - Preparing, administering, and evaluating client responses to medications.
  - Developing and maintaining an up-to-date knowledge base of medications administered, including uses, mechanisms of action, routes of administration, safe dosage range, side effects, adverse responses, precautions, and contraindications.
  - Maintaining knowledge of acceptable practice and skill competency.
  - Determining accuracy of medication prescriptions.
  - Reporting all medication errors.
  - Safeguarding and storing medications.

Medication Category and Classification

- Nomenclature
  - Chemical name – Medication is named by its chemical composition.
  - Generic name – Official or nonproprietary name that is given by the United States Adopted Names Council. Each medication has only one generic name.
  - Trade name – Brand or proprietary name that is given by the company that manufacturers the medication. One medication may have multiple trade names.

- Prescription medications are administered under the supervision of providers. These medications can be habit-forming, have potential harmful effects, and/or require supervision.

  ○ Uncontrolled substances – These medications require monitoring by a provider, but do not pose a risk of abuse and/or addiction. Antibiotics are an example of uncontrolled prescription medications.

  ○ Controlled substances – Medications that have a potential for abuse and dependence are categorized into schedules. Heroin is a medication in Schedule I and has no medical use in the United States. Medications categorized in Schedules II through V have approved applications. Each level has a decreasing risk of abuse and dependence. For example, morphine (Duramorph) is a Schedule II medication that has a greater risk of abuse and dependence than phenobarbital (Luminal), which is a Schedule IV medication.

  ○ The U.S. Food and Drug Administration Pregnancy Risk Category (A, B, C, D, X) classifies medications in terms of their potential harm during pregnancy, with Category A being the safest and Category X the most dangerous. Teratogenesis is most likely to occur during the first trimester. Before administering any medication to a woman who is pregnant or could be pregnant, determine whether or not it is safe for administration during pregnancy.

KNOWLEDGE REQUIRED PRIOR TO MEDICATION ADMINISTRATION	
Medication category/class	› Medications are organized according to pharmacologic action, therapeutic use, body system, chemical makeup, and safe use during pregnancy. For example, lisinopril (Zestril) is classified as an angiotensin-converting enzyme inhibitor (pharmacologic action) and an antihypertensive (therapeutic use).
Mechanism of action	› This is how the medication produces the desired therapeutic effect. For example, glipizide (Glucotrol) is an oral hypoglycemic agent. Glipizide lowers blood glucose levels primarily by stimulating pancreatic islet cells to release insulin.
Therapeutic effect	› This is the preferred and expected effect for which the medication is administered to a specific client. One medication may have more than one therapeutic effect. For example, one client is administered acetaminophen (Tylenol) to lower fever, whereas another client is administered this medication to relieve pain.
Side effects	› Usually expected and inevitable when a medication is administered at a therapeutic dose. For example, morphine (Duramorph) given for pain relief usually results in constipation. Side effects are usually identified according to body system.
Adverse effects	› These are undesired, inadvertent, and unexpected dangerous effects of the medication. Adverse effects are usually identified according to body system.
Toxic effects	› Medications can have specific risks and manifestations of toxicity. For example, clients taking digoxin (Lanoxin) should be monitored for dysrhythmias, a manifestation of cardiotoxicity. Hypokalemia places these clients at greater risk for digoxin toxicity.

KNOWLEDGE REQUIRED PRIOR TO MEDICATION ADMINISTRATION	
Medication interactions	› Medications can interact with each other, resulting in desired or undesired effects. For example, a desired interaction is the beta-blocker atenolol (Tenormin) used concurrently with the calcium channel blocker nifedipine (Procardia) to prevent reflex tachycardia. Medications can also increase or decrease the actions of other medications. Obtain a complete medication history and be knowledgeable of clinically significant interactions.
Precautions/ Contraindications	› Medications may be contraindicated for a client who has a specific disease or condition. For example, tetracyclines can stain developing teeth and should not be administered to children under 8 years of age. › Some medications should be used with caution. For example, vancomycin (Vancocin) is excreted unchanged in the kidneys and should be used cautiously for clients who have renal impairment.
Preparation, dosage, administration	› It is important to know any special considerations for preparation, recommended dosages, and how to administer the medication. For example, morphine (Duramorph) is available in 10 different formulations. Oral doses of morphine are generally higher than parenteral doses due to extensive first-pass effect. Clients who have chronic severe pain, as seen with cancer, are generally given oral doses of morphine.
Nursing implications	› Know how to monitor therapeutic effects, prevent and treat adverse effects, provide for comfort, and instruct clients in the safe use of medications.

Medication Prescriptions

- Each facility has written policies related to medication prescriptions. Policies include which providers can write, receive, and transcribe medication prescriptions.

- Types of medication prescriptions include:

  ○ Routine prescription/standard prescription.

    ▪ A routine/standard prescription identifies medications that are given on a regular schedule. It may or may not have a termination date. Without a specified termination date, the prescription will be in effect until the provider discontinues it or the client is discharged.

    ▪ Certain medications, such as opioids and antibiotics, must be represcribed within a specified amount of time or they will automatically be discontinued.

  ○ Single/one-time prescription.

    ▪ A single/one-time prescription is to be administered once at a specified time or as soon as possible. For example, a one-time prescription instructs the nurse to administer warfarin (Coumadin) 5 mg PO at 1700.

  ○ Stat prescription.

    ▪ A stat prescription is only administered once, and it is administered immediately. For example, a stat prescription instructs the nurse to administer digoxin (Lanoxin) 0.125 mg IV bolus stat.

○ PRN prescription.

▪ A PRN prescription stipulates at what dosage, what frequency, and under what conditions a medication may be administered. The nurse uses clinical judgment to determine the client's need for the medication. For example, a PRN prescription instructs the nurse to administer morphine (Duramorph) 2 mg IV bolus every hour PRN for chest pain.

○ Standing prescriptions.

▪ Standing prescriptions may be written for specific circumstances and/or for specific units. For example, the critical care unit has standing prescriptions to treat a client who has asystole.

- Components of a medication prescription

  ○ The client's full name

  ○ The date and time of the prescription

  ○ The name of the medication (may be generic or brand)

  ○ The dosage of the medication

  ○ The route of administration

  ○ The time and frequency of medication administration – exact times or number of times per day (dictated by facility policy or the specific qualities of the medication)

  ○ The signature of the prescribing provider

- Communicating medication prescriptions

  ○ Origination of medication prescriptions

    ▪ Medication prescriptions are written on the client's medical record or entered into the client's electronic medical record by the provider or a nurse who takes a verbal or telephone prescription from a provider. If the nurse writes a medication prescription on the client's medical record, facility policy specifies how much time the provider has in which to sign the prescription. Medication prescriptions are transcribed to the medication administration record (MAR) by a nurse or other health care provider.

  ○ Taking a telephone prescription

    ▪ Ensure that the prescription is complete and correct by reading it back to the provider: the client's name, the name of the medication, the dosage, the time to be given, the frequency, and the route.

    ▪ To ensure correct spelling, use aids such as "b as in boy." State numbers separately, such as "one, seven" for 17.

    ▪ Remind the provider that the prescription must be signed within the specified amount of time.

    ▪ Write or enter the prescription in the client's medical record.

Q̲S̲ - Medication reconciliation

  ○ The Joint Commission requires policies and procedures for medication reconciliation. The nurse compiles a list of current medications, ensuring that all medications are included with correct dosages and frequency. This list is compared with new medication prescriptions and reconciled to resolve any discrepancies. This list becomes the current list from which medications should be administered. This process takes place upon admission, when transferring between units or facilities, and at discharge.

Preassessment for Medication Therapy

- The following information is obtained before initiating medication therapy, and updated as necessary.
  - Health history
    - Age
    - Diagnosed health problems and the current reason for seeking care
    - All medications currently being taken (prescription and nonprescription): the name, dose, route, and frequency of each medication
    - Any unexpected findings possibly related to medication therapy
    - Use of herbal or "natural" products for medicinal purposes
    - Use of caffeine, tobacco, alcohol, and/or street drugs
    - The client's understanding of the purpose of the medications
    - All known medication and food allergies
  - Physical examination – A systematic physical examination provides a baseline to evaluate therapeutic effects of medication therapy and to detect possible side and adverse medication effects.

Six Rights of Safe Medication Administration

- Right client – Verify the client's identification each time a medication is administered. The Joint Commission requires two client identifiers be used when administering medications. Acceptable identifiers include the client's name, an assigned identification number, telephone number, birth date, or other person-specific identifier. Bar code scanners may be used to identify clients. Check for allergies by asking the client, checking for an allergy bracelet, and checking the medication administration record.

- Right medication – Correctly interpret medication prescription (verify completeness and clarity). Read labels three times: when the container is selected, when removing the dose from container, and when the container is replaced. Leave unit-dose medication in its package until administration.

- Right dose – Calculate the correct medication dose; check a drug reference to ensure the dose is within the usual range. Ask another nurse to verify the dose if uncertain of the calculation.

- Right time – Administer medication on time to maintain a consistent therapeutic blood level. It is generally acceptable to administer the medication ½ hr before or after the scheduled time. Refer to the drug reference or facility policy for exceptions.

- Right route – Most common routes of administration are oral, topical, subcutaneous, intramuscular (IM), and intravenous (IV). Select the correct preparation for the ordered route (otic vs. ophthalmic topical ointment or drops). Know how to administer medication safely and correctly.

- Right documentation – Immediately record pertinent information, including the client's response to the medication. Document the medication after administration, not before.

Additional Considerations

- Assessment – Appropriate data is collected before administering medication (apical heart rate before giving digitalis preparations). Assess the client for physical and psychosocial factors that may affect medication response.

- Education – As part of informed consent, provide accurate information about the medication therapy and its implications (therapeutic response, side/adverse effects). To individualize the teaching, determine what the client already knows about the medication, needs to know about the medication, and wants to know about the medication.

- Evaluation – Determine the effectiveness of the medication based on the client's response, as well as the occurrence of side/adverse effects.

- Medication refusal – Clients have the right to refuse a medication. Determine the reason for refusal, provide information regarding the risk of refusal, notify appropriate health care personnel, and document the refusal and actions taken.

- Resources for medication information
  - Nursing drug handbooks
  - Pharmacology textbooks
  - Professional journals
  - *The Physicians' Desk Reference* (PDR)
  - Professional Web sites

Medication Error Prevention

- Common medication errors
  - Wrong medication or IV fluid
  - Incorrect dose or IV rate
  - Wrong client, route, or time
  - Administration of known allergic medication
  - Omission of dose
  - Incorrect discontinuation of medication or IV fluid

- The Institute for Safe Medication Practices (ISMP) is a nonprofit organization working to educate health care providers and consumers regarding safe medication practices. The ISMP and the U.S. Food and Drug Administration (FDA) identify the most common medical abbreviations that result in misinterpretation, mistakes, and injury. A complete list can be found at the organization's Web site (www.ismp.org).
  - Error-Prone Abbreviation List – Certain abbreviations are associated with a high number of medication errors.

DO NOT USE	USE
MS, MSO$_4$	morphine sulfate
MgSO$_4$	magnesium sulfate
abbreviated medicine names (e.g., SSI, SSRI, HCL, HCT)	full name of drug or spell out sliding scale insulin, sliding scale regular insulin
naked decimal or decimal points without a leading zero (e.g., .5 mg)	smaller units (e.g., 500 micrograms) or a leading zero (e.g., 0.5 mg)
trailing zero (e.g., 1.0 mg, 100.0 g)	without a trailing zero (e.g., 1 mg, 100 g)
u, U or IU	units
μ, μg	mcg or microgram
cc	mL
apothecary units	use metric units
od, O.D., OD	daily or intended time of administration
q.d, qd, Q.D, QD, q1d, i/d	daily
q.o.d., QOD	every other day
Q6PM, etc.	6 PM daily or daily at 6 PM
TIW or tiw	3 times weekly
UD	as directed
HS	half-strength
BT, hs, HS, qhs, qn	bedtime or hour of sleep
SC , SQ, sub q	subcut or subcutaneously
IN	intranasal or NAS
IJ	injection
ss	sliding scale, one half
> or <	"greater than" or "less than"
@	at
& or +	and
/	per
AD, AS, AU	right ear, left ear, both ears
OD, OS, OU	right eye, left eye, both eyes
D/C, dc, d/c	discharge or discontinue

○ Confused Medication Name List – Sound-alike and look-alike medication names.

ESTABLISHED NAME	RECOMMENDED NAME	ESTABLISHED NAME	RECOMMENDED NAME
Acetohexamide	AcetoHEXAMIDE	Hydralazine	HydrALAZINE
Acetazolamide	AcetaZOLAMIDE	Hydromorphone	HYDROmorphone
Bupropion	BuPROPion	Hydroxyzine	HydrOXYzine
Buspirone	BusPIRone	Medroxyprogesterone	MedroxyPROGESTERone
Chlorpromazine	ChlorproMAZINE	Methylprednisolone	MethylPREDNISolone
Chlorpropamide	ChlorproPAMIDE	Methyltestosterone	MethylTESTOSTERone
Clomiphene	ClomiPHENE	Mitoxantrone	MitoXANTRONE
Clomipramine	ClomiPRAMINE	Nicardipine	NiCARdipine
Cyclosporine	CycloSPORINE	Nifedipine	NIFEdipine
Cycloserine	CycloSERINE	Prednisone	PredniSONE
Daunorubicin	DAUNOrubicin	Prednisolone	PrednisoLONE
Doxorubicin	DOXOrubicin	Risperidone	risperiDONE
Dimenhydrinate	DimenhyDRINATE	Ropinirole	rOPINIRole
Diphenhydramine	DiphenhydrAMINE	Sulfadiazine	SulfADIAZINE
Dobutamine	DOBUTamine	Sulfisoxazole	SulfiSOXAZOLE
Dopamine	DOPamine	Tolazamide	TOLAZamide
Glipizide	GlipiZIDE	Tolbutamide	TOLBUTamide
Glyburide	GlyBURIDE	Vinblastine	VinBLAStine
		Vincristine	VinCRIStine

 View Video: Look-Alike, Sound-Alike Medications

○ High-Alert Medication List – The following 30 drugs and drug categories require special safeguards to reduce the risk of errors. Strategies include limiting access; using auxiliary labels/automated alerts; standardizing the prescription, preparation, and administration; and using automated or independent double checks.

  ▪ Class/Category of Medications

    □ Adrenergic agonists, IV (e.g., epinephrine)

    □ Adrenergic antagonists, IV (e.g., propranolol)

    □ Anesthetic agents, general, inhaled and IV (e.g., propofol)

    □ Cardioplegic solutions

    □ Chemotherapeutic agents, parenteral and oral

    □ Dextrose, hypertonic, 20% or greater

    □ Dialysis solutions, peritoneal and hemodialysis

    □ Epidural or intrathecal medications

    □ Glycoprotein IIb/IIIa inhibitors (e.g., eptifibatide)

    □ Hypoglycemics, oral

- □ Inotropic medications, IV (e.g., digoxin, milrinone)
- □ Liposomal forms of drugs (e.g., liposomal amphotericin B)
- □ Moderate sedation agents, IV (e.g., midazolam)
- □ Moderate sedation agents, oral, for children (e.g., chloral hydrate)
- □ Narcotics/opiates, IV and oral (including liquid concentrates, immediate- and sustained- release)
- □ Neuromuscular blocking agents (e.g., succinylcholine)
- □ Radiocontrast agents, IV
- □ Thrombolytics/fibrinolytics, IV (e.g., tenecteplase)
- □ Total parenteral nutrition solutions
  - Specific Medications
    - □ IV amiodarone
    - □ Colchicine injection
    - □ Heparin, low molecular weight, injection
    - □ Heparin, unfractionated, IV
    - □ Insulin, subcutaneous and IV
    - □ IV lidocaine
    - □ Magnesium sulfate injection
    - □ Methotrexate, oral, nononcologic use
    - □ Nesiritide
    - □ Nitroprusside, sodium, for injection
    - □ Potassium chloride for injection concentrate
    - □ Potassium phosphates injection
    - □ Sodium chloride injection, hypertonic, more than 0.9% concentration
    - □ Warfarin
- Use the nursing process to prevent medication errors.
  - ○ Assessment/Data Collection
    - Ensure knowledge of medication to be administered and why the client is receiving it.
    - Obtain information about the client's medical diagnoses and conditions related to medication administration, such as the ability to swallow, allergies, heart, liver, and/or kidney disorders.
      - □ Identify the client's allergies.
      - □ Obtain necessary preadministration data (heart rate, blood pressure) to assess appropriateness of medication and obtain baseline data to evaluate effectiveness of medication.
      - □ Omit or delay doses as indicated by the client's condition.
    - Determine if the medication prescription is complete – To include the client's name, date and time, name of medication, dosage, route of administration, time and frequency, and signature of the prescribing provider.
    - Interpret the medication prescription accurately. Refer to the ISMP lists.

- Question the provider if the prescription is unclear or seems inappropriate for the client's condition. Refuse to administer a medication if it is believed to be unsafe. Notify the charge nurse or supervisor.

- Dosage changes are usually made gradually. Question the provider if abrupt and excessive changes in dosages are made.

- Planning

  - Identify client outcomes for medication administration.

  - Set priorities.

- Implementation

  - Avoid distractions during medication preparation (poor lighting, phones). Interruptions may increase the risk of error.

  - Prepare medications for one person at a time.

  - Check the labels for the medication name and concentration. Read labels carefully. Measure doses accurately, and double-check high-alert medications such as insulin and heparin with a colleague. Check the medication expiration date.

  - Doses are usually one to two tablets or one single-dose vial. Question multiple tablets or vials for a single dose.

  - Follow the six rights of medication administration consistently. Take the MAR to the bedside.

  - Only give medications that have been personally prepared.

  - Encourage clients to become part of the safety net, teaching them about medications and the importance of proper identification before medications are administered. Omit or delay a dose if the client questions the size of the dose or the appearance of the medication.

  - Follow correct procedures for all routes of administration.

  - Communicate clearly both in writing and speaking.

  - Use verbal prescriptions only for emergencies, and follow facility protocol for telephone prescriptions.

  - Omit or delay doses as indicated by the client's condition, and document and report appropriately.

  - Follow all laws and regulations regarding controlled substances when preparing and administering medications. Keep controlled substances in a locked area. Discarding an excess of a controlled substance must be witnessed by a licensed health care provider.

  - Only leave medications at a client's bedside if allowed by facility policy, such as topical medications.

○ Evaluation

- Evaluate the client's response to a medication, and document and report appropriately.

- Recognize side/adverse effects, and document and report appropriately.

- Report all errors, and implement corrective measures immediately.

  □ Complete an unusual occurrence report within the specified time frame, usually 24 hr. This report should include the client's identification, the time and place of the incident, an accurate account of the event, who was notified, what actions were taken, and the signature of the person completing the report. This report does not become a part of the client's permanent record, and the report should not be referenced in another part of the record.

  □ Medication errors can be related to systems, procedures, product design, or practice patterns. Report all errors to assist the facility to learn how errors occur and what changes are needed to avoid similar errors in the future.

APPLICATION EXERCISES

1. A nurse prepares an injection of morphine (Duramorph) to administer to a client who reports pain. Prior to administering the medication, the nurse is called to another room to assist another client onto a bedpan. She asks a second nurse to give the injection. Which of the following actions should the second nurse take?

    A. Offer to assist the client needing the bedpan.

    B. Administer the injection prepared by the other nurse.

    C. Prepare another syringe and administer the injection.

    D. Tell the client needing the bedpan she will have to wait for her nurse.

2. A nurse is preparing to administer a medication to a client. The medication was scheduled for administration at 0900. Which of the following are acceptable administration times for this medication? (Select all that apply.)

    _____ A. 0905

    _____ B. 0825

    _____ C. 1000

    _____ D. 0840

    _____ E. 0935

3. A nurse is working with a newly hired nurse who is administering medications to clients. Which of the following actions by the newly hired nurse indicates an understanding of medication error prevention?

    A. Taking all medications out of the unit-dose wrappers before entering the client's room

    B. Checking with the provider when a single dose requires administration of multiple tablets

    C. Administering a medication, then looking up the usual dosage range

    D. Relying on another nurse to clarify a medication prescription

4. A nurse educator is teaching a module on safe medication administration to newly hired nurses. Which of the following statements by a newly hired nurse indicate understanding of the nurse's responsibility when implementing medication therapy? (Select all that apply.)

    _____ A. "I will observe for medication side effects."

    _____ B. "I will monitor for therapeutic effects."

    _____ C. "I will prescribe the appropriate dose."

    _____ D. "I will change the dose if adverse effects occur."

    _____ E. "I will refuse to give a medication if I believe it is unsafe."

5. A nurse is preparing to administer digoxin (Lanoxin) to a client who states, "I don't want to take that medication. I do not want one more pill." Which of the following responses by the nurse is appropriate in this situation?

    A. "Your physician prescribed it for you, so you really should take it."

    B. "Well, let's just get it over quickly then."

    C. "Okay, I'll just give you your other medications."

    D. "Tell me your concerns with taking this medication."

6. A nurse educator is teaching a module on the six rights of safe medication administration to a group of newly licensed nurses. Use the ATI Active Learning Template: Basic Concept to complete this item to include the following:

    A. Related Content: List the six rights of safe medication administration.

    B. Underlying Principles: List at least three acceptable identifiers that can be used to verify the client's identification.

APPLICATION EXERCISES KEY

1. A. **CORRECT:** The second nurse should offer to assist the client needing the bedpan. This will allow the nurse who prepared the injection to administer it.

    B. INCORRECT: A nurse should only administer medications that he prepared.

    C. INCORRECT: Preparing another syringe will delay the administration of the pain medication.

    D. INCORRECT: Telling the client to wait is not an acceptable option for a client needing a bedpan.

    (N) NCLEX® Connection: Management of Care, Legal Rights and Responsibilities

2. A. **CORRECT:** A medication should be administered within 30 min of the scheduled time. 0905 is within 30 min of a scheduled administration time of 0900.

    B. INCORRECT: 0825 is not within 30 min of a scheduled administration time of 0900.

    C. INCORRECT: 1000 is not within 30 min of a scheduled administration time of 0900.

    D. **CORRECT:** 0840 is within 30 min of a scheduled administration time of 0900.

    E. INCORRECT: 0935 is not within 30 min of a scheduled administration time of 0900.

    (N) NCLEX® Connection: Pharmacological and Parenteral Therapies, Medication Administration

3. A. INCORRECT: The nurse should not take unit-dose medications out of wrappers until at the bedside when performing the third check of medication administration. This prevents errors. The nurse can encourage client involvement and provide teaching at this time.

    B. **CORRECT:** If a single dose requires multiple tablets, it is possible that an error has occurred in the transcription of the medication. This action could prevent a medication error.

    C. INCORRECT: Reviewing usual dosage range prior to adminstration may uncover an inaccurate dosage.

    D. INCORRECT: If the prescription is unclear, the nurse should contact the provider for clarification, not another nurse.

    (N) NCLEX® Connection: Pharmacological and Parenteral Therapies, Medication Administration

4.   A. **CORRECT:** The nurse is responsible for observing for medication side effects. This is within a nurse's scope of practice.

   B. **CORRECT:** The nurse is responsible for monitoring for therapeutic effects. This is within a nurse's scope of practice.

   C. INCORRECT: The provider, not the nurse, is responsible for prescribing the appropriate dose. This is outside of the nurse's scope of practice.

   D. INCORRECT: The provider, not the nurse, is responsible for changing the dose if adverse effects occur. This is outside of the nurse's scope of practice.

   E. **CORRECT:** The nurse is responsible for recognizing if a medication could potentially harm a client. It is within the nurse's scope of practice to refuse to administer the medication and contact the provider.

    NCLEX® Connection: Pharmacological and Parenteral Therapies, Expected Actions/Outcomes

5.   A. INCORRECT: This response is dismissive of the client's concerns.

   B. INCORRECT: The nurse is dismissing the client's concerns about taking the medication by continuing with medication administration.

   C. INCORRECT: Although clients have the right to refuse a medication, the nurse should provide information regarding the risk of refusal instead of proceeding with medication administration.

   D. **CORRECT:** Although clients have the right to refuse a medication, the nurse is correct in determining the reason for refusal by asking the client his concerns. After gathering the client's concerns, the nurse can provide information regarding the risk of refusal and provide information for an informed decision. At that point, if the client still exercises his right to refuse a medication, the nurse should notify appropriate personnel and document the refusal and actions taken.

    NCLEX® Connection: Management of Care, Client Rights

6. *Using the ATI Active Learning Template: Basic Concept*

    A. Related Content: Six Rights of Safe Medication Administration

- Right client – Verify the client's identification each time a medication is given. The Joint Commission requires that the nurse use two client identifiers when administering medications.

- Right medication – Correctly interpret medication prescription (verify completeness and clarity). Read labels three times: when the container is selected, when removing the dose from container, and when the container is replaced.

- Right dose – Calculate the correct medication dose; check a drug reference to ensure the dose is within the usual range. Ask another nurse to verify the dose if uncertain of the calculation.

- Right time – Administer medication on time to maintain a consistent therapeutic blood level. It is generally acceptable to administer the medication 1/2 hr before or after the scheduled time. Refer to the drug reference or facility policy for exceptions.

- Right route – Most common routes of administration are oral, topical, subcutaneous, intramuscular (IM), and intravenous (IV). Select the correct preparation for the ordered route. Know how to administer medication safely and correctly.

- Right documentation – Immediately record pertinent information, including the client's response to the medication. Document the medication after administration, not before.

    B. Underlying Principles

- Acceptable identifiers include the client's name, an assigned identification number, telephone number, birth date, or other person-specific identifier.

- The nurse can use bar code scanners to identify clients.

    (N) NCLEX® Connection: Pharmacological and Parenteral Therapies, Medication Administration

chapter 48

Overview

- Basic medication dose conversion and calculation skills are essential to the provision of safe nursing care.
- Nurses are responsible for administering the correct amount of medication by calculating the appropriate amount of medication to give. Types of calculations required include:
  - Solid oral medication
  - Liquid oral medication
  - Injectable medication
  - Correct dose based on the client's weight
  - IV infusion
- Nurses can use three different methods for dosage calculation. These are ratio and proportion, desired over have, and dimensional analysis.
- Standard conversion factors include:
  - 1 mg = 1,000 mcg
  - 1 g = 1,000 mg
  - 1 kg = 1,000 g
  - 1 oz = 30 mL
  - 1 L = 1,000 mL
  - 1 tsp = 5 mL
  - 1 tbsp = 15 mL
  - 1 tbsp = 3 tsp
  - 1 kg = 2.2 lb
  - 1 gr = 60 mg
- General Rounding Guidelines
  - Rounding up: If the number to the right is equal to or greater than 5, round up by adding 1 to the number on the left.
  - Rounding down: If the number to the right is less than 5, round down by dropping the number, leaving the number to the left as is.
  - For dosages less than 1.0, round to the nearest hundredth.
    - For example (rounding up): 0.746 mL = 0.75 mL. The calculated dose is 0.746 mL. Look at the number in the thousandths place (6). Six is greater than 5. To round to hundredths, add 1 to 4 in the hundredths place and drop the 6. The rounded dose is 0.75 mL.
    - Or (rounding down): 0.743 mL = 0.74 mL. The calculated dose is 0.743 mL. Look at the number in the thousandths place (3). Three is less than 5. To round to the hundredth, drop the 3 and leave the 4 as is. The rounded dose is 0.74 mL.

○ For dosages greater than 1.0, round to the nearest tenth.

- For example (rounding up): 1.38 = 1.4. The calculated dose is 1.38 mg. Look at the number in the hundredths place (8). Eight is greater than 5. To round to the tenth, add 1 to the 3 in the tenth place and drop the 8. The rounded dose is 1.4 mg.

- Or (rounding down): 1.34 mL = 1.3 mL. The calculated dose is 1.34 mL. Look at the number in the hundredths place (4). Four is less than 5. To round to the tenth, drop the 4 and leave the 3 as is. The rounded dose is 1.3 mL.

SOLID DOSAGE

Example: A nurse is preparing to administer phenytoin (Dilantin) 0.2 g PO every 8 hr. The amount available is phenytoin 100 mg/capsule. How many capsules should the nurse administer per dose? (Round the answer to the nearest whole number.)

Using Ratio and Proportion

STEP 1: *What is the unit of measurement to calculate?*
cap

STEP 2: *What is the dose needed? Dose needed = Desired.*
0.2 g

STEP 3: *What is the dose available? Dose available = Have.*
200 mg

STEP 4: *Should the nurse convert the units of measurement?*
Yes (g ≠ mg)
Equivalents:
1 g = 1,000 mg (1 x 1,000)
0.2 g = 200 mg (0.2 x 1,000)

STEP 5: *What is the quantity of the dose available?*
1 cap

STEP 6: *Set up an equation and solve for X.*

$$\frac{Have}{Quantity} = \frac{Desired}{X}$$

$$\frac{100 \text{ mg}}{1 \text{ cap}} = \frac{200 \text{ mg}}{X \text{ cap(s)}}$$

X = 2

STEP 7: *Round if necessary.*

STEP 8: *Reassess to determine whether the amount to give makes sense.*
If there are 100 mg caps and the prescribed amount is 0.2 g (200 mg), it makes sense to give 2 caps. The nurse should administer phenytoin 2 caps PO every 8 hr.

Using Desired Over Have

STEP 1: *What is the unit of measurement to calculate?*
cap

STEP 2: *What is the dose needed? Dose needed = Desired.*
0.2 g

STEP 3: *What is the dose available? Dose available = Have.*
200 mg

STEP 4: *Should the nurse convert the units of measurement?*
Yes (g ≠ mg)
Equivalents:
1 g = 1,000 mg (1 x 1,000)
0.2 g = 200 mg (0.2 x 1,000)

STEP 5: *What is the quantity of the dose available?*
1 cap

STEP 6: *Set up an equation and solve for X.*

$$\frac{Desired \times Quantity}{Have} = X$$

$$\frac{200 \text{ mg} \times 1 \text{ cap}}{100 \text{ mg}} = X \text{ cap(s)}$$

2 = X

STEP 7: *Round if necessary.*

STEP 8: *Reassess to determine whether the amount to give makes sense.*
If there are 100 mg caps and the prescribed amount is 0.2 g (200 mg), it makes sense to give 2 caps. The nurse should administer phenytoin 2 caps PO every 8 hr.

Using Dimensional Analysis

STEP 1: *What is the unit of measurement to calculate?*
cap

STEP 2: *What quantity of the dose is available?*
1 cap

STEP 3: *What is the dose available? Dose available = Have.*
100 mg

STEP 4: *What is the dose needed? Dose needed = Desired.*
0.2 g

STEP 5: *Should the nurse convert the units of measurement?*
Yes (g ≠ mg)
1,000 mg = 1 g

STEP 6: *Set up an equation and solve for X.*

$$X = \frac{Quantity}{Have} \times \frac{Conversion\ (Have)}{Conversion\ (Desired)} \times \frac{Desired}{}$$

$$X\ cap\,(s) = \frac{1\ cap}{100\ mg} \times \frac{1,000\ mg}{1\ g} \times \frac{0.2\ g}{}$$

$$X = 2$$

STEP 7: *Round if necessary.*

STEP 8: *Reassess to determine whether the amount to give makes sense.*
If there are 100 mg caps and the prescribed amount is 0.2 g (200 mg), it makes sense to give 2 caps.
The nurse should administer phenytoin 2 caps PO every 8 hr.

LIQUID DOSAGE

Example: A nurse is preparing to administer erythromycin estolate 0.25 g PO every 6 hr. The amount available is erythromycin estolate oral suspension 250 mg/mL. How many mL should the nurse administer per dose? (Round the answer to the nearest whole number.)

Using Ratio and Proportion

STEP 1: *What is the unit of measurement to calculate?*
mL

STEP 2: *What is the dose needed? Dose needed = Desired.*
0.25 g

STEP 3: *What is the dose available? Dose available = Have.*
250 mg

STEP 4: *Should the nurse convert the units of measurement?*
Yes (g ≠ mg)
Equivalents:
1 g = 1,000 mg (1 x 1,000)
0.25 g = 250 mg (0.25 x 1,000)

STEP 5: *What is the quantity of the dose available?*
1 mL

STEP 6: *Set up an equation and solve for X.*

$$\frac{Have}{Quantity} = \frac{Desired}{X}$$

$$\frac{250\ mg}{1\ mL} = \frac{250\ mg}{X\ mL}$$

$$X = 1$$

STEP 7: *Round if necessary.*

STEP 8: *Reassess to determine whether the amount to give makes sense.*
If there are 250 mg/mL and the prescribed amount is 0.25 g (250 mg), it makes sense to administer 1 mL. The nurse should administer erythromycin estolate oral suspension 1 mL PO every 6 hr.

Using Desired Over Have

STEP 1: *What is the unit of measurement to calculate?*
mL

STEP 2: *What is the dose needed? Dose needed = Desired.*
0.25 g

STEP 3: *What is the dose available? Dose available = Have.*
250 mg

STEP 4: *Should the nurse convert the units of measurement?*
Yes (g ≠ mg)
Equivalents:
1 g = 1,000 mg (1 x 1,000)
0.25 g = 250 mg (0.25 x 1,000)

STEP 5: *What is the quantity of the dose available?*
1 mL

STEP 6: *Set up an equation and solve for X.*

$$\frac{\text{Desired x Quantity}}{\text{Have}} = X$$

$$\frac{250 \text{ mg x 1 mL}}{250 \text{ mg}} = X \text{ mL}$$

1 = X

STEP 7: *Round if necessary.*

STEP 8: *Reassess to determine whether the amount to give makes sense.*
If there are 250 mg/mL and the prescribed amount is 0.25 g (250 mg), it makes sense to administer 1 mL. The nurse should administer erythromycin estolate oral suspension 1 mL PO every 6 hr.

Using Dimensional Analysis

STEP 1: *What is the unit of measurement to calculate?*
mL

STEP 2: *What quantity of the dose is available?*
1 mL

STEP 3: *What is the dose available? Dose available = Have.*
250 mg

STEP 4: *What is the dose needed? Dose needed = Desired.*
0.25 g

STEP 5: *Should the nurse convert the units of measurement?*
Yes (g ≠ mg)

$$\frac{1,000 \text{ mg}}{1 \text{ g}}$$

STEP 6: *Set up an equation and solve for X.*

$$X = \frac{\text{Quantity}}{\text{Have}} \times \frac{\text{Conversion (Have)}}{\text{Conversion (Desired)}} \times \frac{\text{Desired}}{}$$

$$X \text{ mL} = \frac{1 \text{ mL}}{250 \text{ mg}} \times \frac{1,000 \text{ mg}}{1 \text{ g}} \times \frac{0.25 \text{ g}}{}$$

X = 1

STEP 7: *Round if necessary.*

STEP 8: *Reassess to determine whether the amount administer makes sense.*
If there are 250 mg/mL and the prescribed amount is 0.25 g (250 mg), it makes sense to administer 1 mL. The nurse should administer erythromycin estolate oral suspension 1 mL PO every 6 hr.

INJECTABLE DOSAGE

Example: A nurse is preparing to administer heparin 8,000 units subcutaneously every 12 hr. The amount available is heparin injection 10,000 units/mL. How many mL should the nurse administer per dose? (Round the answer to the nearest tenth.)

Using Ratio and Proportion

STEP 1: *What is the unit of measurement to calculate?*
mL

STEP 2: *What is the dose needed? Dose needed = Desired.*
8,000 units

STEP 3: *What is the dose available? Dose available = Have.*
10,000 units

STEP 4: *Should the nurse convert the units of measurement?*
No

STEP 5: *What is the quantity of the dose available?*
1 mL

STEP 6: *Set up an equation and solve for X.*

$$\frac{\text{Have}}{\text{Quantity}} = \frac{\text{Desired}}{X}$$

$$\frac{10,000 \text{ units}}{1 \text{ mL}} = \frac{8,000 \text{ units}}{X \text{ mL}}$$

$$X = 0.8$$

STEP 7: *Round if necessary.*

STEP 8: *Reassess to determine whether the amount to administer makes sense.*
If there are 10,000 units/mL and the prescribed amount is 8,000 units, it makes sense to administer 0.8 mL. The nurse should administer heparin injection 0.8 mL subcutaneously every 12 hr.

Using Desired Over Have

STEP 1: *What is the unit of measurement to calculate?*
mL

STEP 2: *What is the dose needed? Dose needed = Desired.*
8,000 units

STEP 3: *What is the dose available? Dose available = Have.*
10,000 units

STEP 4: *Should the nurse convert the units of measurement?*
No

STEP 5: *What is the quantity of the dose available?*
1 mL

STEP 6: *Set up an equation and solve for X.*

$$\frac{\text{Desired} \times \text{Quantity}}{\text{Have}} = X$$

$$\frac{8,000 \text{ units} \times 1 \text{ mL}}{10,000 \text{ units}} = X \text{ mL}$$

$$0.8 = X$$

STEP 7: *Round if necessary.*

STEP 8: *Reassess to determine whether the amount to administer makes sense.*
If there are 10,000 units/mL and the prescribed amount is 8,000 units, it makes sense to administer 0.8 mL. The nurse should administer heparin injection 0.8 mL subcutaneously every 12 hr.

Using Dimensional Analysis

STEP 1: *What is the unit of measurement to calculate?*
mL

STEP 2: *What quantity of the dose is available?*
1 mL

STEP 3: *What is the dose available? Dose available = Have.*
10,000 units

STEP 4: *What is the dose needed? Dose needed = Desired.*
8,000 units

STEP 5: *Should the nurse convert the units of measurement?*
No

STEP 6: *Set up an equation and solve for X.*

$$X = \frac{\text{Quantity}}{\text{Have}} \times \frac{\text{Conversion (Have)}}{\text{Conversion (Desired)}} \times \frac{\text{Desired}}{}$$

$$X \text{ mL} = \frac{1 \text{ mL}}{10,000 \text{ units}} \times \frac{8,000 \text{ units}}{}$$

$$X = 0.8$$

STEP 7: *Round if necessary.*

STEP 8: *Reassess to determine whether the amount to administer makes sense.*
If there are 10,000 units/mL and the prescribed amount is 8,000 units, it makes sense to administer 0.8 mL. The nurse should administer heparin injection 0.8 mL subcutaneously every 12 hr.

DOSAGES BY WEIGHT

Example: A nurse is preparing to administer cefixime (Suprax) 8 mg/kg/day PO divided in equal doses every 12 hr to a toddler who weighs 22 lb. The amount available is cefixime suspension 100 mg/5 mL. How many mL should the nurse administer per dose? (Round the answer to the nearest whole number.)

Using Ratio and Proportion

STEP 1: *What is the unit of measurement to calculate?*
kg

STEP 2: *Set up an equation and solve for X.*

$$\frac{2.2 \text{ lb}}{1 \text{ kg}} = \frac{\text{Client weight in lb}}{X \text{ kg}}$$

$$\frac{2.2 \text{ lb}}{1 \text{ kg}} = \frac{22 \text{ lb}}{X \text{ kg}}$$

X = 10

STEP 3: *Round if necessary.*

STEP 4: *Reassess to determine whether the equivalent makes sense.*
If 1 kg = 2.2 lb, it makes sense that 22 lb = 10 kg.

STEP 5: *What is the unit of measurement to calculate?*
mg

STEP 6: *Set up an equation and solve for X.*
mg x kg/day = X
8 mg x 10 kg = 80 mg

STEP 7: *Round if necessary.*

STEP 8: *Reassess to determine whether the amount makes sense.* If the prescribed amount is 8 mg/kg/day divided in equal doses every 12 hr and the toddler weighs 10 kg, it makes sense to give 80 mg/day, or 40 mg every 12 hr.

STEP 9: *What is the unit of measurement to calculate?*
mL

STEP 10: *What is the dose needed? Dose needed = Desired.*
40 mg

STEP 11: *What is the dose available? Dose available = Have.*
100 mg

STEP 12: *Should the nurse convert the units of measurement?*
No

STEP 13: *What is the quantity of the dose available?*
5 mL

STEP 14: *Set up an equation and solve for X.*

$$\frac{\text{Have}}{\text{Quantity}} = \frac{\text{Desired}}{X}$$

$$\frac{100 \text{ mg}}{5 \text{ mL}} = \frac{40 \text{ mg}}{X \text{ mL}}$$

X = 2

STEP 15: *Round if necessary.*

STEP 16: *Reassess to determine whether the amount to give makes sense.*
If there are 100 mg/5 mL and the prescribed amount is 40 mg, it makes sense to give 2 mL. The nurse should administer cefixime suspension 2 mL PO every 12 hr.

Using Desired Over Have

STEP 1: *What is the unit of measurement to calculate?*
kg

STEP 2: *Set up an equation and solve for X.*

$$\frac{2.2 \text{ lb}}{1 \text{ kg}} = \frac{\text{Client weight in lb}}{X \text{ kg}}$$

$$\frac{2.2 \text{ lb}}{1 \text{ kg}} = \frac{22 \text{ lb}}{X \text{ kg}}$$

X = 10

STEP 3: *Round if necessary.*

STEP 4: *Reassess to determine whether the equivalent makes sense.*
If 1 kg = 2.2 lb, it makes sense that 22 lb = 10 kg.

STEP 5: *What is the unit of measurement to calculate?*
mg

STEP 6: *Set up an equation and solve for X.*
mg x kg/day = X
8 mg x 10 kg = 80 mg

STEP 7: *Round if necessary.*

STEP 8: *Reassess to determine whether the amount makes sense.*
If the prescribed amount is 8 mg/kg/day divided in equal doses every 12 hr and the toddler weighs 10 kg, it makes sense to give 80 mg/day, or 40 mg every 12 hr.

STEP 9: *What is the unit of measurement to calculate?*
mL

STEP 10: *What is the dose needed? Dose needed = Desired.*
40 mg

STEP 11: *What is the dose available? Dose available = Have.*
100 mg

STEP 12: *Should the nurse convert the units of measurement?*
No

STEP 13: *What is the quantity of the dose available?*
5 mL

STEP 14: *Set up an equation and solve for X.*

$$\frac{\text{Desired x Quantity}}{\text{Have}} = X$$

$$\frac{40 \text{ mg x 5 mL}}{100 \text{ mg}} = X \text{ mL}$$

2 = X

STEP 15: *Round if necessary.*

STEP 16: *Reassess to determine whether the amount to give makes sense.*
If there are 100 mg/5 mL and the prescribed amount is 40 mg, it makes sense to give 2 mL. The nurse should administer cefixime suspension 2 mL PO every 12 hr.

Using Dimensional Analysis

STEP 1: *What is the unit of measurement to calculate?*
kg

STEP 2: *Set up an equation and solve for X.*

$$\frac{2.2 \text{ lb}}{1 \text{ kg}} = \frac{\text{Client weight in lb}}{X \text{ kg}}$$

$$\frac{2.2 \text{ lb}}{1 \text{ kg}} = \frac{22 \text{ lb}}{X \text{ kg}}$$

X = 10

STEP 3: *Round if necessary.*

STEP 4: *Reassess to determine whether the equivalent makes sense.*
If 1 kg = 2.2 lb, it makes sense that 22 lb = 10 kg.

STEP 5: *What is the unit of measurement to calculate?*
mg

STEP 6: *Set up an equation and solve for X.*
mg x kg/day = X
8 mg x 10 kg = 80 mg

STEP 7: *Round if necessary.*

STEP 8: *Reassess to determine whether the amount makes sense.*
If the prescribed amount is 8 mg/kg/day divided in equal doses every 12 hr and the toddler weighs 10 kg, it makes sense to give 80 mg/day, or 40 mg every 12 hr.

STEP 9: *What is the unit of measurement to calculate?*
mL

STEP 10: *What quantity of the dose is available?*
1 mL

STEP 11: *What is the dose available? Dose available = Have.*
100 mg

STEP 12: *What is the dose needed? Dose needed = Desired.*
40 mg

STEP 13: *Should the nurse convert the units of measurement?*
No

STEP 14: *Set up an equation and solve for X.*

$$X = \frac{\text{Quantity}}{\text{Have}} \times \frac{\text{Conversion (Have)}}{\text{Conversion (Desired)}} \times \frac{\text{Desired}}{}$$

$$X \text{ mL} = \frac{5 \text{ mL}}{100 \text{ mg}} \times \frac{40 \text{ mg}}{}$$

X = 2

STEP 15: *Round if necessary.*

STEP 16: *Reassess to determine whether the amount to give makes sense.*
If there are 100 mg/5 mL and the prescribed amount is 40 mg, it makes sense to give 2 mL. The nurse should administer cefixime suspension 2 mL PO every 12 hr.

IV FLOW RATES

- Nurses calculate IV flow rates for large-volume continuous IV infusions and intermittent IV bolus infusions using electronic infusion pumps (mL/hr) and manual IV tubing (gtt/min).

- IV infusions using electronic infusion pumps

  ○ Infusion pumps control an accurate rate of fluid infusion. Infusion pumps are able to deliver a specified amount of fluid during a specified amount of time. For example, an infusion pump can deliver 150 mL in 1 hr or 50 mL in 15 min.

Example: A nurse is preparing to administer dextrose 5% in water (D_5W) 500 mL IV to infuse over 4 hr. The nurse should set the IV infusion pump to deliver how many mL/hr? (Round the answer to the nearest whole number.)

Using Ratio and Proportion, Desired Over Have, and Dimensional Analysis

STEP 1: *What is the unit of measurement to calculate?*
mL/hr

STEP 2: *What is the volume needed? Volume needed = Volume.*
500 mL

STEP 3: *What is the total infusion time? Time available = Time.*
4 hr

STEP 4: *Should the nurse convert the units of measurement?*
No

STEP 5: *Set up an equation and solve for X.*

$$\frac{Volume\ (mL)}{Time\ (hr)} = X$$

$$\frac{500\ mL}{4\ hr} = X\ mL/hr$$

$$125 = X$$

STEP 6: *Round if necessary.*

STEP 7: *Reassess to determine whether the IV flow rate makes sense.*
If the amount prescribed is 500 mL to infuse 4 hr, it makes sense to administer 125 mL/hr. The nurse should set the IV pump to deliver D_5W 500 mL IV at 125 mL/hr.

Example: A nurse is preparing to administer cefotaxime (Claforan) 1 g intermittent IV bolus. Available is cefotaxime 1 g in 100 mL of 0.9% sodium chloride (0.9% NaCl) to infuse over 45 min. The nurse should set the IV infusion pump to deliver how many mL/hr? (Round the answer to the nearest whole number.)

Using Ratio and Proportion, Desired Over Have, and Dimensional Analysis

STEP 1: *What is the unit of measurement to calculate?*
mL/hr

STEP 2: *What is the volume needed? Volume needed = Volume.*
100 mL

STEP 3: *What is the total infusion time? Time available = Time.*
45 min

STEP 4: *Should the nurse convert the units of measurement?*
No (mL = mL)
Yes (min ≠ hr)

$$\frac{1\ hr}{60\ min} = \frac{X\ hr}{45\ min}$$

$$X = 0.75$$

STEP 5: *Set up an equation and solve for X.*

$$\frac{Volume\ (mL)}{Time\ (hr)} = X$$

$$\frac{100\ mL}{0.75\ hr} = X\ mL/hr$$

$$133.3333 = X$$

STEP 6: *Round if necessary.*
133.3333 = 133

STEP 7: *Reassess to determine whether the IV flow rate makes sense.*
If the amount prescribed is 100 mL to infuse over 45 min (0.75 hr), it makes sense to administer 133 mL/hr. The nurse should set the IV pump to deliver cefotaxime 1 g in 100 mL of 0.9% NaCl IV at 133 mL/hr.

- Manual IV infusions
  - If an electronic infusion pump is not available, you can regulate the IV flow rate using the roller clamp on the IV tubing. When setting the flow rate, count the number of drops that fall into the drip chamber over the period of 1 min. Then calculate the flow rate using the drop factor found on the manufacturer's package containing the administration set. The drop factor is the number of drops per milliliter of solution.

Example: A nurse is preparing to administer lactated Ringer's (LR) 1,500 mL IV to infuse over 10 hr. The drop factor of the manual IV tubing is 15 gtt/mL. The nurse should set the manual IV infusion to deliver how many gtt/min? (Round the answer to the nearest whole number.)

Using Ratio and Proportion and Desired Over Have

STEP 1: *What is the unit of measurement to calculate?*
gtt/min

STEP 2: *What is the volume needed?*
Volume needed = Volume.
1,500 mL

STEP 3: *What is the total infusion time? Time available = Time.*
10 hr

STEP 4: *Should the nurse convert the units of measurement?*
No (mL = mL)
Yes (hr ≠ min)

$$\frac{1\ hr}{60\ min} = \frac{10\ hr}{X\ min}$$

X = 600 min

STEP 5: *Set up an equation and solve for X.*

$$\frac{Volume\ (mL)}{Time\ (min)} \times Drop\ factor\ (gtt/mL) = X$$

$$\frac{1,500\ mL}{600\ min} \times 15\ gtt/mL = X\ gtt/min$$

37.5 = X

STEP 6: *Round if necessary.*
37.5 = 38

STEP 7: *Reassess to determine whether the IV flow rate makes sense.*
If the amount prescribed is 1,500 mL to infuse over 10 hr (600 min), it makes sense to administer 38 gtt/min. The nurse should set the manual IV infusion to deliver LR 1,500 mL IV at 38 gtt/min.

Using Dimensional Analysis

STEP 1: *What is the unit of measurement to calculate?*
gtt/min

STEP 2: *What is the quantity of the drop factor that is available?*
15 gtt/mL

STEP 3: *What is the total infusion time? Time available = Time.*
10 hr

STEP 4: *What is the volume needed? Volume needed = Volume.*
1,500 mL

STEP 5: *Should the nurse convert the units of measurement?*
No (mL = mL)
Yes (hr ≠ min)

$$\frac{1\ hr}{60\ min}$$

STEP 6: *Set up an equation and solve for X.*

$$X = \frac{Quantity}{1\ mL} \times \frac{Conversion\ (Have)}{Conversion\ (Desired)} \times \frac{Volume}{Time}$$

$$X\ gtt/min = \frac{15\ gtt}{1\ mL} \times \frac{1\ hr}{60\ min} \times \frac{1,500\ mL}{10\ hr}$$

X = 37.5

STEP 7: *Round if necessary.*
37.5 = 38

STEP 8: *Reassess to determine whether the IV flow rate makes sense.*
If the amount prescribed is 1,500 mL to infuse over 10 hr (600 min), it makes sense to administer 38 gtt/min. The nurse should set the manual IV infusion to deliver LR 1,500 mL IV at 38 gtt/min.

Example: A nurse is preparing to administer ranitidine (Zantac) 150 mg by intermittent IV bolus. Available is ranitidine 150 mg in 100 mL of 0.9% sodium chloride (0.9% NaCl) to infuse over 30 min. The drop factor of the manual IV tubing is 10 gtt/mL. The nurse should set the manual IV infusion to deliver how many gtt/min? (Round the answer to the nearest whole number.)

Using Ratio and Proportion and Desired Over Have

STEP 1: *What is the unit of measurement to calculate?*
gtt/min

STEP 2: *What is the volume needed? Volume needed = Volume.*
100 mL

STEP 3: *What is the total infusion time? Time available = Time.*
30 min

STEP 4: *Should the nurse convert the units of measurement?*
No

STEP 5: *Set up an equation and solve for X.*

$$\frac{\text{Volume (mL)}}{\text{Time (min)}} \times \text{Drop factor (gtt/mL)} = X$$

$$\frac{100 \text{ mL} \times 10 \text{ gtt/mL}}{30 \text{ min}} = X \text{ gtt/min}$$

33.3333 = 33

STEP 6: *Round if necessary.*
33.3333 = 33

STEP 7: *Reassess to determine whether the IV flow rate makes sense.*
If the amount prescribed is 150 mL to infuse over 30 min, it makes sense to administer 33 gtt/min. The nurse should set the manual IV infusion to deliver ranitidine 150 mg in 100 mL of 0.9% NaCl IV at 33 gtt/min.

Using Dimensional Analysis

STEP 1: *What is the unit of measurement to calculate?*
gtt/min

STEP 2: *What is the quantity of the drop factor that is available?*
10 gtt/mL

STEP 3: *What is the total infusion time? Time available = Time.*
30 min

STEP 4: *What is the volume needed? Volume needed = Volume.*
150 mL

STEP 5: *Should the nurse convert the units of measurement?*
No

STEP 6: *Set up an equation and solve for X.*

$$X = \frac{\text{Quantity}}{1 \text{ mL}} \times \frac{\text{Conversion (Have)}}{\text{Conversion (Desired)}} \times \frac{\text{Volume}}{\text{Time}}$$

$$X \text{ gtt/min} = \frac{10 \text{ gtt}}{1 \text{ mL}} \times \frac{150 \text{ mL}}{30 \text{ min}}$$

X = 33.3333

STEP 7: *Round if necessary.*
33.3333 = 33

STEP 8: *Reassess to determine whether the IV flow rate makes sense.*
If the amount prescribed is 150 mL to infuse over 30 min, it makes sense to administer 33 gtt/min. The nurse should set the manual IV infusion to deliver ranitidine 150 mg in 100 mL of 0.9% NaCl IV at 33 gtt/min.

APPLICATION EXERCISES

1. A nurse is preparing to administer methylprednisolone acetate (Depo-Medrol) 10 mg by IV bolus. The amount available is methylprednisolone acetate injection 40 mg/mL. How many mL should the nurse administer? (Round the answer to the nearest tenth.)

2. A nurse is preparing to administer lactated Ringer's (LR) IV 100 mL over 15 min. The nurse should set the IV infusion pump to deliver how many mL/hr? (Round the answer to the nearest whole number.)

3. A nurse is preparing to administer 0.9% sodium chloride (0.9% NaCl) 250 mL IV to infuse over 30 min. The drop factor of the manual IV tubing is 10 gtt/mL. The nurse should set the manual IV infusion to deliver how many gtt/min? (Round the answer to the nearest whole number.)

4. A nurse is preparing to administer metoprolol (Lopressor) 200 mg PO daily. The amount available is metoprolol 100 mg/tab. How many capsules should the nurse administer? (Round the answer to the nearest whole number.)

5. A nurse is preparing to administer kanamycin (Kantrex) 15 mg/kg/day IV bolus divided in equal doses every 8 hr to a school-age child who weighs 66 lb. The amount available is kanamycin injection 1 g/mL. How many mL should the nurse administer per dose? (Round the answer to the nearest tenth.)

6. A nurse is preparing to administer dextrose 5% in water (D_5W) 1,000 mL IV to infuse over 10 hr. The nurse should set the IV infusion pump to deliver how many mL/hr? (Round the answer to the nearest whole number.)

7. A nurse is preparing to administer acetaminophen (Tylenol) 325 mg PO every 4 hr PRN for pain. The amount available is acetaminophen liquid 160 mg/5mL. How many mL should the nurse administer per dose? (Round the answer to the nearest whole number.)

8. A nurse is preparing to administer lactated Ringer's (LR) 1,000 mL to infuse over 4 hr. The drop factor of the manual IV tubing is 20 gtt/mL. The nurse should set the manual IV infusion to deliver how many gtt/min? (Round the answer to the nearest whole number.)

APPLICATION EXERCISES KEY

1. **0.3** mL

Using Ratio and Proportion

STEP 1: *What is the unit of measurement to calculate?*
mL

STEP 2: *What is the dose needed? Dose needed = Desired.*
10 mg

STEP 3: *What is the dose available? Dose available = Have.*
40 mg

STEP 4: *Should the nurse convert the units of measurement?*
No

STEP 5: *What is the quantity of the dose available?*
1 mL

STEP 6: *Set up an equation and solve for X.*

$$\frac{Have}{Quantity} = \frac{Desired}{X}$$

$$\frac{40\ mg}{1\ mL} = \frac{10\ mg}{X\ mL}$$

$$0.25 = X$$

STEP 7: *Round if necessary.*
0.25 = 0.3

STEP 8: *Reassess to determine whether the amount to give makes sense.*
If there are 40 mg/mL and the prescribed amount is 10 mg, it makes sense to administer 0.3 mL. The nurse should administer methylprednisolone acetate injection 0.3 mL by IV bolus.

Using Desired Over Have

STEP 1: *What is the unit of measurement to calculate?*
mL

STEP 2: *What is the dose needed? Dose needed = Desired.*
10 mg

STEP 3: *What is the dose available? Dose available = Have.*
40 mg

STEP 4: *Should the nurse convert the units of measurement?*
No

STEP 5: *What is the quantity of the dose available?*
1 mL

STEP 6: *Set up an equation and solve for X.*

$$\frac{Desired \times Quantity}{Have} = X$$

$$\frac{10\ mg \times 1\ mL}{40\ mg} = X\ mL$$

$$X = 0.25$$

STEP 7: *Round if necessary.*
0.25 = 0.3

STEP 8: *Reassess to determine whether the amount to give makes sense.*
If there are 40 mg/mL and the prescribed amount is 10 mg, it makes sense to administer 0.3 mL. The nurse should administer methylprednisolone acetate injection 0.3 mL by IV bolus.

Using Dimensional Analysis

STEP 1: *What is the unit of measurement to calculate?*
mL

STEP 2: *What quantity of the dose is available?*
1 mL

STEP 3: *What is the dose available? Dose available = Have.*
40 mg

STEP 4: *What is the dose needed? Dose needed = Desired.*
10 mg

STEP 5: *Should the nurse convert the units of measurement?*
No

STEP 6: *Set up an equation and solve for X.*

$$X = \frac{Quantity}{Have} \times \frac{Conversion\ (Have)}{Conversion\ (Desired)} \times Desired$$

$$X\ mL = \frac{1\ mL}{40\ mg} \times \frac{10\ mg}{}$$

$$X = 0.25$$

STEP 7: *Round if necessary.*
0.25 = 0.3

STEP 8: *Reassess to determine whether the amount to give makes sense.*
If there are 40 mg/mL and the prescribed amount is 10 mg, it makes sense to administer 0.3 mL. The nurse should administer methylprednisolone acetate injection 0.3 mL by IV bolus.

Ⓝ NCLEX® Connection: Pharmacological and Parenteral Therapies, Dosage Calculation

2.   **400** mL/hr

Using Ratio and Proportion, Desired Over Have, and Dimensional Analysis

STEP 1: *What is the unit of measurement to calculate?*
mL/hr

STEP 2: *What is the volume needed? Volume needed = Volume.*
100 mL

STEP 3: *What is the total infusion time? Time available = Time.*
15 min

STEP 4: *Should the nurse convert the units of measurement?*
No (mL = mL)
Yes (min ≠ hr)

$$\frac{1\ hr}{60\ min} = \frac{X\ hr}{15\ min}$$

X = 0.25

STEP 5: *Set up an equation and solve for X.*

$$\frac{Volume\ (mL)}{Time\ (hr)} = X$$

$$\frac{100\ mL}{0.25} = X\ mL/hr$$

400 = X

STEP 6: *Round if necessary.*

STEP 7: *Reassess to determine whether the IV flow rate makes sense.*
If the amount prescribed is 100 mL to infuse over 15 min (0.25 hr), it makes sense to administer 400 mL/hr. The nurse should set the IV pump to deliver LR IV 100 mL at 400 mL/hr.

   Ⓝ NCLEX® Connection: Pharmacological and Parenteral Therapies, Dosage Calculation

3.   **83** gtt/min

Using Ratio and Proportion and Desired Over Have

STEP 1: *What is the unit of measurement to calculate?*
gtt/min

STEP 2: *What is the volume needed? Volume needed = Volume.*
250 mL

STEP 3: *What is the total infusion time? Time available = Time.*
30 min

STEP 4: *Should the nurse convert the units of measurement?*
No

STEP 5: *Set up an equation and solve for X.*

$$\frac{Volume\ (mL)}{Time\ (min)} \times Drop\ factor\ (gtt/mL) = X$$

$$\frac{250\ mL}{30\ min} \times 10\ gtt/mL = X\ gtt/min$$

83.3333 = X

STEP 6: *Round if necessary.*
83.3333 = 83

STEP 7: *Reassess to determine whether the IV flow rate makes sense.*
If the amount prescribed is 250 mL to infuse over 30 min it makes sense to administer 83 gtt/min. The nurse should set the manual IV infusion to deliver 0.9% NaCl 250 mL IV at 83 gtt/min.

Using Dimensional Analysis

STEP 1: *What is the unit of measurement to calculate?*
gtt/min

STEP 2: *What is the quantity of the drop factor that is available?*
10 gtt/min

STEP 3: *What is the total infusion time? Time available = Time.*
30 min

STEP 4: *What is the volume needed? Volume needed = Volume.*
250 mL

STEP 5: *Should the nurse convert the units of measurement?*
No

STEP 6: *Set up an equation and solve for X.*

$$X = \frac{Quantity}{1\ mL} \times \frac{Conversion\ (Have)}{Conversion\ (Desired)} \times \frac{Volume}{Time}$$

$$X\ gtt/min = \frac{10\ gtt}{1\ mL} \times \frac{250\ mL}{30\ min}$$

$$X = 83.3333$$

STEP 6: *Round if necessary.*
83.3333 = 83

STEP 7: *Reassess to determine whether the IV flow rate makes sense.*
If the amount prescribed is 250 mL to infuse over 30 min it makes sense to administer 83 gtt/min. The nurse should set the manual IV infusion to deliver 0.9% NaCl 250 mL IV at 83 gtt/min.

(N) NCLEX® Connection: Pharmacological and Parenteral Therapies, Dosage Calculation

4. **2 tab**

Using Ratio and Proportion

STEP 1: *What is the unit of measurement to calculate?*
tab

STEP 2: *What is the dose needed? Dose needed = Desired.*
200 mg

STEP 3: *What is the dose available? Dose available = Have.*
100 mg

STEP 4: *Should the nurse convert the units of measurement?*
No

STEP 5: *What is the quantity of the dose available?*
1 tab

STEP 6: *Set up an equation and solve for X.*

$$\frac{Have}{Quantity} = \frac{Desired}{X}$$

$$\frac{100\ mg}{1\ tab} = \frac{200\ mg}{X\ tab\,(s)}$$

$$X = 2$$

STEP 7: *Round if necessary.*

STEP 8: *Reassess to determine whether the amount to give makes sense.*
If there is 100 mg/tab and the prescribed amount is 200 mg, it makes sense to give 2 tabs. The nurse should administer metoprolol 2 tabs PO daily.

Using Desired Over Have

STEP 1: *What is the unit of measurement to calculate?*
tab

STEP 2: *What is the dose needed? Dose needed = Desired.*
200 mg

STEP 3: *What is the dose available? Dose available = Have.*
100 mg

STEP 4: *Should the nurse convert the units of measurement?*
No

STEP 5: *What is the quantity of the dose available?*
1 tab

STEP 6: *Set up an equation and solve for X.*

$$\frac{Desired \times Quantity}{Have} = X$$

$$\frac{200\ mg \times 1\ tab}{100\ mg} = X\ tab\,(s)$$

$$2 = X$$

STEP 7: *Round if necessary.*

STEP 8: *Reassess to determine whether the amount to give makes sense.*
If there is 100 mg/tab and the prescribed amount is 200 mg, it makes sense to give 2 tabs. The nurse should administer metoprolol 2 tabs PO daily.

Using Dimensional Analysis

STEP 1: *What is the unit of measurement to calculate?*
tab

STEP 2: *What quantity of the dose is available?*
1 tab

STEP 3: *What is the dose available? Dose available = Have.*
100 mg

STEP 4: *What is the dose needed? Dose needed = Desired.*
200 mg

STEP 5: *Should the nurse convert the units of measurement?*
No

STEP 6: *Set up an equation and solve for X.*

$$X = \frac{Quantity}{Have} \times \frac{Conversion\ (Have)}{Conversion\ (Desired)} \times \frac{Desired}{}$$

$$X\ tab\ (s) = \frac{1\ tab}{100\ mg} \times 200\ mg$$

$$X = 2$$

STEP 7: *Round if necessary.*

STEP 8: *Reassess to determine whether the amount to give makes sense.*
If there is 100 mg/ tab and the prescribed amount is 200 mg, it makes sense to give 2 tabs. The nurse should administer metoprolol 2 tabs PO daily.

(N) NCLEX® Connection: Pharmacological and Parenteral Therapies, Dosage Calculation

5. **0.2** mL

Using Ratio and Proportion

STEP 1: *What is the unit of measurement to calculate?*
kg

STEP 2: *Set up an equation and solve for X.*

$$\frac{2.2\ lb}{1\ kg} = \frac{Client\ weight\ in\ lb}{X\ kg}$$

$$\frac{2.2\ lb}{1\ kg} = \frac{66\ lb}{X\ kg}$$

$$X = 30$$

STEP 3: *Round if necessary.*

STEP 4: *Reassess to determine whether the equivalent makes sense.*
If 1 kg = 2.2 lb, it makes sense that 66 lb = 30 kg.

STEP 5: *What is the unit of measurement to calculate?*
mg

STEP 6: *Set up an equation and solve for X.*
mg x kg/day = X
15 mg x 30 kg = 450 mg

STEP 7: *Round if necessary.*

STEP 8: *Reassess to determine whether the amount makes sense.*
If the prescribed amount is 15 mg/kg/day divided in equal doses every 8 hr and the school-age child weighs 30 kg, it makes sense to give 450 mg/day, or 150 mg every 8 hr.

STEP 9: *What is the unit of measurement to calculate?*
mL

STEP 10: *What is the dose needed? Dose needed = Desired.*
150 mg

STEP 11: *What is the dose available? Dose available = Have.*
1 g

STEP 12: *Should the nurse convert the units of measurement?*
Yes (g ≠ mg)
1 g = 1,000 mg (1 x 1,000)

STEP 13: *What is the quantity of the dose available?*
1 mL

STEP 14: *Set up an equation and solve for X.*

$$\frac{Have}{Quantity} = \frac{Desired}{X}$$

$$\frac{1,000\ mg}{1\ mL} = \frac{150\ mg}{X\ mL}$$

$$X = 0.15$$

STEP 15: *Round if necessary.*
0.15 = 0.2

STEP 16: *Reassess to determine whether the amount to give makes sense.*
If there is 1 g (1,000 mg)/mL and the prescribed amount is 150 mg, it makes sense to give 0.2 mL. The nurse should administer kanamycin injection 0.2 mL IV bolus every 8 hr.

Using Desired Over Have

STEP 1: *What is the unit of measurement to calculate?*
kg

STEP 2: *Set up an equation and solve for X.*

$$\frac{2.2\ \text{lb}}{1\ \text{kg}} = \frac{\text{Client weight in lb}}{X\ \text{kg}}$$

$$\frac{2.2\ \text{lb}}{1\ \text{kg}} = \frac{66\ \text{lb}}{X\ \text{kg}}$$

X = 30

STEP 3: *Round if necessary.*

STEP 4: *Reassess to determine whether the equivalent makes sense.*
If 1 kg = 2.2 lb, it makes sense that 66 lb = 30 kg.

STEP 5: *What is the unit of measurement to calculate?*
mg

STEP 6: *Set up an equation and solve for X.*
mg x kg/day = X
15 mg x 30 kg = 450 mg

STEP 7: *Round if necessary.*

STEP 8: *Reassess to determine whether the amount makes sense.*
If the prescribed amount is 15 mg/kg/day divided in equal doses every 8 hr and the school-age child weighs 30 kg, it makes sense to give 450 mg/day, or 150 mg every 8 hr.

STEP 9: *What is the unit of measurement to calculate?*
mL

STEP 10: *What is the dose needed? Dose needed = Desired.*
150 mg

STEP 11: *What is the dose available? Dose available = Have.*
1 g

STEP 12: *Should the nurse convert the units of measurement?*
Yes (g ≠ mg)
1 g = 1,000 mg (1 x 1,000)

STEP 13: *What is the quantity of the dose available?*
1 mL

STEP 14: *Set up an equation and solve for X.*

$$\frac{\text{Desired x Quantity}}{\text{Have}} = X$$

$$\frac{150\ \text{mg}\ \ \text{x}\ 1\ \text{mL}}{1,000\ \text{mg}} = X\ \text{mL}$$

0.15 = X

STEP 15: *Round if necessary.*
0.15 = 0.2

STEP 16: *Reassess to determine whether the amount to give makes sense.*
If there is 1 g (1,000 mg)/mL and the prescribed amount is 150 mg, it makes sense to give 0.2 mL. The nurse should administer kanamycin injection 0.2 mL IV bolus every 8 hr.

Using Dimensional Analysis

STEP 1: *What is the unit of measurement to calculate?*
kg

STEP 2: *Set up an equation and solve for X.*

$$\frac{2.2\ lb}{1\ kg} = \frac{Client\ weight\ in\ lb}{X\ kg}$$

$$\frac{2.2\ lb}{1\ kg} = \frac{66\ lb}{X\ kg}$$

X = 30

STEP 3: *Round if necessary.*

STEP 4: *Reassess to determine whether the equivalent makes sense.*
If 1 kg = 2.2 lb, it makes sense that 66 lb = 30 kg.

STEP 5: *What is the unit of measurement to calculate?*
mg

STEP 6: *Set up an equation and solve for X.*
mg x kg/day = X
15 mg x 30 kg = 450 mg

STEP 7: *Round if necessary.*

STEP 8: *Reassess to determine whether the amount makes sense.*
If the prescribed amount is 15 mg/kg/day divided in equal doses every 8 hr and the school-age child weighs 30 kg, it makes sense to give 450 mg/day, or 150 mg every 8 hr.

STEP 9: *What is the unit of measurement to calculate?*
mL

STEP 10: *What quantity of the dose is available?*
1 mL

STEP 11: *What is the dose available?*
Dose available = Have.
1 g

STEP 12: *What is the dose needed?*
Dose needed = Desired.
150 mg

STEP 13: *Should the nurse convert the units of measurement?*
Yes (g ≠ mg)
1 g = 1,000 mg (1 x 1,000)

STEP 14: *Set up an equation and solve for X.*

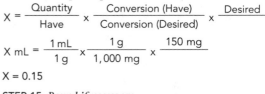

$$X = \frac{Quantity}{Have} \times \frac{Conversion\ (Have)}{Conversion\ (Desired)} \times \frac{Desired}{}$$

$$X\ mL = \frac{1\ mL}{1\ g} \times \frac{1\ g}{1,000\ mg} \times \frac{150\ mg}{}$$

X = 0.15

STEP 15: *Round if necessary.*
0.15 = 0.2

STEP 16: *Reassess to determine whether the amount to give makes sense.*
If there is 1 g (1,000 mg)/ mL and the prescribed amount is 150 mg, it makes sense to give 0.2 mL. The nurse should administer kanamycin injection 0.2 mL IV bolus every 8 hr.

(N) NCLEX® Connection: Pharmacological and Parenteral Therapies, Dosage Calculation

6.   **100** mL/hr

Using Ratio and Proportion, Desired Over Have, and Dimensional Analysis

STEP 1: *What is the unit of measurement to calculate?*
mL/hr

STEP 2: *What is the volume needed? Volume needed = Volume.*
1,000 mL

STEP 3: *What is the total infusion time? Time available = Time.*
10 hr

STEP 4: *Should the nurse convert the units of measurement?*
No

STEP 5: *Set up an equation and solve for X.*

$$\frac{Volume\ (mL)}{Time\ (hr)} = X$$

$$\frac{1,000\ mL}{10} = X\ mL/hr$$

100 = X

STEP 6: *Round if necessary.*

STEP 7: *Reassess to determine whether the IV flow rate makes sense.*
If the amount prescribed is D₅W 1,000 mL IV to infuse over 10 hr it makes sense to administer 100 mL/hr. The nurse should set the IV pump to deliver D₅W 1,000 mL at 100 mL/hr.

(N) NCLEX® Connection: Pharmacological and Parenteral Therapies, Dosage Calculation

7.　**10** mL

Using Ratio and Proportion

STEP 1: *What is the unit of measurement to calculate?*
mL

STEP 2: *What is the dose needed? Dose needed = Desired.*
325 mg

STEP 3: *What is the dose available? Dose available = Have.*
160 mg

STEP 4: *Should the nurse convert the units of measurement?*
No

STEP 5: *What is the quantity of the dose available?*
5 mL

STEP 6: *Set up an equation and solve for X.*

$$\frac{Have}{Quantity} = \frac{Desired}{X}$$

$$\frac{160 \text{ mg}}{5 \text{ mL}} = \frac{325 \text{ mg}}{X \text{ mL}}$$

X = 10.1562

STEP 7: *Round if necessary.*
10.1562 = 10

STEP 8: *Reassess to determine whether the amount to administer makes sense.*
If there are 160 mg/5 mL and the prescribed amount is 325 mg, it makes sense to administer 10 mL. The nurse should administer acetaminophen liquid 10 mL PO every 4 hr PRN for pain.

Using Desired Over Have

STEP 1: *What is the unit of measurement to calculate?*
mL

STEP 2: *What is the dose needed? Dose needed = Desired.*
325 mg

STEP 3: *What is the dose available? Dose available = Have.*
160 mg

STEP 4: *Should the nurse convert the units of measurement?*
No

STEP 5: *What is the quantity of the dose available?*
5 mL

STEP 6: *Set up an equation and solve for X.*

$$\frac{Desired \times Quantity}{Have} = X$$

$$\frac{325 \text{ mg} \times 5 \text{ mL}}{160 \text{ mg}} = X \text{ mL}$$

10.1562 = X

STEP 7: *Round if necessary.*
10.1562 = 10

STEP 8: *Reassess to determine whether the amount to administer makes sense.*
If there are 160 mg/5 mL and the prescribed amount is 325 mg, it makes sense to administer 10 mL. The nurse should administer acetaminophen liquid 10 mL PO every 4 hr PRN for pain.

Using Dimensional Analysis

STEP 1: *What is the unit of measurement to calculate?*
mL

STEP 2: *What quantity of the dose is available?*
5 mL

STEP 3: *What is the dose available? Dose available = Have.*
160 mg

STEP 4: *What is the dose needed? Dose needed = Desired.*
325 mg

STEP 5: *Should the nurse convert the units of measurement?*
No

STEP 6: *Set up an equation and solve for X.*

$$X = \frac{Quantity}{Have} \times \frac{Conversion (Have)}{Conversion (Desired)} \times \frac{Desired}{}$$

$$X \text{ mL} = \frac{5 \text{ mL}}{160 \text{ mg}} \times \frac{325 \text{ mg}}{}$$

X = 10.1562

STEP 7: *Round if necessary.*
10.1562 = 10

STEP 8: *Reassess to determine whether the amount to administer makes sense.*
If there are 160 mg/5 mL and the prescribed amount is 325 mg, it makes sense to administer 10 mL. The nurse should administer acetaminophen liquid 10 mL PO every 4 hr PRN for pain.

Ⓝ NCLEX® Connection: Pharmacological and Parenteral Therapies, Dosage Calculation

8. **83** gtt/min

Using Ratio and Proportion and Desired Over Have

STEP 1: *What is the unit of measurement to calculate?*
gtt/min

STEP 2: *What is the volume needed? Volume needed = Volume.*
1,000 mL

STEP 3: *What is the total infusion time? Time available = Time.*
12 hr

STEP 4: *Should the nurse convert the units of measurement?*
No (mL = mL)
Yes (hr ≠ min)

$$\frac{1 \text{ hr}}{60 \text{ min}} = \frac{4 \text{ hr}}{X \text{ min}}$$

X = 240 min

STEP 5: *Set up an equation and solve for X.*

$$\frac{\text{Volume (mL)}}{\text{Time (min)}} \times \text{Drop factor (gtt/mL)} = X$$

$$\frac{1,000 \text{ mL}}{240 \text{ min}} \times 20 \text{ gtt/mL} = X \text{ gtt/min}$$

83.3333 = X

STEP 6: *Round if necessary.*
83.3333 = 83

STEP 7: *Reassess to determine whether the IV flow rate makes sense.*
If the amount prescribed is 1,000 mL to infuse over 4 hr (240 min) it makes sense to administer 83 gtt/min. The nurse should set the manual IV infusion to deliver LR 1,000 mL IV at 83 gtt/min.

Using Dimensional Analysis

STEP 1: *What is the unit of measurement to calculate?*
gtt/min

STEP 2: *What is the quantity of the drop factor that is available?*
20 gtt/min

STEP 3: *What is the total infusion time? Time available = Time.*
4 hr

STEP 4: *What is the volume needed? Volume needed = Volume.*
1,000

STEP 5: *Should the nurse convert the units of measurement?*
No (mL = mL)
Yes (hr ≠ min)

$$\frac{1 \text{ hr}}{60 \text{ min}}$$

STEP 6: *Set up an equation and solve for X.*

$$X = \frac{\text{Quantity}}{1 \text{ mL}} \times \frac{\text{Conversion (Have)}}{\text{Conversion (Desired)}} \times \frac{\text{Volume}}{\text{Time}}$$

$$X \text{ gtt/min} = \frac{20 \text{ gtt}}{1 \text{ mL}} \times \frac{1 \text{ hr}}{60 \text{ min}} \times \frac{100 \text{ mL}}{45 \text{ min}}$$

83.3333 = X

STEP 7: *Round if necessary.*
83.3333 = 83

STEP 8: *Reassess to determine whether the IV flow rate makes sense.*
If the amount prescribed is 1,000 mL to infuse over 4 hr (240 min), it makes sense to administer 83 gtt/min. The nurse should set the manual IV infusion to deliver LR 1,000 mL IV at 83 gtt/min.

Ⓝ NCLEX® Connection: Pharmacological and Parenteral Therapies, Dosage Calculation

chapter 49

Overview

- Intravenous (IV) therapy involves administering fluids via an intravenous catheter for the purpose of administering medications, supplementing fluid intake, or providing fluid replacement, electrolytes, or nutrients.

- Large-volume IV infusions are administered on a continuous basis.

- An IV medication infusion may be mixed in a large volume of fluid and given as a continuous IV infusion or mixed in a small amount of solution and given intermittently. It can also be administered as an IV bolus, in which the medication is given in a small amount of solution, concentrated or diluted, and injected over a short time (1 to 2 min) in emergent and nonemergent situations.

Indications and Risk Factors

- Advantages and Disadvantages of IV Therapy

ADVANTAGES	DISADVANTAGES
› Rapid absorption and onset of action › Maintains constant therapeutic blood levels › Less irritation to subcutaneous and muscle tissue	› Circulatory fluid overload is possible if the volume of solution is large and/or if the infusion rate is rapid. › Immediate absorption leaves no time to correct errors. › Solution and IV catheter can cause irritation to the lining of the vein. › Failure to maintain surgical asepsis can lead to local infection and septicemia.

Description of Procedure

- The provider prescribes the type of IV fluid, the volume to be infused, and either the rate at which the IV fluid should be infused or the total amount of time it should take for the fluid to be infused. The nurse regulates the IV infusion to insure the appropriate amount is administered. This can be done with an IV pump or manually.

- Large-volume IV infusions are administered on a continuous basis, such as 0.9% sodium chloride IV to infuse at 100 mL/hr or 0.9% sodium chloride 1,000 mL to be given IV over 3 hr.

- A fluid bolus is a large amount of IV fluid given in a short period of time, usually less than 1 hr. A fluid bolus is given to rapidly replace fluid loss that could be caused by dehydration, shock, hemorrhage, burns, or trauma.

  ○ A large-gauge angiocatheter (18-gauge or larger) is needed to maintain the rapid rate necessary to give a fluid bolus to an adult.

- IV medication infusions may be administered in the following ways:
  - The medication is mixed in a large volume of fluid (500 to 1,000 mL) and administered as a continuous IV infusion. Potassium chloride or vitamins can be administered this way.
  - The medication is provided in premixed solution bags or can be added to the IV bag by the pharmacist.
  - Volume-controlled infusions
    - Some medications, such as antibiotics, are administered intermittently in a small amount of solution (25 to 250 mL) through a continuous IV system, or with saline or heparin lock systems.
    - The medications infuse for short periods of time and are administered on a scheduled basis.
    - These infusions can be administered by a secondary ("piggyback") IV bag or bottle or tandem setup, volume-control administration set, or by mini-infusion pump.
  - IV bolus dose administration
    - The medications are typically in small amounts of solution, concentrated or diluted, that can be injected over a short time (1 to 2 min) in emergent and nonemergent situations.
    - Some medications are administered directly into the peripheral IV or access port to achieve an immediate medication level in the bloodstream, such as with pain medication.
    - Make sure medications are prepared according to the recommended concentration and administered according to the safe recommended rate.
    - Use extreme caution and observe for complications such as redness, burning, or increasing pain.
- Types of IV Access
  - IV access can be via a peripheral or central vein (central venous access device).
  - Central venous access devices can be peripherally inserted or directly inserted into the jugular or subclavian vein.

Guidelines for Safe IV Medication Administration

- Certain medications, such as potassium chloride, can cause serious adverse reactions. They should be infused on an IV pump for accurate dosage control, and never administered by IV bolus.
- Never administer IV medication through tubing that is infusing blood, blood products, or parenteral nutritional solutions.
- Verify the compatibility of medications before infusing a medication through tubing that is infusing another medication.
- Needlestick Prevention
  - Be familiar with IV insertion equipment.
  - Avoid using needles when needleless systems are available.
  - Use protective safety devices when available.
  - Dispose of needles immediately in designated puncture-resistant receptacles.
  - Do not break, bend, or recap needles.

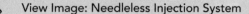

M View Image: Needleless Injection System

Special Considerations

- Older adult clients, clients taking anticoagulants, or clients who have fragile veins
  - Avoid tourniquets.
  - Use a blood pressure (BP) cuff instead.
  - Do not slap the extremity to visualize veins.
  - Avoid rigorous friction while cleaning the site.
- Edema in extremities
  - Apply digital pressure over the selected vein to displace edema.
  - Apply pressure with swab of cleaning solution.
  - Cannulation must be quick.
- Obese clients may require the use of anatomical landmarks to find veins.
- Preventing IV Infections
  - Perform hand hygiene before and after handling the IV system.
  - Use standard precautions.
  - Change IV sites according to facility policy (usually 72 hr).
  - Change continuous infusion tubing no more frequently than every 96 hr, and change intermittent infusion tubing every 24 hr according to facility policy.
  - Remove catheters as soon as they are no longer clinically indicated.
  - Change the catheter if any break in surgical aseptic technique is suspected, such as emergency insertions.
  - Use a sterile needle/catheter for each insertion attempt.
  - Avoid writing on IV bags with pens or markers, because ink can contaminate the solution.
  - Change tubing immediately if contamination is known or suspected.
  - Fluids should not hang more than 24 hr unless it is a closed system (pressure bags for hemodynamic monitoring).
  - Wipe all ports with alcohol or an antiseptic swab before connecting IV lines or inserting a syringe to prevent the introduction of micro-organisms into the system.
  - Never disconnect tubing for convenience or to position the client.

Preprocedure

- Equipment
  - IV start kit if available to include:
    - Tourniquet, sterile drape, antiseptic swabs, transparent dressing, small roll of sterile tape, 2x2 or 4x4 gauze sponge, and safety positioning device.
  - Correct size catheter
    - 16-gauge for trauma clients, rapid fluid volume
    - 18-gauge for surgical clients, rapid blood administration
    - 22- to 24-gauge for all other clients (children, adults)

- ○ Correct tubing
- ○ Prefilled syringe containing 1 to 3 mL of 0.9% sodium chloride solution
- ○ Infusion pump, if indicated
- ○ Clean gloves
- ○ Scissors or electric shaver for hair removal
- Nursing Actions
  - ○ Check the provider's prescription (solution, rate).
  - ○ Assess the client for allergies to products used in initiating and maintaining IV therapy (latex, tape).
  - ○ Follow the six rights of medication administration (including compatibilities of all IV solutions).
  - ○ Perform hand hygiene.
  - ○ Examine the solution to be infused for clarity, leaks, and expiration date.
  - ○ Don clean gloves.
  - ○ Assess extremities and veins. If hair removal is needed, clip it with scissors or shave it with an electric shaver.
- Client Education
  - ○ Identify the client and explain the procedure.
  - ○ Place the client in a comfortable position.

Intraprocedure

- Nursing Actions
  - ○ Apply a clean tourniquet or BP cuff (especially for older adults) 4 to 6 inches above the proposed insertion site to compress only venous blood flow.
  - ○ Select the vein by choosing:
    - ▪ Distal veins first on the nondominant hand.
    - ▪ A site that is not painful or bruised and will not interfere with activity.
    - ▪ A vein that is resilient with a soft, bouncy sensation when palpated.
    - ▪ Additional methods to enhance venous access include gravity, fist clenching, friction with cleaning solution, and heat.
    - ▪ Avoid:
      - ▫ Varicose veins that are permanently dilated and tortuous.
      - ▫ Veins in the inner wrist with bifurcations, in flexion areas, near valves (appearing as bumps), in lower extremities, and in the antecubital fossa (except for emergency access).
      - ▫ Veins in the back of the hand.
      - ▫ Veins that are sclerosed or hard.
      - ▫ Veins in an extremity with impaired sensitivity (scar tissue, paralysis), lymph nodes removed, recent infiltration, a PICC line, or an arteriovenous fistula/graft.
  - ○ Untie the tourniquet or deflate the BP cuff.

○ Cleanse the area at the site using friction in a circular motion from the middle and outwardly with chlorhexidine or cleaning agent per facility protocol. Allow it to air dry for 1 to 2 min.

○ Remove the cover from the catheter, grasp the plastic hub, and examine the device for smooth edges.

○ Retie the tourniquet or reinflate the BP cuff.

○ Anchor the vein below the site of insertion.

○ Pull the skin taut and hold it.

○ Warn the client of a sharp, quick stick.

○ Insert the catheter into the skin with the bevel up at an angle of 10° to 30° using a steady, smooth motion.

○ Advance the catheter through the skin and into the vein, maintaining a 10° to 30° angle. Flashback of blood will confirm placement in the vein.

○ Lower the hub of the catheter close to the skin to prepare for threading it into the vein approximately 0.25 in.

○ Loosen the needle from the catheter and pull back slightly on the needle so that it no longer extends past the tip of the catheter.

○ Use the thumb and index finger to advance the catheter into the vein until the hub rests against the insertion site.

○ Stabilize the IV catheter with one hand and release the tourniquet or BP cuff with the other.

○ Apply pressure approximately 1.25 in (3 cm) above the insertion site with the middle finger and stabilize the catheter with the index finger.

○ Remove the needle and activate the safety device.

○ Maintain pressure above the IV site and connect the appropriate equipment to the hub of the IV catheter.

○ Apply a dressing per facility protocol. The dressing is usually left in place until the catheter is removed, unless it becomes damp, loose, or soiled.

○ Avoid encircling the entire extremity with tape, and taping under the sterile dressing.

○ If a continuous IV infusion is prescribed, regulate IV infusion rate according to the prescription.

○ Dispose of used equipment properly.

○ Document in the chart:

   ▪ The date and time of insertion.

   ▪ The insertion site and appearance.

   ▪ The catheter size.

   ▪ The type of dressing.

   ▪ The IV fluid and rate (if applicable).

   ▪ The number, locations, and conditions of site-attempted catheterizations.

   ▪ The client's response.

   ▪ Sample documentation: 6/1/2013, 1635, #22-gauge IV catheter inserted into left wrist cephalic vein (1 attempt) with sterile occlusive dressing applied. IV 5% dextrose in lactated Ringer's infusing at 100 mL/hr per infusion pump without redness or edema at the site. Tolerated without complications. S. Velez, RN

Postprocedure

- Nursing Actions
  - Maintaining patency of IV access
    - Do not stop a continuous infusion or allow blood to back up into the catheter for any length of time. Clots can form at the tip of the needle or catheter and can be lodged against the vein wall, blocking the flow of fluid.
    - Instruct the client not to manipulate the flow rate device, change the settings on the IV pump, or lie on the tubing.
    - Make sure the IV insertion site dressing is not too tight.
    - Flush intermittent IV catheters with the appropriate solution after every medication administration or every 8 to 12 hr when not in use, per facility policy.
    - Monitor the site and infusion rate at least every hour.
  - Discontinuing IV therapy
    - Check the prescription/prepare equipment.
    - Perform hand hygiene.
    - Don clean gloves.
    - Clamp the IV tubing.
    - Remove the tape and dressing, stabilizing the IV catheter.
    - Apply a sterile gauze pad over the site without putting pressure on the vein. Do not use alcohol.
    - Using the other hand, withdraw the catheter by pulling it straight back from the site, keeping the hub parallel to the skin.
    - Elevate the extremity and apply pressure for 2 to 3 min.
    - Assess the site.
    - Apply tape over the gauze.
    - Use a pressure dressing, if needed.
    - Assess the catheter for intactness.
    - Dispose of catheter in designated puncture-resistant receptacle, and IV solution and equipment in appropriate location.
    - Document.

Complications

- Complications require notification of the provider and documentation. All IV infusions should be restarted with new tubing and catheters.

FINDINGS	TREATMENT	PREVENTION
Infiltration or extravasation		
› Pallor, local swelling at the site, decreased skin temperature around the site, damp dressing, slowed rate of infusion	› Stop the infusion and remove the catheter. › Elevate the extremity. › Encourage active range of motion. › Apply warm or cold compress depending on solution infusing. › Restart the infusion proximal to the site or in another extremity.	› Carefully select the site and catheter. › Secure the catheter.
Phlebitis/thrombophlebitis		
› Edema; throbbing, burning, or pain at the site; increased skin temperature; erythema; red line up the arm with a palpable band at the vein site; slowed rate of infusion	› Promptly discontinue the infusion and remove the catheter. › Elevate the extremity. › Apply warm compresses three to four times/day. › Restart the infusion proximal to the site or in another extremity. › Culture the site and catheter if drainage is present.	› Rotate sites at least every 72 hr. › Avoid the lower extremities. › Use hand hygiene. › Use surgical aseptic technique.
Hematoma		
› Ecchymosis at site	› Do not apply alcohol. › Apply pressure after IV catheter removal. › Use warm compress and elevation after the bleeding stops.	› Minimize tourniquet time. › Remove the tourniquet before starting the IV infusion. › Maintain pressure after IV catheter removal.
Fluid overload		
› Distended neck veins, increased BP, tachycardia, shortness of breath, crackles in the lungs, edema; additional assessment findings depend on the solution being used for IV therapy	› Stop infusion. › Raise the head of the bed. › Assess vital signs and oxygen saturation. › Adjust the rate as prescribed. › Administer diuretics if prescribed.	› Use an infusion pump. › Monitor I&O.

FINDINGS	TREATMENT	PREVENTION
Cellulitis		

› Pain; warmth; edema; induration; red streaking; fever, chills, and malaise	› Discontinue the infusion and remove the catheter.
	› Elevate the extremity.
	› Apply warm compresses three to four times/day.
	› Obtain a specimen for culture at the site and prepare the catheter for culture if drainage is present.
	› Administer:
	  » Antibiotics
	  » Analgesics
	  » Antipyretics
		› Rotate sites at least every 72 hr.
		› Avoid the lower extremities.
		› Use hand hygiene.
		› Use surgical aseptic technique.

Catheter embolus		
› Missing catheter tip when discontinued; severe pain at the site with migration, or absence of findings if no migration	› Place the tourniquet high on the extremity to limit venous flow. › Prepare for removal under x-ray or via surgery. › Save the catheter after removal to determine the cause.	› Do not reinsert the stylet into the catheter.

APPLICATION EXERCISES

1. A nurse on the IV team is conducting an education program for a newly hired nurse. After discussing complications of IV therapy, which of the following statements by the nurse indicates an understanding of clinical manifestations of infiltration? (Select all that apply.)

_____ A. "The temperature around the IV site is cooler."

_____ B. "The rate of the infusion increases."

_____ C. "The skin at the IV site is red."

_____ D. "The IV dressing is damp."

_____ E. "The tissue around the venipuncture site is swollen."

2. A nurse is teaching a newly licensed nurse on the proper procedure for inserting an IV catheter for a preoperative client. Which of the following statements by the nurse indicates understanding of the procedure?

A. "I will thread the needle all the way into the vein until the hub rests against the insertion site after I see a flashback of blood."

B. "I will insert the needle into the client's skin with the bevel up at an angle of 10° to 30°."

C. "I will apply pressure approximately 1.25 inches below the insertion site prior to removing the needle."

D. "I will choose the antecubital fossa vein for IV insertion due to its size and easily accessible location."

3. A nurse is caring for a client receiving dextrose 5% in 0.9% sodium chloride IV at 120 mL/hr. Which of the following statements by the client should alert the nurse to suspect fluid overload? (Select all that apply.)

_____ A. "I feel lightheaded."

_____ B. "I feel as though my heart is racing."

_____ C. "I feel a little short of breath."

_____ D. "The nurse's aide told me that my blood pressure was 150/90."

_____ E. "I think my ankles are less swollen."

4. A nurse educator is teaching a module about preventing IV infections during new employee orientation. Which of the following statements by a newly hired nurse indicates understanding of the teaching?

    A. "I will leave the IV catheter in my client after the IV antibiotics are completed."

    B. "As long as I am working with the same client, I can use the same IV catheter for my second insertion attempt."

    C. "If my client needs to use the rest room, it would be safer to disconnect his IV infusion as long as I clean the injection port thoroughly with an antiseptic swab."

    D. "I will change continuous infusion tubing no more frequently than every 96 hours and change intermittent infusion tubing every 24 hours."

5. A nurse is assessing a client who is receiving IV therapy and reports pain in his arm, chills, and "not feeling well." The nurse notes warmth, edema, induration, and red streaking on the client's arm close to the IV insertion site. Which of the following actions should the nurse plan to do first?

    A. Obtain a specimen for culture.

    B. Apply a warm compress.

    C. Administer analgesics.

    D. Discontinue the infusion.

6. A nurse educator is teaching a module on required documentation following insertion of an IV catheter to a group of newly hired nurses. What information should the nurse educator include in the teaching? Use the ATI Active Learning Template: Basic Concept to complete this item. In the section Related Content, list the seven recommended components of documentation following insertion of an IV catheter.

APPLICATION EXERCISES KEY

1. A. **CORRECT:** A decrease in skin temperature around the site is a clinical manifestation of infiltration due to the IV solution entering the subcutaneous tissue around the venipuncture site.

   B. INCORRECT: When infiltration occurs, the rate of infusion may slow or stop, not increase as the solution is no longer infusing directly into the vein. This occurs due to dislodgment of the catheter or rupture of the vein.

   C. INCORRECT: When infiltration occurs, the skin around the IV site is pale, not red, because the solution is no longer infusing directly into the vein and enters the subcutaneous tissue around the venipuncture site.

   D. **CORRECT:** A damp IV dressing is a common finding of infiltration due to the IV solution entering the subcutaneous tissue and leaking out through the venipuncture site.

   E. **CORRECT:** Swollen tissue around the venipuncture site is a clinical manifestation of infiltration due to the IV solution entering the subcutaneous tissue and causing swelling, as the fluid is no longer infusing into the vein.

   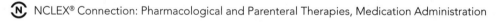 NCLEX® Connection: Pharmacological and Parenteral Therapies, Medication Administration

2. A. INCORRECT: After seeing a flashback of blood, the nurse lowers the hub close to the skin to prepare for threading the needle into the vein, then loosens the needle from the catheter and pulls back slightly on the needle so that it no longer extends past the tip of the catheter. Use the thumb and index finger to advance the catheter into the vein until the hub rests against the insertion site. Inserting the needle all the way into the vein could puncture the vein.

   B. **CORRECT:** The nurse inserts the catheter into the skin with the bevel up at an angle of 10° to 30° using a steady, smooth motion. This is the optimal angle to prevent puncture of the posterior vein wall.

   C. INCORRECT: The nurse applies pressure approximately 1.25 inch above the insertion site to reduce the backflow of blood into the vein prior to removing the needle.

   D. INCORRECT: The nurse should not use the antecubital fossa vein for IV insertion, except for emergency access, because mobility of the client's arm is limited.

   NCLEX® Connection: Pharmacological and Parenteral Therapies, Parenteral/Intravenous Therapies

3. A. INCORRECT: A clinical manifestation of fluid overload is hypertension. Lightheadness is a clinical manifestation of hypotension.

   B. **CORRECT:** A clinical manifestation of fluid overload is tachycardia due to the increased blood volume, which causes the heart rate to increase.

   C. **CORRECT:** A clinical manifestation of fluid overload is shortness of breath or dyspnea due to the increased amount of fluid entering the air spaces in the lungs, which reduces the amount of circulating oxygen.

   D. **CORRECT:** A clinical manifestation of fluid overload is hypertension due to the increased blood volume, which causes the blood pressure to increase.

   E. INCORRECT: A clinical manifestation of fluid overload is edema. If the client's ankles are less swollen, this is an indication that the edema is decreasing.

    NCLEX® Connection: Physiological Adaptations, Fluid and Electrolyte Imbalances

4. A. INCORRECT: It is recommended to remove catheters as soon as they are no longer clinically indicated to eliminate a portal of entry for pathogens or bacteria.

   B. INCORRECT: It is recommended to use a sterile needle/catheter for each insertion attempt for client safety and prevention of infection.

   C. INCORRECT: It is not recommended to disconnect tubing for convenience because this increases the risk of bacteria entering the system.

   D. **CORRECT:** It is recommended to change the primary intermittent tubing set every 24 hr and change continuous infusion tubing no more frequently than every 96 hr to prevent the entry of pathogens or bacteria into the client's bloodstream.

    NCLEX® Connection: Pharmacological and Parenteral Therapies, Medication Administration

5. A. INCORRECT: Although it is recommended to obtain a specimen for culture as a component in the treatment of cellulitis, it is not the first action the nurse should take.

   B. INCORRECT: Although it is recommended to apply a warm compress as a component in the treatment of cellulitis, it is not the first action the nurse should take.

   C. INCORRECT: Although it is recommended to administer analgesics as prescribed as a component in the treatment of cellulitis, it is not the first action the nurse should take.

   D. **CORRECT:** The greatest risk to the client is infection. The first action the nurse should perform in the treatment of cellulitis is to stop the infusion and remove the catheter because the catheter may be the source of infection.

    NCLEX® Connection: Pharmacological and Parenteral Therapies, Medication Administration

6. *Using the ATI Active Learning Template: Basic Concept*

- Related Content
  - Date and time of insertion
  - Insertion site and appearance
  - Catheter size
  - Type of dressing
  - IV fluid and rate (if applicable)
  - Number, locations and conditions of site-attempted catheterizations
  - Client's response

Ⓝ NCLEX® Connection: Pharmacological and Parenteral Therapies, Parenteral/Intravenous Therapies

UNIT 4 PHYSIOLOGICAL INTEGRITY
SECTION: PHARMACOLOGICAL AND PARENTERAL THERAPIES

CHAPTER 50 **Adverse Effects, Interactions, and Contraindications**

Overview

- To ensure safe medication administration and prevent errors, nurses must know why a medication is prescribed and the intended therapeutic effect. In addition, nurses must be aware of potential adverse effects, interactions, contraindications, and precautions.

- Every medication has the potential to cause adverse effects. Adverse effects are undesired, inadvertent, and unexpected dangerous effects of the medication. Adverse effects can range from mild to severe, and some can be potentially life-threatening.

- Medications are chemicals that affect the body. When more than one medication is given, there is a potential for an interaction. In addition, medications can interact with foods.

- Contraindications and precautions of specific medications refer to client conditions that make it unsafe or potentially harmful to administer these medications.

Adverse Medication Effects

- These effects are classified according to body systems.

ADVERSE MEDICATION EFFECTS	NURSING IMPLICATIONS/INTERVENTIONS
› Central nervous system (CNS) effects – May result from either CNS stimulation (excitement) or CNS depression.	› Implement seizure precautions if the client is at risk for seizures due to CNS stimulation. › If CNS depression is likely, advise clients not to drive or participate in other activities that can be dangerous.
› Extrapyramidal symptoms (EPSs) (abnormal body movements) – May include involuntary fine motor tremors, rigidity, uncontrollable restlessness, and acute dystonias (spastic movements and/ or muscle rigidity affecting the head, neck, eyes, facial area, and limbs). These may occur within a few hours or may take months to develop.	› EPSs are more often associated with medications affecting the CNS, such as those used to treat mental health disorders.
› Anticholinergic effects – Many medications have adverse effects that are a result of muscarinic receptor blockade. Most effects are seen in the eye, smooth muscle, exocrine glands, and the heart.	› Teach clients how to manage these effects. For example, dry mouth may be relieved by sipping on liquids; photophobia can be managed by use of sunglasses; and urinary retention may be reduced by urinating before taking the medication.

ADVERSE MEDICATION EFFECTS	NURSING IMPLICATIONS/INTERVENTIONS
› Cardiovascular effects – Cardiovascular effects may involve blood vessels and the heart.	› Antihypertensives can cause orthostatic hypotension. › Instruct clients about indications of postural hypotension (lightheadedness, dizziness). If these occur, advise the client to sit or lie down. Postural hypotension can be minimized by getting up and changing positions slowly.
› Gastrointestinal (GI) effects – GI effects may result from local irritation of the GI tract. Stimulation of the vomiting center also results in adverse effects.	› Many medications, such as NSAIDs, may cause GI upset. If appropriate, advise the client to take with food.
› Hematologic effects – Relatively common and potentially life-threatening with some groups of medications.	› Bone marrow depression/suppression is generally associated with anticancer medications and hemorrhagic disorders with anticoagulants and thrombolytics. Educate clients taking an anticoagulant about indications of bleeding, such as bruising, discolored urine/stool, petechiae, and bleeding gums. Tell clients to notify the provider if any of these are present.
› Hepatotoxicity – Because most medications are metabolized in the liver, the liver is particularly vulnerable to drug-induced injury. Damage to liver cells can impair metabolism of many medications, causing medication accumulation in the body and producing adverse effects. Many medications can alter normal values of liver function tests with no obvious clinical signs of liver dysfunction.	› When two or more medications that are hepatotoxic are combined, the risk for liver damage is increased. › Liver function tests are indicated when a client starts a medication known to be hepatotoxic and periodically thereafter.
› Nephrotoxicity – May occur with a number of medications, but is primarily the result of certain antimicrobial agents and NSAIDs. Impaired kidney function may interfere with medication excretion, leading to medication accumulation and adverse effects.	› Certain types of medications, such as aminoglycosides, may cause kidney damage. › Monitor serum creatinine and BUN levels of clients taking a medication known to be nephrotoxic.
› Toxicity – An adverse medication effect that is considered severe and may be life threatening. It may be caused by an excessive dose, but can also occur at therapeutic dose levels.	› An overdose of certain medications, such as acetaminophen (Tylenol), can result in toxicity, which can lead to liver damage. › The antidote acetylcysteine (Mucomyst) is effective in minimizing liver damage due to acetaminophen toxicity. › There is a greater risk of toxicity and liver damage with chronic alcohol use.

ADVERSE MEDICATION EFFECTS	NURSING IMPLICATIONS/INTERVENTIONS
› Allergic reaction – When an individual develops an immune response to a medication. The individual has been previously exposed to the medication and has developed antibodies.	› Allergic reactions range from minor to serious. Mild rashes and hives are commonly treated with diphenhydramine (Benadryl). › Before administering any medications, obtain a complete medication and allergy history.
› Anaphylactic reaction – A life-threatening immediate allergic reaction that causes respiratory distress, severe bronchospasm, and cardiovascular collapse.	› Treat with epinephrine, bronchodilators, and antihistamines. › Provide respiratory support and notify the provider.
› Immunosuppression – A decreased or absent immune response.	› Glucocorticoids depress the immune response and increase the risk for infection. › Monitor clients taking glucocorticoids for indications of infection.

Medication-Medication Interactions

CONSEQUENCES OF MEDICATION-MEDICATION INTERACTIONS	
Type of Interaction	Nursing Implications/Interventions
› Increased therapeutic effects	› Some medications may be given together to increase therapeutic effect. For example, clients who have asthma are instructed to use albuterol (Proventil), a beta$_2$-adrenergic agonist inhaler, 5 min prior to using fluticasone propionate (Flovent), a glucocorticoid inhaler, in order to increase the absorption of fluticasone propionate.
› Increased adverse effects	› Clients may take two medications that have the same adverse effects. Taking these two medications together increases the risk of these adverse effects. Diazepam (Valium) and hydrocodone bitartrate 5 mg/acetaminophen 500 mg (Vicodin) both have CNS depressant effects. When these medications are used together, the client has an increased risk for CNS depression.
› Decreased therapeutic effects	› One medication can increase the metabolism of a second medication and therefore decrease the serum level and effectiveness of the second medication. Phenytoin (Dilantin) increases hepatic medication-metabolizing enzymes that affect warfarin (Coumadin) and thereby decreases the serum level and the effect of warfarin.
› Decreased adverse effects	› One medication can be given to counteract the adverse effects of another medication. Ondansetron hydrochloride (Zofran), an antiemetic, may be administered to counteract the adverse effects of nausea and vomiting for a client receiving chemotherapy.
› Increased serum levels, leading to toxicity	› One medication can decrease the metabolism of a second medication and therefore increase the serum level of the second medication. This may lead to toxicity. Fluconazole (Diflucan), an antifungal, inhibits hepatic medication-metabolizing enzymes that affect aripiprazole (Abilify), an antipsychotic, and thereby increases serum levels of aripiprazole.

OVER-THE-COUNTER (OTC) MEDICATIONS	
Interactions	Nursing Implications/Interventions
› Ingredients in OTC medications may interact with other OTC or prescription medications. › Inactive ingredients such as dyes, alcohol, or preservatives may cause adverse reactions. › The potential for overdose exists because of the use of several preparations (including prescription medications) with similar ingredients.	› Obtain a complete medication history that includes both prescribed and OTC medications. › Instruct clients to follow the manufacturer's recommendations for dosage.
› Interactions of certain prescription and OTC medications can interfere with therapeutic effects.	› Clients are advised to use caution and to check with their provider before using any OTC preparations such as antacids, laxatives, decongestants, or cough syrups. For example, antacids can interfere with the absorption of ranitidine (Zantac) and other medications. Advise clients to take antacids 1 hr apart from other medications.

Medication-Food Interactions

- Food may alter medication absorption and may contain substances that react with certain medications.
  - Consuming foods with tyramine while taking monoamine oxidase inhibitors (MAOIs) can lead to hypertensive crisis. Clients taking an MAOI should be aware of such foods and avoid them.
  - Vitamin K can decrease the therapeutic effects of warfarin (Coumadin) and place clients at risk for developing blood clots. Clients taking warfarin should maintain a consistent intake of dietary vitamin K to avoid sudden fluctuations that could affect the action of warfarin.
  - Tetracycline (Tetracyn) can interact with a chelating agent such as milk, and form an insoluble, unabsorbable compound. Instruct clients not to take tetracycline within 2 hr of consuming any dairy products.
  - Grapefruit juice seems to act by inhibiting presystemic medication metabolism in the small bowel, thus increasing absorption of certain oral medications such as nifedipine (Procardia), a calcium channel blocker. This combination can result in increased effects or intensified adverse reactions. Instruct clients not to drink grapefruit juice if they are taking such a medication.

Contraindications and Precautions

- Take extra precautions for a client who is at greater risk of developing an adverse reaction to a medication. For example, morphine (Duramorph) depresses respiratory function, so it should be used with caution for clients who have asthma or impaired respiratory function.
- Contraindications to specific medications are present depending on the client's physical status, health, and allergy history. For example, penicillins are contraindicated for a client who has an allergy to this medication. Pregnancy or health conditions such as kidney disease also indicate contraindications to certain medications.

- The U.S. Food and Drug Administration places medications in categories based on risk to a fetus.

  ○ Category A: There is no evidence of risk to fetus during pregnancy based on adequate and well-controlled studies. Ferrous sulfate (Feosol), an iron supplement, is a Category A medication.

  ○ Category B: There is no evidence of risk to animal fetus based on studies but there are no adequate and well-controlled studies in pregnant women. Or there is evidence of risk to animal fetus, but controlled studies in pregnant women show no evidence of risk to the fetus. Esomeprazole magnesium (Nexium), an antiulcer, is a Category B medication.

  ○ Category C: Adverse effects have been demonstrated on animal fetuses, but there are no adequate and well-controlled studies in pregnant women. Or there have not been any studies done in animals or pregnant women. The use of these medications during pregnancy may be warranted based on the potential benefits. Glipizide (Glucotrol), an antidiabetic, is a Category C medication.

  ○ Category D: Adverse effects have been demonstrated on human fetuses based on data from investigational or marketing experience, but use of the medication during pregnancy may be warranted based on the potential benefits. Sorafenib (Nexavar), an antineoplastic, is a Category D medication.

  ○ Category X: Adverse effects have been demonstrated on animal and human fetuses based on studies and data from investigational or marketing experience. The use of the medication is contraindicated during pregnancy because the risks outweigh the potential benefits. Estradiol (Estrace), an estrogen replacement, is a Category X medication.

APPLICATION EXERCISES

1. A nurse is assessing a client who takes haloperidol (Haldol) for the treatment of schizophrenia. Which of the following findings should the nurse document as extrapyramidal symptoms (EPSs)? (Select all that apply.)

_____ A. Orthostatic hypotension

_____ B. Fine motor tremors

_____ C. Acute dystonias

_____ D. Decreased level of consciousness

_____ E. Uncontrollable restlessness

2. A nurse is providing teaching about managing anticholinergic effects for a client who has a new prescription for oxybutynin (Ditropan XL). Which of the following are appropriate to include in the teaching? (Select all that apply.)

_____ A. Take frequent sips of water.

_____ B. Wear sunglasses when exposed to sunlight.

_____ C. Use a soft toothbrush when brushing teeth.

_____ D. Take the medication with an antacid.

_____ E. Urinate prior to taking the medication.

3. A nurse is reviewing the reported medications of a client who was recently admitted. The medications include cimetidine (Tagamet) and imipramine hydrochloride (Tofranil). Knowing that cimetidine decreases the metabolism of imipramine hydrochloride, the nurse should identify that this combination is likely to result in which of the following effects?

A. Decreased therapeutic effects of cimetidine

B. Increased risk of imipramine hydrochloride toxicity

C. Decreased risk of adverse effects of cimetidine

D. Increased therapeutic effects of imipramine hydrochloride

4. A nurse in an outpatient clinic is caring for a client who states she is trying to get pregnant. The client currently takes a Category D pregnancy risk medication for the control of seizures. Which of the following statements by the nurse is appropriate?

    A. "This medication is prescribed if necessary but is known to cause adverse effects to the fetus."

    B. "This medication has evidence indicating that it is safe to take during pregnancy and will not harm the fetus."

    C. "This medication cannot be taken during pregnancy because the risk outweighs the potential benefits."

    D. "This medication hasn't been studied in pregnant women but is believed to be safe for the fetus."

5. A nurse in an outpatient surgical center is admitting a client for a laparoscopic procedure. The client has a prescription for preoperative diazepam (Valium). Prior to administering the medication, which of the following actions is the highest priority?

    A. Teaching the client about the purpose of the medication

    B. Administering the medication to the client at the prescribed time

    C. Identifying the client's medication allergies

    D. Documenting the client's anxiety level

6. A nurse is providing teaching for a client who has a new prescription for warfarin (Coumadin) for the prevention of venous thrombosis. Use the ATI Active Learning Template: Medication and the Pharmacology Review Module to complete this item to include the following sections:

    A. Side/Adverse Effects: Identify two adverse effects of warfarin.

    B. Nursing Interventions:
      • Identify at least two nursing interventions that are appropriate for the identified adverse effects.
      • Identify at least three contraindications for warfarin.

    C. Medication/Food Interactions:
      • Identify two medication interactions that increase the client's risk for bleeding.
      • Identify two medication interactions that decrease the effectiveness of warfarin.

    D. Client Education: Identify at least three foods that the client should avoid or limit while taking warfarin, and discuss the rationale for avoiding or limiting these foods.

APPLICATION EXERCISES KEY

1. A. INCORRECT: Orthostatic hypotension is an adverse effect, but it is not an EPS.

    B. **CORRECT:** Fine motor tremors are an EPS.

    C. **CORRECT:** Acute dystonias are an EPS.

    D. INCORRECT: Decreased level of consciousness is an adverse effect, but it is not an EPS.

    E. **CORRECT:** Uncontrollable restlessness is an EPS.

    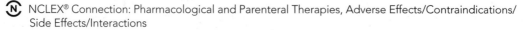 NCLEX® Connection: Pharmacological and Parenteral Therapies, Adverse Effects/Contraindications/ Side Effects/Interactions

2. A. **CORRECT:** Taking frequent sips of water will help relieve the anticholinergic effect of dry mouth.

    B. **CORRECT:** Wearing sunglasses will help relieve the anticholinergic effect of photophobia.

    C. INCORRECT: Anticholinergic effects do not increase the client's risk for bleeding.

    D. INCORRECT: Taking the medication with an antacid will not decrease anticholinergic effects.

    E. **CORRECT:** Urinating prior to taking the medication will help relieve the anticholinergic effect of urinary retention.

    (N) NCLEX® Connection: Pharmacological and Parenteral Therapies, Medication Administration

3. A. INCORRECT: A medication that increases the metabolism of a second medication can decrease the effectiveness of the second medication.

    B. **CORRECT:** A medication that decreases the metabolism of a second medication increases the serum level of the second medication, increasing the risk for toxicity.

    C. INCORRECT: A medication that decreases the metabolism of a second medication does not decrease the risk for adverse effects.

    D. INCORRECT: A medication that decreases the metabolism of a second medication does not increase the medication's therapeutic effects.

    (N) NCLEX® Connection: Pharmacological and Parenteral Therapies, Medication Administration

4. A. **CORRECT:** Category D medications are known to cause adverse effects on human fetuses. However, the use during pregnancy may be warranted based on the potential benefits.

    B. INCORRECT: Category A medications are safe to take during pregnancy and will not harm the fetus.

    C. INCORRECT: Category X medications cannot be taken during pregnancy.

    D. INCORRECT: Category B medications are believed to be safe for the fetus even though they may not have undergone controlled studies in pregnant women.

    (N) NCLEX® Connection: Pharmacological and Parenteral Therapies, Medication Administration

5. A. INCORRECT: Client education is an important action, but it does not address the greatest risk to the client and is therefore not the priority action.

    B. INCORRECT: Administering the medication at the prescribed time is an important action, but it does not address the greatest risk to the client and is therefore not the priority action.

    C. **CORRECT:** The greatest risk to this client is an allergic reaction. The priority action is to identify the client's allergies prior to medication administration.

    D. INCORRECT: Documenting the client's anxiety level is an important action, but it does not address the greatest risk to the client and is therefore not the priority action.

    Ⓝ NCLEX® Connection: Pharmacological and Parenteral Therapies, Medication Administration

6. *Using the ATI Active Learning Template: Medication*

    A. Side/Adverse Effects
    - Hemorrhage
    - Hepatitis
    - Toxicity

    B. Nursing Interventions
    - Hemorrhage
      ○ Monitor vital signs.
      ○ Advise clients to monitor for indications of bleeding.
      ○ Monitor PT and INR levels and compare to baseline values.
      ○ Have vitamin K (Mephyton) available as an antidote.
    - Hepatitis
      ○ Monitor liver enzymes and compare to baseline values.
      ○ Assess for jaundice.
    - Toxicity
      ○ Administer vitamin K.
      ○ Administer fresh frozen plasma or whole blood.
    - Contraindications
      ○ Pregnancy
      ○ Thrombocytopenia or bleeding disorders
      ○ During or following surgery of the eye, brain, or spinal cord; lumbar puncture; or regional anesthesia
      ○ Vitamin K deficiencies
      ○ Liver disorders
      ○ Alcohol use disorder

    C. Medication/Food Interactions
    - Medications that increase the risk for bleeding
      ○ Heparin, aspirin, acetaminophen, glucocorticoids, sulfonamides, parenteral cephalosporins
    - Medications that decrease the effectiveness of Coumadin
      ○ Phenobarbital, carbamazepine (Tegretol), phenytoin (Dilantin), oral contraceptives

    D. Client Education
    - The client should avoid or limit foods high in vitamin K that can decrease the anticoagulant effects of Coumadin.
      ○ Dark green leafy vegetables, cabbage, broccoli, Brussels sprouts, mayonnaise, canola and soybean oil

    Ⓝ NCLEX® Connection: Pharmacological and Parenteral Therapies, Medication Administration

chapter 51

Overview

- Various factors may affect how clients respond to medications. It is important for nurses to recognize these factors in order to individualize nursing care when administering medications.

Factors Affecting Medication Dosages and Responses

- Body Weight – Because medications are absorbed and distributed in body tissue, individuals who have a greater body mass may require larger doses.

- Age – Liver and kidney function are immature in young children and often decreased in older adults, which may require proportionately smaller medication doses.

- Gender – Females may respond differently to medications than males due to a higher proportion of body fat and the effects of female hormones.

- Genetics – Genetic factors such as missing enzymes can alter the metabolism of certain medications, thus enhancing or reducing medication action.

- Biorhythmic Cycles – Responses to certain medications vary with the biologic rhythms of the body. For example, hypnotic medications work better when given at the usual sleep time than at other times.

- Tolerance – Responsiveness to a medication is reduced, and is either congenital (genetic factors) or acquired (stimulation of liver enzymes or other physiologic variations). Cross-tolerance may occur with other chemically similar medications.

- Accumulation – An increased medication concentration occurs in the body due to the inability to metabolize or excrete a medication rapidly enough, resulting in a toxic medication effect. For older adults, decreased kidney function is the major cause of medication accumulation leading to toxicity.

- Psychological Factors – Emotional state and expectations can influence the effects of a medication. The placebo effect describes positive medication effects influenced by psychological factors.

- Medical Conditions

  ○ Inadequate gastric acid inhibits the absorption of medications that require an acid medium to dissolve.

  ○ Diarrhea causes oral medications to pass through the gastrointestinal tract too quickly to be absorbed.

  ○ Vascular insufficiency prevents distribution of a medication to affected tissue.

  ○ Liver disease/failure impairs medication metabolism, which may cause toxicity.

  ○ Kidney disease/failure prevents or delays medication excretion, which may cause toxicity.

Pharmacology and Children

- While most medications administered to adults are useful for children, the dosages are different. Pediatric dosages often are based on body weight or body surface area (BSA). Neonates (younger than 1 month old) and infants (1 month to 1 year old) have immature liver and kidney function, alkaline gastric juices, and an immature blood-brain barrier. Certain medication dosages are based on age due to a greater risk for decreased skeletal bone growth, acute cardiopulmonary failure, or hepatic toxicity.

- Additional pharmacokinetic factors specific to children
  - Decreased gastric acid production and slower gastric emptying time
  - Decreased first-pass medication metabolism
  - Increased absorption of topical medications (greater body surface area and thinner skin)
  - Lower blood pressure (more blood flow to the liver and brain and less to the kidneys)
  - Higher body water content (dilutes water-soluble medications)
  - Decreased serum protein-binding sites (until age 1 year). This can result in an increase in the serum level of protein-binding medications.

- Be particularly alert when administering medications to children due to the risk for medication errors.
  - Dosages are usually based on weight or BSA.
  - Most medications are not tested on children.
  - Adult medication forms and concentrations may require dilution, calculation, preparation, and administration of very small doses.
  - Limited sites exist for IV medication administration.

Pharmacology and Older Adults (65+ Years)

- Physiologic changes associated with aging that affect pharmacokinetics
  - Increased gastric pH (alkaline)
  - Decreased gastrointestinal motility and gastric emptying time
  - Decreased blood flow through the cardiovascular system, liver, and kidneys
  - Decreased hepatic enzyme function
  - Decreased kidney function and glomerular filtration rate
  - Decreased protein-binding sites
  - Decreased body water, increased body fat, and decreased lean body mass
- Other factors affecting medication therapy for older adults
  - Impaired memory or altered mental state
  - Changes in vision and hearing
  - Decreased mobility and dexterity
  - Poor adherence
  - Reduced financial resources
  - Polypharmacy – The practice of taking several medications simultaneously (prescribed and/or over-the-counter [OTC]) with diminished bodily functions and some medical conditions. This can contribute to the potential for medication toxicity.

- Nursing interventions for older adults
  - Decreasing the risk of adverse medication effects.
    - Obtain a complete medication history and include all OTC medications.
    - Make sure the medication therapy starts at the lowest possible dose.
    - Assess/monitor for therapeutic and adverse effects.
    - Assess/monitor for medication-medication and medication-food interactions.
    - Document findings.
    - Notify the provider of adverse effects.
  - Promoting adherence.

    - Give clear and concise instructions, verbally and in writing.
    - Ensure that the dosage form is appropriate. Administer liquid forms to clients who have difficulty swallowing pills or tablets.
    - Provide clearly marked containers that are easy to open.
    - Assist the client to set up a daily calendar with the use of pill containers.
    - Suggest that the client obtain assistance from a friend, neighbor, or relative.

Pharmacology – Pregnancy and Lactation

- Pregnancy – Any medication ingested by a woman who is pregnant will be distributed to the fetus as well. Medications are classified according to potential harm to the fetus. Most medications are considered potentially harmful to the fetus, so the benefits of maternal medication administration are weighed against possible fetal risk. Medications are used during pregnancy most commonly as nutritional supplements (iron, vitamins, minerals) and for the treatment of nausea, vomiting, gastric acidity, and mild discomforts. Management of chronic medical conditions such as diabetes mellitus or hypertension is done in conjunction with careful maternal-fetal monitoring. Live-virus vaccines (measles, mumps, polio, rubella, yellow fever) are contraindicated due to possible teratogenic effects.
- Lactation – Most medications are secreted in breast milk. Avoid all medications with an extended half-life or those that are known to be harmful to the infant. For medications that are safe, administer immediately after breastfeeding to minimize medication concentration in the next feeding.

APPLICATION EXERCISES

1. A nurse is providing teaching to an older adult client to promote adherence with medication administration. Which of the following instructions should the nurse include? (Select all that apply.)

_____ A. Adjust dosages according to daily weight.

_____ B. Place pills in daily pill holders.

_____ C. Provide liquid forms if the client has difficulty swallowing pills.

_____ D. Ask a relative to assist periodically.

_____ E. Request child-guard caps on medication containers.

2. A charge nurse is leading a peer group discussion about factors affecting medication dosages and responses. Which of the following statements by a fellow nurse indicates the need for further teaching?

A. "Clients who have a higher BMI may require larger doses of medications."

B. "Client tolerance to medication is a result of decreased metabolism."

C. "Clients who have a placebo effect can have increased effectiveness of medication."

D. "Client gender can affect responsiveness to medications."

3. A nurse is preparing medications for a preschool-age client. Which of the following factors should the nurse recognize as altering how children are affected by a medication? (Select all that apply.)

_____ A. Increased gastric acid production

_____ B. Lower blood pressure

_____ C. Higher body water content

_____ D. Increased absorption of topical medications

_____ E. Increased gastric emptying time

4. A nurse is providing medication teaching for a client who is lactating. Which of the following is appropriate to include to minimize secretion in breast milk?

A. Drink a full glass of milk with each dose of medication.

B. Recommend medications that have an extended half-life.

C. Take each prescribed dose right after breastfeeding.

D. Pump breast milk and freeze prior to feeding to the infant.

5. A nurse in an outpatient clinic is providing teaching to a client who is in her first trimester of pregnancy. Which of the following statements is appropriate for the nurse to include?

    A. "You will need to have a rubella vaccine if not received prior to pregnancy."

    B. "You can safely take over-the-counter medications."

    C. "You should avoid any vitamin preparations containing iron."

    D. "Your provider can prescribe medication for nausea if needed."

6. A nurse is preparing to administer medications to an older adult client who has vascular insufficiency and impaired kidney function. Use the ATI Active Learning Template: Basic Concept to complete this item to include the following sections:

    A. Underlying Principles:

- Discuss medication considerations related to vascular insufficiency.
- Discuss medication considerations related to impaired kidney function.
- Identify at least four additional physiologic changes associated with aging that impact pharmacokinetics.

    B. Nursing Interventions: Identify at least three interventions to decrease the risk of adverse effects.

APPLICATION EXERCISES KEY

1. A. INCORRECT: Adjustment of dosages is prescribed by the provider. Instructing the client to base dosages according to daily weight increases the risk for error in medication administration.

    B. **CORRECT:** Organizing medications in daily pill holders promotes medication adherence.

    C. **CORRECT:** Providing a form of medication that is easier for the client to swallow promotes medication adherence.

    D. **CORRECT:** Including the client's support system promotes medication adherence.

    E. INCORRECT: The older adult client may have difficulty opening child-guard caps. Request easy-open containers from the pharmacy.

    (N) NCLEX® Connection: Pharmacological and Parenteral Therapies, Medication Administration

2. A. INCORRECT: Clients who have a greater body mass may require larger doses of medications.

    B. **CORRECT:** This statement requires further teaching. Tolerance refers to a reduced responsiveness to medication. Accumulation refers to increased medication concentration in the body due to decreased metabolism.

    C. INCORRECT: The placebo effect describes positive medication effects influenced by psychological factors.

    D. INCORRECT: Client gender can affect responses to medication.

    (N) NCLEX® Connection: Physiological Adaptations, Pathophysiology

3. A. INCORRECT: Children have decreased gastric acid production.

    B. **CORRECT:** Children have a lower blood pressure.

    C. **CORRECT:** Children have a higher body water content.

    D. **CORRECT:** Children have an increased absorption of topical medications.

    E. INCORRECT: Children have a slower gastric emptying time.

    (N) NCLEX® Connection: Health Promotion and Maintenance, Developmental Stages and Transitions

4. A. INCORRECT: The intake of food or fluid with medication does not affect secretion of the medication into the breast milk.

    B. INCORRECT: The client should avoid medications that have an extended half-life due to increased secretion in breast milk.

    C. **CORRECT:** Taking medication immediately after breastfeeding helps minimize medication concentration in the next feeding.

    D. INCORRECT: Pumping and freezing breast milk does not affect the secretion of the medication into the breast milk.

    Ⓝ NCLEX® Connection: Health Promotion and Maintenance, Developmental Stages and Transitions

5. A. INCORRECT: Live-virus vaccines, including rubella, are contraindicated during pregnancy due to possible teratogenic effects.

    B. INCORRECT: Most medications, including over-the-counter, are considered potentially harmful to the fetus. The client should avoid any medications unless prescribed by her provider.

    C. INCORRECT: Nutritional supplements that include iron are commonly used during pregnancy to support the health of the mother and fetus.

    D. **CORRECT:** Providers can prescribe medications for the treatment of nausea and other discomforts of pregnancy.

    Ⓝ NCLEX® Connection: Health Promotion and Maintenance, Developmental Stages and Transitions

6. *Using the ATI Active Learning Template: Basic Concept*
    A. Underlying Principles
        - Vascular insufficiency prevents distribution of a medication to affected tissue. The nurse should document and monitor for the medication's effectiveness and report concerns to the provider.
        - Impaired kidney function prevents or delays medication excretion, which increases the risk for toxicity. Decreased kidney function is the major cause of medication accumulation leading to toxicity.
        - Physiologic changes
            - Increased gastric pH
            - Decreased gastrointestinal motility and gastric emptying time
            - Decreased hepatic enzyme function
            - Decreased protein-binding sites
            - Decreased body water
            - Increased body fat, decreased lean body mass
            - Impaired memory or altered mental state
            - Decreased mobility and dexterity
    B. Nursing Interventions
        - Obtain a complete medication history and include all OTC medications.
        - Make sure medication therapy starts at the lowest possible dose.
        - Assess/monitor for therapeutic and adverse effects.
        - Assess/monitor for medication-medication and medication-food interactions.
        - Notify the provider of adverse effects.

    Ⓝ NCLEX® Connection: Physiological Adaptations, Illness Management

UNIT 4   Physiological Integrity

SECTION: REDUCTION OF RISK POTENTIAL

› Specimen Collection for Glucose Monitoring
› Airway Management
› Nasogastric Intubation and Enteral Feedings

NCLEX® CONNECTIONS

When reviewing the chapters in this unit, keep in mind the relevant sections of the NCLEX® outline, in particular:

Client Needs: Basic Care and Comfort	Client Needs: Reduction of Risk Potential	Client Needs: Physiological Adaptation

› Relevant topics/tasks include:
  » Nutrition and Oral Hydration
    › Provide client nutrition through continuous or intermittent tube feedings.
	› Relevant topics/tasks include:
	  » Laboratory Values
	    › Obtain specimens other than blood for diagnostic testing.
	  » Potential for Alterations in Body Systems
	    › Identify the client's potential for skin breakdown.
	  » Potential for Complications of Diagnostic Tests/Treatments/Procedures
	    › Position the client to prevent complications following tests/treatments/procedures.
		› Relevant topics/tasks include:
		  » Fluid and Electrolyte Imbalances
		    › Manage the care of the client with a fluid and electrolyte imbalance.

chapter **52**

Overview

Q
EBP

- Monitoring blood glucose levels is an essential component in the care of clients who have diabetes mellitus.

- Blood glucose testing is the preferred method of monitoring blood glucose levels.

- Urine testing is not an effective measure of glucose level as glucose levels must be greater than 220 mg/dL before glucose appears in the urine.

- Clients who are able and willing to continue monitoring independently can learn how to self-monitor blood glucose levels. Required abilities include the following:

  - Alertness or the ability to comprehend and give a return demonstration of the process

  - Adequate finger dexterity

  - Adequate visual acuity

Blood Glucose Testing

- For blood glucose testing, clients who have diabetes mellitus use a glucometer or a blood glucose meter with small test strips to "read" the blood sample. These systems require proper calibration, storage of supplies, and matching of lot numbers.

- Indications

  - Regular testing is necessary for clients who have diabetes mellitus to manage the disease by maintaining safe blood glucose levels.

- Interpretation of Findings

  - Usually, a blood glucose level greater than 250 mg/dL indicates hyperglycemia.

  - Usually, a blood glucose level less than 70 mg/dL indicates hypoglycemia.

  - Poor storage of glucose test strips can lead to falsely high and low readings. Typically, these test strips come in a vial to store at room temperature or as the manufacturer directs.

- Preprocedure

  - Nursing Actions

    - Check the client's record and prescription

      - Frequency and type of test

        - Testing times vary based on the goals of management and the complexity of the client's hypoglycemic medication schedule.

      - Results from previous tests – norms and ranges

      - Actions according to results

- Review the client's medication profile.
  - Note anticoagulant usage, history of bleeding disorders, and low platelet count.
  - Note the times and dose of hypoglycemic agents.
  - Note the use of corticosteroids, oral contraceptives, beta blockers, antipsychotics, and other medications that can elevate blood glucose levels.
- Gather materials and prepare the equipment.
  - Blood glucose meter
  - Reagent strip compatible with the meter
  - Washcloth and soap or antiseptic swab
  - Clean gloves
  - Sterile lancet
  - Cotton ball
- Review the meter and the manufacturer's instructions.
- Check the strip solution's expiration date.
- Some meters require calibration; others requiring zeroing of the timer. Follow the manufacturer's directions.
- Explain the procedure to the client.
- Evaluate the selected puncture site.
  - Integrity of the skin (to avoid areas of bruising, open lesions)
  - Compromised circulation
- Perform hand hygiene and put on gloves.
- Intraprocedure
  - Nursing Actions
    - Select a site from which to collect the blood sample.
      - Outer edge of a fingertip (most common site)
      - Alternate site (heel, palm, arm, thigh)
    - Rotate sites to avoid ongoing tenderness.
    - Wrap the site in a warm, moist towel to enhance circulation, especially when it has been difficult to obtain an adequate sample.
    - Cleanse the site with warm water and soap or an antiseptic swab (not alcohol), and allow it to dry. Alcohol can interfere with results.
    - Hold the finger in a dependent position before puncturing to improve blood flow.
    - Pierce the skin using a sterile lancet (or a lancet injector device) and holding it perpendicular to the skin.
    - Wipe away the first drop of blood with a cotton ball.

- Place a drop of blood on the test strip.
    - Follow the manufacturer's procedure for applying blood to the strip.
    - If necessary, gently milk the finger to squeeze out a drop. (Forceful milking or squeezing can cause pain, bruising, and scarring.) Do not touch the site directly to stimulate bleeding.
    - Hold the test strip next to the blood on the fingertip.
    - Do not smear blood onto the strip because this can cause an inaccurate reading.

- Allow the meter to process the reading. (Time varies with the meter.)
- Apply a cotton ball over the puncture site.
- Note the reading, turn off the meter, and dispose of the cotton ball, test strip, and gloves.
- Postprocedure
    - Nursing Actions
        - Perform hand hygiene.
        - Document the meter's reading.
        - Check the prescription for medication or treatment actions and implement.

Urine Glucose Testing

- Indications
    - Clients who have diabetes mellitus perform urine glucose testing at home at times of acute illness or stress to identify the presence of ketones.
- Interpretation of Findings
    - If the test is positive for ketones, it indicates uncontrolled blood glucose.
- Preprocedure
    - Nursing Actions
        - If testing urine, evaluate the client's ability to urinate.
        - Verify the prescription for frequency and actions to take based on the results.
        - Gather materials and prepare the equipment.
            - Urine specimen cup
            - Chemical reagent strips, container with glucose reading scale
            - Clean gloves
            - Towelette or soap and washcloth
        - Check the strip's expiration date.
        - Explain the procedure.
        - Perform hand hygiene, and put on clean gloves.

- Intraprocedure
  - Nursing Actions
    - Assist the client with urine sample collection.
    - Dip the reagent strip into the urine sample.
    - Compare the strip's color change with the ranges on the container within the instructed time (usually 1 to 5 seconds).
- Postprocedure
  - Nursing Actions
    - Dispose of the remaining urine sample, test strip, and gloves.
    - Perform hand hygiene.
    - Check the prescription for medication or treatment actions, and implement.

APPLICATION EXERCISES

1. A nurse is assessing a client's ability to learn self-monitoring of blood glucose using a glucometer. Which of the following abilities should the nurse confirm that the client has before proceeding with teaching? (Select all that apply.)

_____ A. Finger dexterity

_____ B. Visual acuity

_____ C. Color vision

_____ D. Basic literacy

_____ E. Demonstration ability

2. A client has an admission blood glucose reading of 260 mg/dL and no documented history of diabetes mellitus. While the nurse reviews the client's medication history, which of the following types of medications should alert the nurse to the possibility that the client has developed an adverse effect of pharmacologic therapy? (Select all that apply.)

_____ A. Diuretics

_____ B. Corticosteroids

_____ C. Oral anticoagulants

_____ D. Opioid analgesics

_____ E. Antipsychotics

3. A nurse is teaching a client who just found out she has type 1 diabetes mellitus how to check her blood glucose levels. Which of the following instructions should the nurse give the client for transferring her blood onto the reagent portion of the test strip?

A. Smear the blood onto the strip.

B. Squeeze the blood onto the strip.

C. Touch the puncture to stimulate bleeding.

D. Hold the test strip next to the blood on the fingertip.

4. A nurse attempts to collect a capillary blood specimen via finger stick to test the glucose level of a client who has diabetes mellitus. The nurse is unable to obtain an adequate drop of blood for the reagent strip. Which of the following actions should the nurse take?

    A. Puncture another finger to obtain a capillary specimen.

    B. Test the client's urine with a urine reagent strip.

    C. Wrap the client's hand in a warm, moist cloth.

    D. Perform a venipuncture to obtain a venous sample.

5. A nurse is teaching self-monitoring of blood glucose (SMBG) to a client who has diabetes mellitus. Which of the following instructions should the nurse include? (Select all that apply.)

    _____ A. Perform SMBG once daily at bedtime.

    _____ B. Wipe his hand with an alcohol swab.

    _____ C. Hold his hand in a dependent position prior to the puncture.

    _____ D. Place the puncturing device perpendicular to the site.

    _____ E. Prick the outer edge of his fingertip for the blood sample.

6. A nurse is teaching a group of nursing students how to perform urine glucose testing. Use the ATI Active Learning Template: Diagnostic Procedure to complete this item. Under Nursing Actions (pre, intra, post), list the steps of the procedure in the three phases.

APPLICATION EXERCISES KEY

1. A. **CORRECT:** To use a glucometer to monitor blood glucose, the client has to have the manual dexterity to cleanse and puncture his finger, collect the blood, insert the strip into the meter, and otherwise operate the meter.

    B. **CORRECT:** To use a glucometer to monitor blood glucose, the client has to have the ability to see the digital reading of the results.

    C. INCORRECT: Clients who have color blindness might have difficulty interpreting the colors on a reagent strip for urine glucose testing, but they should be able to perform blood glucose testing accurately.

    D. INCORRECT: For basic use of a glucometer to monitor blood glucose, the client needs only to recognize numerals. Reading skills are not necessary.

    E. **CORRECT:** For the nurse to verify that the client has learned to use a glucometer accurately and safely, the client must be able to give the nurse a return demonstration of the procedure.

    Ⓝ NCLEX® Connection: Reduction of Risk Potential, Therapeutic Procedures

2. A. **CORRECT:** Diuretics can cause hyperglycemia, especially in clients who have diabetes mellitus, and also can cause many electrolyte imbalances.

    B. **CORRECT:** Corticosteroids, or glucocorticoids, can cause hyperglycemia and glycosuria.

    C. INCORRECT: Anticoagulants are unlikely to raise blood glucose levels. However, they could possibly cause excessive bleeding during blood sampling for glucose testing.

    D. INCORRECT: Opioid analgesics cause many adverse effects, including respiratory depression, but they are unlikely to raise blood glucose levels.

    E. **CORRECT:** Antipsychotics, particularly atypical antipsychotics, can cause new-onset diabetes mellitus.

    Ⓝ NCLEX® Connection: Pharmacological and Parenteral Therapies, Adverse Effects/Contraindications/ Side Effects/Interactions

3. A. INCORRECT: Smearing the blood can cause inaccurate results.

    B. INCORRECT: The client should milk her finger gently to squeeze out a drop of blood. Forceful milking or squeezing can cause pain, bruising, and scarring.

    C. INCORRECT: Touching the puncture could transfer micro-organisms to the wound.

    D. **CORRECT:** Holding the pad of the strip next to the puncture allows the blood to flow until the amount on the strip is adequate. Too little blood can result in falsely low readings.

     NCLEX® Connection: Reduction of Risk Potential, Therapeutic Procedures

4. A. INCORRECT: If the previous problem was due to inadequate peripheral circulation, the nurse might have the same unsuccessful result.

    B. INCORRECT: Unless the client's blood glucose level is significantly elevated, urine testing will not provide useful information.

    C. **CORRECT:** Warming the finger with a warm, moist cloth promotes blood flow in preparation for the next finger stick.

    D. INCORRECT: It is inappropriate to request a laboratory procedure after a single attempt at obtaining a glucometer reading.

     NCLEX® Connection: Reduction of Risk Potential, Therapeutic Procedures

5. A. INCORRECT: Generally, the timing and frequency of SMBG testing correlates with the client's medication schedule. It might be as often as before each meal and at bedtime. Monitoring once a day at bedtime does not provide enough information to monitor blood glucose control effectively.

    B. INCORRECT: The client should wash his hand with warm water and soap. Alcohol can alter the blood glucose reading.

    C. **CORRECT:** The dependent position increases blood flow to the fingers.

    D. **CORRECT:** Holding the lancet perpendicular to the skin ensures the correct piercing depth.

    E. **CORRECT:** The outer edge of the fingertip is an appropriate site for blood sampling. The client may also use a heel, palm, arm, or thigh.

     NCLEX® Connection: Reduction of Risk Potential, Therapeutic Procedures

6. *Using ATI Active Learning Template: Diagnostic Procedure*
   - Nursing Actions
     - Preprocedure
       - Evaluate the client's ability to urinate.
       - Verify the prescription for frequency and actions to take based on the results.
       - Gather materials and prepare equipment: urine specimen cup, chemical reagent strips, container with the glucose reading scale, clean gloves, towelette or soap and washcloth.
       - Check the strip's expiration date.
       - Explain the procedure.
       - Perform hand hygiene, and put on clean gloves.
     - Intraprocedure
       - Assist the client with urine sample collection.
       - Dip the reagent strip into the urine sample.
       - Compare the strip's color change with the ranges on the container within the instructed time (usually 1 to 5 seconds).
     - Postprocedure
       - Dispose of the remaining urine sample, test strip, and gloves.
       - Perform hand hygiene.
       - Check the prescription for medication or treatment actions, and implement.

Ⓝ NCLEX® Connection: Reduction of Risk Potential, Therapeutic Procedures

chapter 53

Overview

- Managing airway compromise includes respiratory assessment along with measuring vital signs, including oxygen saturation via pulse oximetry and administration of oxygen.

- Oxygen helps maintain adequate cellular oxygenation for clients who have many acute and chronic respiratory problems (hypoxemia, cystic fibrosis, asthma) or are at risk for developing hypoxia (respiratory illness, circulatory impairment).

- Maintaining a patent airway is a nursing priority. It involves mobilizing secretions, suctioning the airway, and managing artificial airways (endotracheal tubes, tracheostomy tubes) to promote adequate gas exchange and lung expansion.

PULSE OXIMETRY AND OXYGEN THERAPY

Overview

- A pulse oximeter is a device with a sensor probe that attaches securely to the fingertip, toe, bridge of nose, earlobe, or forehead with a clip or band.

- A pulse oximeter measures pulse saturation (SpO_2) via a wave of infrared light that measures light absorption by oxygenated and deoxygenated hemoglobin in arterial blood. SpO_2 reliably reflects the percent of saturation of hemoglobin (SaO_2).

- Oxygen is a tasteless and colorless gas that accounts for 21% of atmospheric air.

- Oxygen flow rates vary to maintain an SpO_2 of 95% to 100% using the lowest amount of oxygen to achieve the goal without risking complications.

- The fraction of inspired oxygen (FiO_2) is the percentage of oxygen the client receives.

Pulse Oximetry

- Noninvasive measurement of the oxygen saturation of the blood for monitoring respiratory status when assessment findings include any of the following:
  - Increased work of breathing
  - Wheezing
  - Coughing
  - Cyanosis
  - Changes in respiratory rate or rhythm
  - Adventitious breath sounds
  - Restlessness, irritability, confusion

- Interpretation of Findings
  - The expected reference range is 95% to 100%. Acceptable levels range from 91% to 100%. Some illness states may even allow for 85% to 89%. Readings below 90% reflect hypoxemia.

  - Values may be slightly lower for older adult clients and clients who have dark skin.
  - Additional reasons for low readings include hypothermia, poor peripheral blood flow, too much light (sun, infrared lamps), low hemoglobin levels, movement, edema, and nail polish.
  - Interventions
    - For readings below 90% (indicating hypoxemia):
      - Confirm probe placement.
      - Confirm that the oxygen delivery system is functioning and that the client is receiving the prescribed oxygen levels.
      - Place the client in semi-Fowler's or Fowler's position promote chest expansion and to maximize ventilation.
      - Encourage deep breathing.
      - Remain with the client and provide emotional support to decrease anxiety.

Oxygen Therapy

- Oxygen is a therapeutic gas that treats hypoxemia (low levels of arterial oxygen). Administering and adjusting it requires a provider's prescription.
  - Clinical manifestations of hypoxemia include:

EARLY	LATE
› Tachypnea	› Stupor
› Tachycardia	› Cyanotic skin, mucous membranes
› Restlessness, anxiety, confusion	› Bradypnea
› Pale skin, mucous membranes	› Bradycardia
› Elevated blood pressure	› Hypotension
› Use of accessory muscles, nasal flaring, tracheal tugging, adventitious lung sounds	› Cardiac dysrhythmias

- Nursing Actions
  - Monitor respiratory rate and pattern, level of consciousness, SpO_2, and arterial blood gases.
  - Provide oxygen therapy at the lowest liter flow that will correct hypoxemia.
  - Make sure the mask creates a secure seal over the nose and mouth.
  - Assess/monitor hypoxemia and hypercarbia (elevated levels of CO_2): restlessness, hypertension, and headache.
  - Auscultate the lungs for breath sounds and adventitious sounds, such as crackles and wheezes.
  - Assess/monitor oxygenation status with pulse oximetry and arterial blood gases (ABGs).
  - Promote oral hygiene.
  - Encourage turning, coughing, deep breathing, and the use of incentive spirometry and suctioning.
  - Promote rest and decrease environmental stimuli.
  - Provide emotional support.
  - Assess nutritional status; provide supplements.

- ○ Assess skin integrity; provide moisture and pressure-relief devices.
- ○ Assess and document the response to oxygen therapy.
- ○ Titrate oxygen to maintain the recommended oxygen saturation.
- ○ Discontinue supplemental oxygen gradually.
- ○ Monitor for respiratory depression (decreased respiratory rate and level of consciousness).
- ○ Low-flow oxygen delivery systems deliver varying amounts of oxygen based on the delivery method and the client's breathing pattern.

View Images

| › Nasal Cannula | › Simple Mask | › Venturi Mask |
| › Nonrebreather Mask | › Face Tent | |

LOW-FLOW OXYGEN DELIVERY SYSTEMS

NASAL CANNULA

Description	› A length of tubing with two small prongs for insertion into the nares
Fraction of Inspired Oxygen (FIO)	› It delivers an FIO_2 of 24% to 44% at a flow rate of 1 to 6 L/min.
Advantages	› It is a safe, simple, and easy-to-apply method. › It is comfortable and well-tolerated. › The client is able to eat, talk, and ambulate.
Disadvantages	› The FIO_2 varies with the flow rate, and rate and depth of the client's breathing. › Extended use may lead to skin breakdown and dry mucous membranes. › It is easily dislodged.
Nursing Interventions	› Assess the patency of the nares. › Ensure that the prongs fit in the nares properly. › Use water-soluble gel to prevent dry nares. › Provide humidification for flow rates of 4 L/min and above.

SIMPLE FACE MASK

Description	› Covers the client's nose and mouth
Fraction of Inspired Oxygen (FIO)	› It delivers an FIO_2 of 40% to 60% at flow rates of 5 to 8 L/min. › The minimum flow rate is 5 L/min to ensure flushing of CO_2 from the mask.
Advantages	› A face mask is easy to apply and may be more comfortable than a nasal cannula. › It is a simple delivery method. › It is more comfortable than a nasal cannula. › It provides humidified oxygen.
Disadvantages	› Flow rates of 5 L/min or lower may result in rebreathing of CO_2. › Clients who have anxiety or claustrophobia do not tolerate it well. › Eating, drinking, and talking are impaired.
Nursing Interventions	› Assess proper fit to ensure a secure seal over the nose and mouth. › Make sure the client wears a nasal cannula during meals. › Use with caution for clients who have a high risk of aspiration or airway obstruction.

LOW-FLOW OXYGEN DELIVERY SYSTEMS

PARTIAL REBREATHER MASK

Description	› Covers the client's nose and mouth
Fraction of Inspired Oxygen (FIO)	› It delivers an FiO_2 of 40% to 70% at flow rates of 6 to 11 L/min.
Advantages	› The mask has a reservoir bag attached with no valve, which allows the client to rebreathe up to $1/3$ of exhaled air together with room air.
Disadvantages	› Complete deflation of the reservoir bag during inspiration causes CO_2 buildup. › The FiO_2 varies with the client's breathing pattern. › Clients who have anxiety or claustrophobia do not tolerate it well. › Eating, drinking, and talking are impaired.
Nursing Interventions	› Keep the bag from deflating by adjusting the oxygen flow rate to keep the reservoir bag inflated. › Assess proper fit to ensure a secure seal over nose and mouth. › Make sure the client uses a nasal cannula during meals. › Use with caution for clients who have a high risk of aspiration or airway obstruction.

NASAL CANNULA

Description	› Covers the client's nose and mouth
Fraction of Inspired Oxygen (FIO)	› It delivers an FiO_2 of 60% to 80% at flow rates of 10 to 15 L/min to keep the reservoir bag $2/3$ full during inspiration and expiration.
Advantages	› It delivers the highest O_2 concentration possible (except for intubation). › A one-way valve situated between the mask and reservoir allows the client to inhale maximum O_2 from the reservoir bag. The two exhalation ports have flaps covering them that prevent room air from entering the mask.
Disadvantages	› The valve and flap on the mask must be intact and functional during each breath. › It is poorly tolerated by clients who have anxiety or claustrophobia. › Eating, drinking, and talking are impaired. › Use with caution for clients who have a high risk of aspiration or airway obstruction.
Nursing Interventions	› Perform an hourly assessment of the valve and flap. › Assess proper fit to ensure a secure seal over the nose and mouth. › Make sure the client uses a nasal cannula during meals.

HIGH-FLOW OXYGEN DELIVERY SYSTEMS	
VENTURI MASK	
Description	› covers the client's nose and mouth
Fraction of inspired oxygen (FiO$_2$)	› It delivers an FiO$_2$ of 24% to 60% at flow rates of 4 to 12 L/min via different size adaptors.
Advantages	› It delivers the most precise oxygen concentration. › Humidification is not required. › It is best for clients who have chronic lung disease.
Disadvantages	› Use is expensive. › Eating, drinking, and talking are impaired.
Nursing Interventions	› Assess frequently to ensure an accurate flow rate. › Make sure the tubing is free of kinks.
AEROSOL MASK	
Description	› Face tent (fits loosely around the face and neck) › Tracheostomy collar (a small mask that covers the surgically created opening of the trachea)
Fraction of inspired oxygen (FiO$_2$)	› They deliver an FiO$_2$ of 24% to 100% at flow rates of at least 10 L/min. › They provide high humidification with oxygen delivery.
Advantages	› Use with clients who do not tolerate masks well. › Useful for clients who have facial trauma, burns, and thick secretions.
Disadvantages	› High humidification requires frequent monitoring.
Nursing Interventions	› Empty condensation from the tubing often. › Ensure adequate water in the humidification canister. › Make sure the tubing does not pull on the tracheostomy.

- Complications

  ○ Oxygen toxicity

    ▪ Oxygen toxicity may result from high concentrations of oxygen (typically above 50%), long durations of oxygen therapy (typically more than 24 to 48 hr), and the severity of lung disease.

    ▪ Manifestations include a nonproductive cough, substernal pain, nasal stuffiness, nausea, vomiting, fatigue, headache, sore throat, and hypoventilation.

    ▪ Nursing Actions

      □ Use the lowest level of oxygen necessary to maintain an adequate SpO$_2$.

      □ Monitor ABGs and notify the provider if SpO$_2$ levels are outside the expected reference range.

      □ Decrease the FiO$_2$ as the client's SpO$_2$ improves.

- ○ Oxygen-induced hypoventilation

  - Oxygen-induced hypoventilation may develop in clients who have chronic obstructive pulmonary disease (COPD) who have chronic hypoxemia and hypercarbia. Clients who have COPD rely on low levels of arterial oxygen as their primary drive for breathing. Providing supplemental oxygen at high levels can decrease or eliminate their respiratory drive.

  - Nursing Actions

    - □ Monitor the client's respiratory rate and pattern, level of consciousness, and SpO$_2$.

    - □ Provide oxygen therapy at the lowest liter flow that corrects hypoxemia.

    - □ If the client tolerates it, use a Venturi mask to deliver precise oxygen levels.

    - □ Notify the provider of impending respiratory depression such as a decreased respiratory rate and a decreased level of consciousness.

- ○ Combustion

  - Oxygen is combustible.

  - Nursing Actions

    - □ Post "No Smoking" or "Oxygen in Use" signs to alert others of the fire hazard.

    - □ Know where to find the closest fire extinguisher.

    - □ Educate about the fire hazard of smoking with oxygen use.

    - □ Have clients wear a cotton gown because synthetic or wool fabrics can generate static electricity.

    - □ Ensure that all electric devices (razors, hearing aids, radios) are working well.

    - □ Make sure all electric machinery (monitors, suction machines) is grounded.

    - □ Do not use volatile, flammable materials (alcohol, acetone) near clients receiving oxygen.

SPECIMEN COLLECTION AND AIRWAY CLEARANCE

Overview

- Mucosal secretion buildup or aspiration of emesis can obstruct a client's airway.

  - ○ Adequate hydration and coughing help the client maintain airway patency.

  - ○ Clients at risk for developing airway compromise include: infants, clients who have neuromuscular disorders, clients who are quadriplegic, and clients who have cystic fibrosis.

  - ○ Nursing interventions that mobilize secretions and maintain airway patency include assistance with coughing, hydration, positioning, humidification, nebulizer therapy, chest physiotherapy, and suctioning.

  - ○ These interventions promote adequate gas exchange and lung expansion.

- Collect sputum specimens by suctioning during coughing.

- Indications that clients need help maintaining airway clearance include hypoxemia (restlessness, irritability, tachypnea, tachycardia, cyanosis, decreased level of consciousness, decreased SpO$_2$ levels), adventitious breath sounds, visible secretions, and absence of spontaneous cough.

- Whenever possible, encourage coughing. Coughing is more effective than artificial suctioning at moving secretions into the upper trachea and laryngopharynx.

- Humidification of oxygen moistens the airways, which loosens and mobilizes pulmonary secretions.

- Nebulization breaks up medications (bronchodilators, mucolytic agents) into minute particles that disperse throughout the respiratory tract and improves clearance of pulmonary secretions.

- Chest physiotherapy (CPT) involves the use of chest percussion, vibration, and postural drainage to help mobilize secretions. Chest percussion and vibration facilitate movement of secretions into the central airways. For postural drainage, one or more positions allow gravity to assist with the removal of secretions from specific areas of the lung.

- Early-morning postural drainage mobilizes secretions that have accumulated through the night.

- Suction orally, nasally, or endotracheally, not routinely but only when clients need it.

- Maintain surgical asepsis when performing any form of tracheal suctioning to avoid bacterial contamination of the airway.

Sputum Specimen Collection

- Collection of sputum for analysis
- Indications
  - For cytology to identify aberrant cells or cancer
  - For culture and sensitivity to grow and identify micro-organisms and the antibiotics effective against them
  - To identify acid-fast bacillus (AFB) to diagnose tuberculosis (TB) (requires three consecutive morning samples)
- Interpretation of Findings
  - Presence of bacteria indicating infection
  - Presence of cancer cells
- Nursing Actions
  - Obtain specimens early in the morning.
  - Wait 1 to 2 hr after the client eats to obtain a specimen to decrease the likelihood of emesis or aspiration.
  - Perform chest physiotherapy to help mobilize secretions.
  - Use a sterile specimen container, a label, a laboratory requisition slip, a biohazard bag for delivery of the specimen to the laboratory, clean gloves, and a mask and goggles if necessary.
  - Use a container with a preservative to obtain a specimen for cytology.
  - Use a sterile container for routine cultures and acid-fast bacillus (AFB) testing.
  - If a client cannot cough effectively and expectorate sputum into the container, collect the specimen by endotracheal suctioning.
  - Older adult clients have a weak cough reflex and decreased muscle strength, making it difficult for them to expectorate. They may require suctioning for sputum specimen collection.

Chest Physiotherapy

- The use of a set of techniques that loosen respiratory secretions and move them into the central airways where coughing or suctioning can remove them.
- Percussion – the use of cupped hands to clap rhythmically on the chest to break up secretions
- Vibration – the use of a shaking movement during exhalation to help remove secretions
- Postural drainage – the use of various positions to allow secretions to drain by gravity
- Chest physiotherapy is for clients who have thick secretions and are unable to clear their airways. It is contraindicated for clients who are pregnant; have a rib, chest, head, or neck injury; have increased intracranial pressure; have had recent abdominal surgery; have a pulmonary embolism; or have bleeding disorders or osteoporosis.
- Nursing Actions
  - Schedule treatments 1 hr before meals or 2 hr after meals and at bedtime to decrease the likelihood of vomiting or aspirating.
  - Administer a bronchodilator medication or nebulizer treatment 30 min to 1 hr prior to postural drainage.
  - Offer the client an emesis basin and facial tissues.
  - Ensure proper positioning to promote drainage of specific areas of the lungs.
    - Both lobes in general: high Fowler's
    - Apical segments of both lobes: sitting on the side of the bed
    - Right upper lobe, anterior segment: supine with head elevation
    - Right upper lobe, posterior segment: on the left side with a pillow under the right side of the chest
    - Right middle lobe, anterior segment: three-quarters supine with dependent lung in Trendelenburg
    - Right middle lobe, posterior segment: prone with thorax and abdomen elevation
    - Right lower lobe, lateral segment: on the left side in Trendelenburg
    - Left upper lobe, anterior segment: supine with head elevation
    - Left upper lobe, posterior segment: on the right side with a pillow under the left side of the chest
    - Left lower lobe, lateral segment: on the right side in Trendelenburg
    - Both lower lobes, anterior segments: supine in Trendelenburg
    - Both lower lobes, posterior segments: prone in Trendelenburg
  - Apply manual percussion to the chest wall using cupped hands or a special device.
  - Place hands on the affected area, tense hand and arm muscles, and move the heel of the hands to create vibrations as the client exhales. Have the client cough after each set of vibrations.
  - Have the client remain in each position for 10 to 15 min to allow time for percussion, vibration, and postural drainage.
  - Discontinue the procedure if the client reports faintness or dizziness.
  - Note that older adult clients have decreased respiratory muscle strength and chest wall compliance, which puts them at risk for aspiration. They require more frequent position changes and other interventions to promote mobility of secretions.

Suctioning

- Suction orally, nasally, or endotracheally when clients have early signs of hypoxemia, such as restlessness, tachypnea, tachycardia, decreased SpO_2 levels, adventitious breath sounds, audible or visible secretions, cyanosis, absence of spontaneous cough.

 View Image: Tracheal Suctioning

- Nursing Actions
  - Don the required personal protective equipment.
  - Assist the client to high-Fowler's or Fowler's position for suctioning if possible.
  - Encourage the client to breathe deeply and cough in an attempt to clear the secretions without artificial suction.
  - Obtain baseline breath sounds and vital signs, including SaO_2 by pulse oximeter. May monitor SaO_2 continually during the procedure.
  - For oropharyngeal suctioning, use a Yankauer or tonsil-tipped rigid suction catheter and move the catheter around the mouth, gum line, and pharynx.
  - For nasopharyngeal and nasotracheal suctioning, use a flexible catheter and lubricate the distal 6 to 8 cm (2 to 3 in) with water-soluble lubricant.
  - For endotracheal suctioning, use a suction catheter with an outer diameter of no more than 1 cm (0.5 in) of the internal diameter of the endotracheal tube.
    - Hyperoxygenate the client using a bag-valve-mask (BVM) or specialized ventilator function with an FiO_2 of 100%.
  - Use medical asepsis for suctioning the mouth.
  - Use surgical asepsis for all other types of suctioning.
  - Use suction pressure no higher than 120 to 150 mm Hg.
  - Limit each suction attempt to no longer than 10 to 15 seconds to avoid hypoxemia and the vagal response. Limit suctioning to two to three attempts.
  - Additional guidelines for nasopharyngeal and nasotracheal suctioning
    - Insert the catheter into the naris during inhalation.
    - Do not apply suction while inserting the catheter.
    - Follow the natural course of the naris and slightly slant the catheter downward while advancing it.
    - Advance the catheter the approximate distance from the tip of the nose to the base of the earlobe.
    - Apply suction intermittently by covering and releasing the suction port with the thumb for 10 to 15 seconds.
    - Apply suction only while withdrawing the catheter and rotating it with the thumb and forefinger.
    - Do not perform more than two passes with the catheter. Allow at least 1 min between passes for ventilation and oxygenation.

○ Additional guidelines for endotracheal suctioning

- Remove the bag or ventilator from the tracheostomy or endotracheal tube and insert the catheter into the lumen of the airway. Advance the catheter until resistance is met. The catheter should reach the level of the carina (location of bifurcation into the mainstem bronchi).

- Pull the catheter back 1 cm (0.4 in) prior to applying suction to prevent mucosal damage.

- Apply suction intermittently by covering and releasing the suction port with the thumb for 10 to 15 seconds.

- Apply suction only while withdrawing the catheter and rotating it with the thumb and forefinger.

- Reattach the BVM or ventilator and administer 100% oxygen.

- Do not reuse the suction catheter.

ARTIFICIAL AIRWAYS AND TRACHEOSTOMY CARE

Overview

- A tracheotomy is a sterile surgical incision into the trachea through the skin and muscles for the purpose of establishing an airway.

- A tracheotomy can be an emergency or a scheduled surgical procedure; it can be temporary or permanent.

- A tracheostomy is the stoma/opening that results from a tracheotomy to provide and secure a patent airway.

- Artificial airways can be placed orotracheally, nasotracheally, or through a tracheostomy to assist with respiration.

- Tracheostomy tubes vary in their composition (plastic, steel, silicone), number of parts, size (long vs. short), and shape (50° to 90° angles).

- There is no standard tracheostomy sizing system; however, the diameter of the tracheostomy tube must be smaller than the trachea.

- The outside cannula has a flange or neck plate that sits against the skin of the neck and has holes on each side for attaching ties around the neck to stabilize the tracheostomy tube.

- Airflow in and out of a tracheostomy without air leakage (a cuffed tracheostomy tube) bypasses the vocal cords, resulting in an inability to produce sound or speech.

- Uncuffed tubes and fenestrated tubes, in place or capped, allow speech. Clients who have a cuffed tube can be off mechanical ventilation, can breathe around the tube, and can use a special valve to allow for speech. The cuff is deflated and the valve occludes the opening.

- Indications for a tracheostomy include acute or chronic upper airway obstruction, edema, anaphylaxis, burns, trauma, head/neck surgery, copious secretions, obstructive sleep apnea refractory to conventional therapy, and the need for long-term mechanical ventilation or reconstruction after laryngeal trauma or laryngeal cancer surgery.

ARTIFICIAL AIRWAY TUBE TYPES	
CHARACTERISTICS	**NURSING CONCERNS**
Single lumen (cannula)	
› Long, single-cannula tube › For clients who have long or thick necks	› Do not use with clients who have excessive secretions.
Double lumen (cannula)	
› An outer cannula fits into the stoma and keeps the airway open. › An inner cannula fits snugly into the outer cannula and locks into place. › An obturator is a thin, solid tube the provider places inside the tracheostomy and uses as a guide for inserting the outer cannula, and removes immediately after outer cannula insertion.	› This device allows removing, cleaning, reusing, discarding, and replacing the inner cannula with a disposable inner cannula. › It is useful for clients who have excessive secretions.
Cuffed tube	
› It has a balloon that inflates around the outside of the distal segment of the tube to protect the lower airway by producing a seal between the upper and lower airway.	› A cuffed tube permits mechanical ventilation. › Cuffs do not hold the tube in place. › Cuff pressures must be monitored to prevent tracheal tissue necrosis. › The client is unable to speak.
Cuffless tube	
› It has no balloon and is for clients who have long-term airway-management needs.	› The client must be at low risk for aspiration. › Cuffless tubes are not for clients on mechanical ventilation. › This device allows the client to speak.
Fenestrated tube – with cuff	
› It has one large or multiple openings (fenestrations) in the posterior wall of the outer cannula with a balloon around the outside of the distal segment of the tube. › Also has an inner cannula	› This device allows for mechanical ventilation. › Removing the inner cannula allows the fenestrations to permit air to flow through the openings. › This device allows the client to speak.
Fenestrated tube – without cuff	
› It has one larger or multiple openings (fenestrations) in the posterior wall of the outer cannula with no balloon. › Also has an inner cannula	› The holes in the tube help wean the client from the tracheostomy. › Removing the inner cannula allows the fenestrations to permit air to flow through the openings. › This device allows the client to speak.

- Nursing Actions
  - ○ Keep the following at the bedside – two extra tracheostomy tubes (one the client's size and one size smaller, in case of accidental decannulation), the obturator for the existing tube, an oxygen source, suction catheters and a suction source, and a BVM.
  - ○ Provide methods to communicate with staff (paper and pen, dry-erase board).
  - ○ Provide an emergency call system and a call light.
  - ○ Provide adequate humidification and hydration to thin secretions and reduce the risk of mucous plugs.
  - ○ Give oral care every 2 hr.
  - ○ Provide tracheostomy care every 8 hr to reduce the risk of infection and skin breakdown.
    - ▪ Suction the tracheostomy tube, if necessary, using sterile suctioning supplies.
    - ▪ Remove soiled dressings and excess secretions.
    - ▪ Apply the oxygen source loosely if the client's SpO$_2$ decreases during the procedure.
    - ▪ Use cotton-tipped applicators and gauze pads to clean exposed outer cannula surfaces. Use the facility-approved solution. Clean in a circular motion from the stoma site outward.
    - ▪ Use surgical asepsis to remove and clean the inner cannula (with the facility-approved solution). Use a new inner cannula if it is disposable.
    - ▪ Clean the stoma site and then the tracheostomy plate.
    - ▪ Place a fresh dressing under and around the tracheostomy holder and plate.
    - ▪ Replace tracheostomy ties if they are wet or soiled. Secure the new ties before removing the soiled ones to prevent accidental decannulation.
    - ▪ If a knot is needed, tie a square knot that is visible on the side of the neck. Check that one or two fingers fit between the tie and the neck.
  - ○ Change nondisposable tracheostomy tubes every 6 to 8 weeks or per protocol.
  - ○ Reposition the client every 2 hr to prevent atelectasis and pneumonia.
  - ○ Minimize dust in the room; do not shake bedding.
  - ○ If the client is permitted to eat, position him upright and tip his chin to his chest to enable swallowing. Assess for aspiration.

Complications

- Accidental Decannulation
    - Accidental decannulation in the first 72 hr after surgery is an emergency because the tracheostomy tract has not matured, and replacement may be difficult.
        - Ventilate the client with a BVM. Call for assistance.
    - Nursing Actions
        - Always keep the tracheostomy obturator and two spare tracheostomy tubes at the bedside.
        - If accidental decannulation occurs after the first 72 hr:
            - Immediately hyperextend the neck and with the obturator inserted into the tracheostomy tube, quickly and gently replace the tube and remove the obturator.
            - Secure the tube.
            - Assess tube placement by auscultating for bilateral breath sounds.
        - If unable to replace the tracheostomy tube, administer oxygen through the stoma. If unable to administer oxygen through the stoma, occlude the stoma and administer oxygen through the nose and mouth.
- Damage to the Trachea
    - Tracheal wall necrosis is tissue damage that results when the pressure of the inflated cuff impairs blood flow to the tracheal wall.
    - Tracheal stenosis is the narrowing of the tracheal lumen due to scar formation resulting from irritation of the tracheal mucosa from the tracheal tube cuff.
        - Keep the cuff pressure between 14 and 20 mm Hg.
        - Check the cuff pressure at least once every 8 hr.
        - Keep the tube in the midline position and prevent pulling or traction on the tracheostomy tube.

APPLICATION EXERCISES

1. A nurse is assessing a client who has an acute respiratory infection that puts her at risk for hypoxemia. Which of the following findings are early indications that should alert the nurse that the client is developing hypoxemia? (Select all that apply.)

_____ A. Restlessness

_____ B. Tachypnea

_____ C. Bradycardia

_____ D. Confusion

_____ E. Pallor

2. A nurse is caring for a client who is having difficulty breathing. The client is lying in bed and is already receiving oxygen therapy via nasal cannula. Which of the following interventions is the nurse's priority?

A. Increase the oxygen flow.

B. Assist the client to Fowler's position.

C. Promote removal of pulmonary secretions.

D. Obtain a specimen for arterial blood gases.

3. A nurse is preparing to perform endotracheal suctioning for a client. Which of the following are appropriate guidelines for the nurse to follow? (Select all that apply.)

_____ A. Apply suction while withdrawing the catheter.

_____ B. Perform suctioning on a routine basis, every 2 to 3 hr.

_____ C. Maintain medical asepsis during suctioning.

_____ D. Use a new catheter for each suctioning attempt.

_____ E. Limit suctioning to two to three attempts.

4. A nurse is caring for a client who has a tracheostomy. Which of the following actions should the nurse take each time he provides tracheostomy care? (Select all that apply.)

_____ A. Apply the oxygen source loosely if the SpO_2 decreases during the procedure.

_____ B. Use surgical asepsis to remove and clean the inner cannula.

_____ C. Clean the outer surfaces in a circular motion from the stoma site outward.

_____ D. Replace the tracheostomy ties with new ties.

_____ E. Cut a slit in gauze squares to place beneath the tube holder.

5. A provider is discharging a client with a prescription for home oxygen therapy via nasal cannula. Client and family teaching by the nurse should include which of the following instructions? (Select all that apply.)

_____ A. Apply petroleum jelly around and inside the nares.

_____ B. Remove the nasal cannula during mealtimes.

_____ C. Check the position of the cannula frequently.

_____ D. Report any nasal stuffiness, nausea, or fatigue.

_____ E. Post "no smoking" signs in a prominent location.

6. A nurse is reviewing with a group of nursing students how to perform postural drainage. Use the ATI Active Learning Template: Nursing Skill to complete this item. Under Nursing Actions (pre, intra, post), list the specific positions that facilitate secretion drainage from at least eight specific lung areas.

APPLICATION EXERCISES KEY

1.   A. **CORRECT:** Restlessness is an early manifestation of hypoxemia, along with tachycardia, elevated blood pressure, use of accessory muscles, nasal flaring, tracheal tugging, and adventitious lung sounds.

    B. **CORRECT:** Tachypnea is an early manifestation of hypoxemia, along with tachycardia, elevated blood pressure, use of accessory muscles, nasal flaring, tracheal tugging, and adventitious lung sounds.

    C. INCORRECT: Bradycardia is a late manifestation of hypoxemia, along with stupor, cyanotic skin and mucous membranes, bradypnea, hypotension, and cardiac dysrhythmias.

    D. **CORRECT:** Confusion is an early manifestation of hypoxemia, along with tachycardia, elevated blood pressure, use of accessory muscles, nasal flaring, tracheal tugging, and adventitious lung sounds.

    E. **CORRECT:** Pallor is an early manifestation of hypoxemia, along with tachycardia, elevated blood pressure, use of accessory muscles, nasal flaring, tracheal tugging, and adventitious lung sounds.

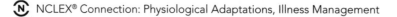 NCLEX® Connection: Physiological Adaptations, Illness Management

2.   A. INCORRECT: The client may need more oxygen, as hypoxemia may be the cause of his difficulty breathing. However, administering oxygen and adjusting the fraction of inspired oxygen requires the provider's prescription after a careful assessment of the client's oxygenation status. There is a higher priority given the nature of the client's distress.

    B. **CORRECT:** The priority action the nurse should take when using the airway, breathing, circulation (ABC) approach to care delivery is to relieve the client's dyspnea (difficulty breathing). Fowler's position facilitates maximal lung expansion and thus optimizes breathing. With the client in this position, the nurse can better assess and determine the cause of the client's dyspnea.

    C. INCORRECT: The client may need suctioning or expectoration, as pulmonary secretions may be the cause of his difficulty breathing. However, there is a higher priority given the nature of the client's distress.

    D. INCORRECT: It is important to check the client's oxygenation status, and in many nursing situations, assessment precedes action, but there is a higher priority given the nature of the client's distress.

    ⊙ NCLEX® Connection: Physiological Adaptations, Illness Management

3. A. **CORRECT:** The nurse should apply suction pressure only while withdrawing the catheter, not while inserting it.

    B. INCORRECT: The nurse should not suction routinely, because suctioning is not without risk. It can cause mucosal damage, bleeding, and bronchospasm.

    C. INCORRECT: Endotracheal suctioning requires surgical asepsis.

    D. **CORRECT:** The nurse should not reuse the suction catheter unless an inline suctioning system is in place.

    E. **CORRECT:** To prevent hypoxemia, the nurse should limit each suctioning session to two to three attempts and allow at least 1 min between passes for ventilation and oxygenation.

    Ⓝ NCLEX® Connection: Physiological Adaptations, Alterations in Body Systems

4. A. **CORRECT:** The nurse must be prepared to provide supplemental oxygen in response to any decline in oxygen saturation while performing tracheostomy care.

    B. **CORRECT:** The nurse should use a sterile disposable tracheostomy cleaning kit or sterile supplies and maintain surgical asepsis throughout this part of the procedure.

    C. **CORRECT:** This helps move mucus and contaminated material away from the stoma for easy removal.

    D. INCORRECT: To help keep the skin clean and dry, the nurse should replace the tracheostomy ties if they are wet or soiled. There is a risk of tube dislodgement with replacing the ties, so he should not replace them routinely.

    E. INCORRECT: The nurse should use a commercially prepared tracheostomy dressing with a slit in it. Cutting gauze squares can loosen lint or gauze fibers the client could aspirate.

    Ⓝ NCLEX® Connection: Reduction of Risk Potential, Potential for Complications of Diagnostic Tests/ Treatments/Procedures

5.   A.   INCORRECT: Protecting the nares from the drying effects of oxygen therapy is important, but the client should use water-based lubricant.

    B.   INCORRECT: A nasal cannula does not interfere with eating. The client should keep it in place during meals.

    C.   **CORRECT:** A disadvantage of this oxygen delivery device is that it dislodges easily. The client should form the habit of checking its position periodically and readjusting it as necessary.

    D.   **CORRECT:** Oxygen toxicity is a complication of oxygen therapy, usually from high concentrations or long durations. Manifestations include a nonproductive cough, substernal pain, nasal stuffiness, nausea, vomiting, fatigue, headache, sore throat, and hypoventilation. The client should report any of these promptly.

    E.   **CORRECT:** Oxygen is combustible and thus increases the risk of fire injuries. No one in the house should smoke or use any device that might generate sparks in the area where the oxygen is in use.

    Ⓝ   NCLEX® Connection: Reduction of Risk Potential, Therapeutic Procedures

6.   *Using the ATI Active Learning Template: Nursing Skill*
*   Nursing Actions
    ◦   Both lobes in general: high Fowler's
    ◦   Apical segments of both lobes: sitting on the side of the bed
    ◦   Right upper lobe, anterior segment: supine with head elevation
    ◦   Right upper lobe, posterior segment: on the left side with a pillow under the right side of the chest
    ◦   Right middle lobe, anterior segment: three-quarters supine with dependent lung in Trendelenburg
    ◦   Right middle lobe, posterior segment: prone with thorax and abdomen elevation
    ◦   Right lower lobe, lateral segment: on the left side in Trendelenburg
    ◦   Left upper lobe, anterior segment: supine with head elevation
    ◦   Left upper lobe, posterior segment: on the right side with a pillow under the left side of the chest
    ◦   Left lower lobe, lateral segment: on the right side in Trendelenburg
    ◦   Both lower lobes, anterior segments: supine in Trendelenburg
    ◦   Both lower lobes, posterior segments: prone in Trendelenburg

    Ⓝ   NCLEX® Connection: Physiological Adaptations, Alterations in Body Systems

FUNDAMENTALS FOR NURSING

UNIT 4   **PHYSIOLOGICAL INTEGRITY**
               SECTION: REDUCTION OF RISK POTENTIAL

CHAPTER 54   Nasogastric Intubation and Enteral Feedings

Overview

- Nasogastric intubation is the insertion of a nasogastric (NG) tube to manage gastrointestinal dysfunction and provide enteral nutrition via NG, jejunal, or gastric tubes.

Nasogastric Intubation

- An NG tube is a hollow, flexible, cylindrical device inserted through the nasopharynx into the stomach.
- Indications
  - Decompression
    - Removal of gases or stomach contents to relieve distention, nausea, or vomiting
    - Tube types – Salem sump, Miller-Abbott, Levin
  - Feeding
    - Alternative to oral route for administering nutritional supplements
    - Tube types – Duo, Levin, Dobhoff
  - Lavage
    - Washing out the stomach to treat active bleeding, ingestion of poison, gastric dilation
    - Tube types – Ewald, Levin, Salem sump
  - Compression
    - Applied pressure using an internal balloon to prevent hemorrhage
    - Tube type – Sengstaken-Blakemore

  M   View Images
        › Enteral Feeding Tube   › Sengstaken-Blakemore Tube

- Preprocedure
  - Nursing Actions
    - Review the prescription and purpose, plan for drainage or suction, and understand the need for placement for diagnostic purposes.
    - Identify the client, and explain the procedure.
    - Evaluate the client's ability to assist and/or cooperate.
    - Establish a means of communication to signal distress, such as the client raising a hand.
    - Perform hand hygiene.

- Set up the equipment.
  - □ NG tube – selected according to the indication
  - □ Tape or use a commercial fixation device to secure the dressing
  - □ Clean gloves
  - □ Water-soluble lubricant
  - □ Topical anesthetic
  - □ Cup of water and straw
  - □ Catheter-tipped syringe, usually 30 to 60 mL
  - □ Basin – to prepare for gag-induced nausea
  - □ pH test strip or meter – to measure gastric secretions for acidity
  - □ Stethoscope
  - □ Disposable towel – to maintain a clean environment
  - □ Clamp or plug – to close the tubing after insertion
  - □ Suction apparatus – if attaching tube to continuous or intermittent suction
  - □ Gauze square – to cleanse the outside of the tubing after insertion
  - □ Safety pin and elastic band or commercial device – to secure the tubing and prevent accidental removal
  - Position a disposable towel and basin.
  - Provide privacy.
- Intraprocedure
  - ○ Nursing Actions
    - Auscultate for bowel sounds, and palpate the abdomen for distention, pain, and rigidity.
    - Raise bed to horizontal level comfortable for nurse.
    - Assist the client to high-Fowler's position (if possible).
    - Assess the nares for the best route to determine how to avoid a septal deviation or other obstruction during the insertion process.
    - Use correct procedure for tube insertion, wearing clean gloves, and evaluate client outcome.
    - Placement check
      - □ Aspirate gently to collect gastric contents, testing pH (4 or less is expected), and assess odor, color, and consistency.
      - □ Confirm placement with an x-ray.
      - □ Injecting air into the tube and then listening over the abdomen is not an acceptable practice.
    - If the tube is not in the stomach, advance it 5 cm, and repeat the placement check.
    - Clamp the nasogastric tube, or connect it to the appropriate suction device.
    - If the client vomits, clear the airway, and provide comfort prior to continuing.
    - Salem sump tubing has a blue pigtail for negative air release. Do not insert any substance into the blue pigtail because it will break the seal and the tubing will leak.

- Postprocedure
    - Nursing Actions
        - The insertion and maintenance of a nasogastric tube is a nursing responsibility, but measuring output, providing comfort, and giving oral care can be delegated.
        - Removal is done wearing clean gloves.
            - Inform the client of the prescription and process, emphasizing that removal is less stressful than placement.
            - Measure and record any drainage, assessing it for color, consistency, and odor.
            - Ensure comfort.
            - Document all relevant information.
                - Tubing removal and condition of the tube
                - Volume and description of the drainage
                - Abdominal assessment, including inspection, auscultation, palpation, and percussion
                - Last and next bowel movement and urine output
- Complications
    - Excoriation of nares and stomach
        - Apply lubricant to the nares as needed.
        - Assess the color of the drainage. Report dark, "coffee-ground," or blood-streaked drainage immediately.
        - Consider switching the tube to the other naris.
    - Discomfort
        - Rinse the mouth with water for dryness.
        - Throat lozenges may help.
        - Provide oral hygiene frequently.
    - Occlusion of the NG tube leading to distention
        - Irrigate the tube per facility protocol to unclog blockages. Use tap water with enteral feedings. Have the client change position in case the tube is against the stomach wall.
        - Verify that suction equipment functions properly.

Enteral Feedings

- Enteral feeding is a method of providing nutrients to clients who cannot consume foods orally.
    - Enteral formulas
        - Polymeric – (1 to 2 kcal/mL) milk-based, blenderized foods
            - Whole-nutrient formulas, either commercial or from the dietary department
            - Use only for clients whose gastrointestinal (GI) tract can absorb whole nutrients
        - Modular formulas – (3.8 to 4 kcal/mL) single macronutrient preparation
            - Not nutritionally complete
            - Supplement to other foods

- Elemental formulas – (1 to 3 kcal/mL) predigested nutrients
  - Not nutritionally complete
  - Easier for a partially dysfunctional GI tract to absorb
- Specialty formulas – (1 to 2 kcal/mL) for meeting specific nutritional needs
  - Not nutritionally complete
  - Primarily for clients who have hepatic failure, respiratory disease, or HIV infection
- Enteral access tubes
  - Nasogastric or nasointestinal
    - Therapy duration less than 4 weeks
    - Inserted via the nose
  - Gastrostomy or jejunostomy
    - Therapy duration longer than 4 weeks
    - Inserted surgically
  - Percutaneous endoscopic gastrostomy (PEG) or jejunostomy (PEJ)
    - Therapy duration longer than 4 weeks
    - Inserted endoscopically
  - Gastroparesis, esophageal reflux, or a history of aspiration pneumonia generally requires intestinal placement.
- Indications
  - Critical illness/trauma
  - Neurological and muscular disorders – brain neoplasm, cerebrovascular accident, dementia, myopathy, Parkinson's disease
  - Cancer that affects the head and neck, upper GI tract
  - Gastrointestinal disorders – enterocutaneous fistula, inflammatory bowel disease, mild pancreatitis
  - Respiratory failure with prolonged intubation
  - Inadequate oral intake
- Nursing Actions
  - Preparation of the Client
    - Review the client's prescription.
      - Generally, the provider and dietary staff consult to determine the type of tube feeding formula.
    - Set up the equipment.
      - Feeding bag
      - Tubing
      - 30- to 60-mL syringe (compatible with the tubing)
      - Stethoscope
      - pH indicator strip
      - Infusion pump (if not a gravity drip)

- Appropriate enteral formula
- Irrigant solution: sterile or tap water, according to facility policy
- Clean gloves
- Supplies for blood glucose (if protocol or prescription indicates)
- Suction equipment to use in case of aspiration

○ Ongoing Care

  ▪ Prepare the formula, tubing, and infusion device.
    - Check expiration dates, and note the content of the formula.
    - Ensure that the formula is at room temperature.
    - Set up the feeding system via gravity or pump.
    - Mix or shake the formula, fill the container, prime the tubing, and clamp it.
  ▪ Assist the client to Fowler's position, or elevate the head of the bed to a minimum of 30°.
  ▪ Auscultate for bowel sounds.
  ▪ Monitor tube placement.
    - Check gastric contents for pH. A good indication of appropriate placement is obtaining gastric contents with a pH between 0 and 4.
    - Aspirate for residual volume.
    - Note the appearance of the aspirate.
    - Return aspirated contents, or follow the facility's protocol.
  ▪ Flush the tubing with at least 30 mL of tap water.
  ▪ Administer the formula.
    - Intermittent feeding
      ▸ Prepare the formula and a 60-mL syringe.
      ▸ Remove the plunger from the syringe.
      ▸ Hold the tubing above the instillation site.
      ▸ Open the stopcock on the tubing, and insert the barrel of the syringe with the end up.
      ▸ Fill the syringe with 40 to 50 mL of formula.
      ▸ If using a feeding bag, fill the bag with the total amount of formula for one feeding, and hang it to drain via gravity until empty (about 30 to 45 min).
      ▸ If using a syringe, hold it high enough for the formula to empty gradually via gravity.
      ▸ Continue to refill the syringe until the amount for the feeding is instilled. Follow with at least 30 mL of tap water to flush the tube and prevent clogging.
    - Continuous-drip feeding
      ▸ Connect the feeding bag system to the feeding tube.
      ▸ If using a pump, program the instillation rate as prescribed, and set the total volume to instill.
      ▸ Start the pump.
      ▸ Flush the enteral tubing with at least 30 mL of irrigant, usually tap water, every 4 to 6 hr, and check tube placement again.

- Monitor intake and output, and include 24-hr totals.
- Monitor capillary blood glucose every 6 hr until the client tolerates maximum administration rate for 24 hr.
- An infusion pump is required for intestinal tube feedings.
- Follow the manufacturer's recommendations for formula hang time. Refrigerate unused formula, and discard after 24 hr.

- Check gastric residual every 4 to 8 hr. Facility protocol specifies the actions to take based on the amount of residual.
- Delegation of this skill to assistive personnel is inappropriate.
- Complications
    - When gastric residual exceeds 250 mL for each of two consecutive assessments
        - Withhold the feeding.
        - Notify the provider.
        - Maintain semi-Fowler's position.
        - Recheck residual in 1 hr.
    - Diarrhea three times or more in a 24-hr period
        - Notify the provider.
        - Confer with the dietitian.
        - Provide skin care and protection.
    - Nausea or vomiting
        - Withhold the feeding.
        - Turn the client to the side.
        - Notify the provider.
        - Check the tube's patency.
        - Aspirate for residual.
        - Auscultate for bowel sounds.
        - Obtain a chest x-ray.
    - Aspiration of formula
        - Withhold the feeding.
        - Turn the client to the side.
        - Suction the airway.
        - Provide oxygen if indicated.
        - Monitor vital signs for elevated temperature.
        - Monitor for decreased oxygen saturation or increased respiratory rate.
        - Auscultate breath sounds for increased congestion.
        - Notify the provider.
        - Obtain a chest x-ray.
    - Skin irritation around the tubing site
        - Provide a skin barrier for any drainage at the site.
        - Monitor the tube's placement.

APPLICATION EXERCISES

1. A nurse is delivering an enteral feeding to a client who has an NG tube in place for intermittent feedings. When the nurse pours water into the syringe after the formula drains from the syringe, the client asks the nurse why the water is necessary. Which of the following is an appropriate response by the nurse?

    A. "Water helps clear the tube so it doesn't get clogged."

    B. "Flushing helps make sure the tube stays in place."

    C. "This will help you get enough fluids."

    D. "Adding water makes the formula less concentrated."

2. A nurse is preparing to instill an enteral feeding to a client who has an NG tube in place. Which of the following is the nurse's highest assessment priority before performing this procedure?

    A. Check how long the feeding container has been open.

    B. Verify the placement of the NG tube.

    C. Confirm that the client does not have diarrhea.

    D. Make sure the client is alert and oriented.

3. A nurse is caring for a client who is receiving continuous enteral feedings. Which of the following nursing interventions is the highest priority when the nurse suspects aspiration of the feeding?

    A. Auscultate breath sounds.

    B. Stop the feeding.

    C. Obtain a chest x-ray.

    D. Initiate oxygen therapy.

4. A nurse is caring for a client in a long-term care facility who is receiving enteral feedings via an NG tube. Which of the following is an appropriate nursing action prior to administering the tube feeding? (Select all that apply.)

    _____ A. Auscultate bowel sounds.

    _____ B. Assist the client to an upright position.

    _____ C. Test the pH of gastric aspirate.

    _____ D. Warm the formula to body temperature.

    _____ E. Discard any residual gastric contents.

5. A nurse is preparing to insert an NG tube for a client who requires gastric decompression. Which of the following actions should the nurse perform before beginning the procedure? (Select all that apply.)

_____ A. Review a signal the client can use if feeling any distress.

_____ B. Lay a towel across the client's chest.

_____ C. Administer oral pain medication.

_____ D. Obtain a Dobhoff tube for insertion.

_____ E. Have a petroleum-based lubricant available.

6. A nurse is teaching a group of nursing students about administering enteral feedings. Use the ATI Active Learning Template: Nursing Skill to complete this item.

A. Indications: List at least four indications for enteral feedings.

B. Nursing Actions (Intraprocedure): List the steps of administering an enteral feeding.

APPLICATION EXERCISES KEY

1. A. **CORRECT:** Flushing the tube after instilling the feeding helps keep the NG tube patent by clearing any excess formula from the tube so that it doesn't clump and clog the tube.

    B. INCORRECT: Tape or a securing device, not flushing the tube with water, helps maintain the position of the NG tube.

    C. INCORRECT: If the client requires additional fluids, the small amount the nurse uses for flushing the NG tube will not be adequate.

    D. INCORRECT: If the formula is supposed to be less concentrated, the dietary staff will prepare it according to the client's prescription before the nurse instills it.

    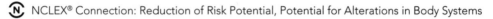 NCLEX® Connection: Reduction of Risk Potential, Potential for Alterations in Body Systems

2. A. INCORRECT: Checking that the container has not exceeded its expiration date, either for having it open or for opening it, is important. However, there is a higher assessment priority among these options.

    B. **CORRECT:** The greatest risk to the client receiving enteral feedings is injury from aspiration. Therefore, the priority nursing assessment before initiating an enteral feeding is to verify proper placement of the NG tube.

    C. INCORRECT: Assessing the client for any possible complications of enteral feedings, such as diarrhea, is important. However, there is a higher assessment priority among these options.

    D. INCORRECT: Determining the client's level of consciousness is an assessment parameter that is ongoing and should precede any procedure. However, there is a higher assessment priority among these options.

     NCLEX® Connection: Reduction of Risk Potential, Potential for Complications of Diagnostic Tests/ Treatments/Procedures

3. A. INCORRECT: Listening to the client's breath sounds is important whenever there is suspicion of aspiration. However, there is a higher assessment priority among these options.

    B. **CORRECT:** The greatest risk to the client is aspiration pneumonia. Therefore, the first action the nurse should take is to stop the feeding so that no more formula can enter the lungs.

    C. INCORRECT: Obtaining a chest x-ray is important whenever there is suspicion of aspiration. However, there is a higher assessment priority among these options.

    D. INCORRECT: Initiating oxygen therapy is important whenever there is suspicion of aspiration. However, there is a higher assessment priority among these options.

    NCLEX® Connection: Reduction of Risk Potential, Potential for Complications of Diagnostic Tests/ Treatments/Procedures

4.   A. **CORRECT:** If the nurse cannot hear bowel sounds, the client's gastrointestinal tract might not be able to absorb nutrients. The nurse should then withhold feedings and notify the provider.

B. **CORRECT:** The optimal position for enteral feeding is upright, and never lower than 30° of elevation of the head of the bed. Upright positioning helps prevent aspiration.

C. **CORRECT:** Before administering enteral feedings, the nurse should verify the placement of the NG tube. The only reliable method is x-ray confirmation, which is impractical prior to every feeding. Testing the pH of gastric aspirate is an acceptable method between x-ray confirmations.

D. INCORRECT: The enteral formula should be at room temperature, not body temperature.

E. INCORRECT: Unless the volume of gastric contents is more than 250 mL or the facility has other guidelines in place, the nurse should return the residual to the client's stomach.

Ⓝ NCLEX® Connection: Reduction of Risk Potential, Potential for Complications of Diagnostic Tests/ Treatments/Procedures

5.   A. **CORRECT:** Before inserting an NG tube, it is important to establish a means for the client to communicate that she wants to stop the procedure.

B. **CORRECT:** Placing a disposable towel across the client's chest provides for a clean environment.

C. INCORRECT: Oral pain medication is not administered prior to the procedure because the purpose of the procedure is to remove stomach contents.

D. INCORRECT: The type of tube to be used for gastric decompression is a Salem sump, Miller-Abbott, or Levin. A Dobhoff tube is used for feeding.

E. INCORRECT: A water-based lubricant is used to reduce complications related to aspiration.

Ⓝ NCLEX® Connection: Reduction of Risk Potential, Potential for Complications of Diagnostic Tests/ Treatments/Procedures

6. *Using the ATI Active Learning Template: Nursing Skill*

A. Indications

- Critical illness/trauma
- Neurological and muscular disorders – brain neoplasm, cerebrovascular accident, dementia, myopathy, Parkinson's disease
- Gastrointestinal disorders – enterocutaneous fistula, inflammatory bowel disease, mild pancreatitis
- Respiratory failure with prolonged intubation
- Inadequate oral intake

B. Nursing Actions (Intraprocedure)

- Prepare the formula and a 60-mL syringe.
- Remove the plunger from the syringe.
- Hold the tubing above the instillation site.
- Open the stopcock on the tubing, and insert the barrel of the syringe with the end up.
- Fill the syringe with 40 to 50 mL of formula.
- If using a feeding bag, fill the bag with the total amount of formula for one feeding, and hang it to drain via gravity until empty (about 30 to 45 min).
- If using a syringe, hold it high enough for the formula to empty gradually via gravity.
- Continue to refill the syringe until the amount for the feeding is instilled.
- Follow with at least 30 mL of tap water to flush the tube and prevent clogging.

Ⓝ NCLEX® Connection: Reduction of Risk Potential, Potential for Complications of Diagnostic Tests/Treatments/Procedures

---

UNIT 4   ## Physiological Integrity

SECTION: PHYSIOLOGICAL ADAPTATION

› Pressure Ulcers, Wounds, and Wound Management
› Bacterial, Viral, Fungal, and Parasitic Infections
› Fluid and Electrolyte Imbalances

NCLEX® CONNECTIONS

When reviewing the chapters in this unit, keep in mind the relevant sections of the NCLEX® outline, in particular:

Client Needs: Reduction of Risk Potential
› Relevant topics/tasks include:
» Changes/Abnormalities in Vital Signs
› Assess and respond to changes in the client's vital signs.
» Potential for Complications of Diagnostic Tests/ Treatments/Procedures
› Perform a focused assessment and reassessment.

Client Needs: Physiological Adaptation
› Relevant topics/tasks include:
» Alterations in Body Systems
› Monitor wounds for signs and symptoms of infection.
» Fluid and Electrolyte Imbalances
› Identify signs and symptoms of the client's fluid and/or electrolyte imbalance.
» Medical Emergencies
› Perform emergency care procedures.
» Pathophysiology
› Understand general principles of pathophysiology.

chapter 55

Overview

- Wounds are a result of injury to the skin. Although there are many different methods and degrees of injury, the basic phases of healing are essentially the same for most wounds.
- A pressure ulcer (formerly called a decubitus ulcer) is a specific type of tissue injury from unrelieved pressure that results in ischemia and damage to the underlying tissue.

Wound Healing and Management

- Stages of Wound Healing
  - The inflammatory stage begins with the injury and lasts 3 to 6 days. Initial care involves the following.
    - Controlling bleeding with vasoconstriction and retraction of blood vessels, and with clot formation.
    - Delivering oxygen, white blood cells, and nutrients to the area via the blood supply.
  - The proliferative stage lasts the next 3 to 24 days. Effects to the wound include:
    - Replacing lost tissue with connective or granulated tissue.
    - Contracting the wound's edges.
    - Resurfacing of new epithelial cells.
  - The maturation or remodeling stage involves the strengthening of the collagen scar and the restoration of a more normal appearance. It can take more than 1 year to complete, depending on the extent of the original wound.
- Healing Processes

TYPE OF HEALING	CHARACTERISTICS	WOUND TYPE
Primary intention	› Little or no tissue loss › Edges approximated, as with a surgical incision	› Heals rapidly › Low risk of infection › No or minimal scarring
Secondary intention	› Loss of tissue › Wound edges widely separated (pressure ulcers, open burn areas)	› Longer healing time › Increase for risk of infection › Scarring
Tertiary intention	› Widely separated › Deep › Spontaneous opening of a previously closed wound › Risk of infection	› Extensive drainage and tissue debris › Closed later › Long healing time

- Factors Affecting Wound Healing
  - An increase in age delays healing because of:
    - Loss of skin turgor.
    - Skin fragility.
    - A decrease in peripheral circulation and oxygenation.
    - Slower tissue regeneration.
    - A decrease in absorption of nutrients.
    - A decrease in collagen.
    - Impaired function of the immune system.
  - Overall wellness – A compound fracture of the femur in a client who has a chronic illness can be difficult to heal.
  - Immune function is the body's ability to fight infection by destroying invading pathogens. A decrease in leukocyte count will delay healing.
  - Some medications (anti-inflammatory and antineoplastic) interfere with the body's ability to respond to and prevent infection.
  - Nutrition provides energy and elements for wound healing.
  - Tissue perfusion provides circulation that delivers nutrients for tissue repair and infection control.
  - Adequate Hgb levels are essential for oxygen delivery to healing tissues.
  - Obesity – Fatty tissue lacks blood supply.
  - Chronic diseases, such as diabetes mellitus and cardiovascular disorders, place additional stress on the body's healing mechanisms.
  - Chronic stress further impedes healing.
  - Smoking impairs oxygenation and clotting.
  - Wound stress, such as from vomiting or coughing, puts pressure on the suture line and disrupts the wound healing process.
- General Principles of Wound Management
  - Wounds impair skin integrity.
  - Inflammation is a localized protective response to injury or destruction of tissue.
  - Wounds heal by various processes and in stages.
  - Wound infections result from the invasion of pathogenic micro-organisms.
  - Principles of wound care include assessment, cleansing, and protection.

Assessment/Data Collection

- Appearance
  - Note the color of open wounds.
    - Red – Healthy regeneration of tissue
    - Yellow – Presence of purulent drainage and slough
    - Black – Presence of eschar that hinders healing and requires removal

- ○ Assess the length, width, and depth, any undermining, any sinus tracts or tunnels, and any redness or swelling. Use a clock face with 12:00 toward the client's head to document the location of sinus tracts.
- ○ Closed wounds – Skin edges should be well-approximated.
- Drainage is a result of the healing process and occurs during the inflammatory and proliferative phases of healing.
  - ○ Note the amount of drainage from a drain or on a dressing.
  - ○ Note the integrity of the surrounding skin.
  - ○ With each cleansing, observe the skin around a drain for irritation and breakdown.
  - ○ The character of drainage is its consistency, color, and odor.
    - ▪ Serous drainage is the portion of the blood (serum) that is watery and clear or slightly yellow in appearance.
    - ▪ Sanguineous drainage contains serum and red blood cells. It is thick and appears reddish. Brighter drainage indicates fresh bleeding; darker drainage indicates older drainage.
    - ▪ Serosanguineous drainage contains both serum and blood. It is watery and appears blood-streaked or blood-tinged.
    - ▪ Purulent drainage is the result of infection. It is thick and contains white blood cells, tissue debris, and bacteria. It may have a foul odor, and its color reflects the type of organism present (green for a *Pseudomonas aeruginosa* infection).
- Wound closure (staples, sutures, wound-closure strips [Steri-strips])
- Status of any drains or tubes
- Pain
  - ○ Note the location, quality, intensity, timing, setting, associated symptoms, and aggravating/relieving factors.

Nursing Interventions

- Provide adequate hydration and meet protein and calorie needs.
  - ○ Encourage an intake of 2,000 to 3,000 mL of fluid/day, from food and beverage sources if not contraindicated (heart and renal failure).
  - ○ Provide education about good sources of protein (meat, fish, poultry, eggs, dairy products, beans, nuts, whole grains).
  - ○ Note if serum albumin levels are low (below 3.5 g/dL), because a lack of protein increases the risk for a delay in wound healing and infection.
  - ○ Provide nutritional support (vitamin and mineral supplements, nutritional supplements, and enteral and parenteral nutrition). Most adult clients need at least 1,500 kcal/day for nutritional support.
- Perform wound cleansing.
  - ○ For clean wounds, such as a surgical incision, cleanse from the least contaminated (the incision) toward the most contaminated (the surrounding skin).
  - ○ Use gentle friction when cleansing or applying solutions to the skin to avoid bleeding or further injury to the wound.
  - ○ Although the provider might prescribe other mild cleansing agents, isotonic solutions remain the preferred cleansing agents.

- ○ Never use the same gauze to cleanse across an incision or wound more than once.
- ○ Do not use cotton balls and other products that shed fibers.
- ○ If irrigating, use a piston syringe or a sterile straight catheter for deep wounds with small openings. Apply 5 to 8 psi of pressure. A 30- to 60-mL syringe with a 19-gauge needle provides approximately 8 psi. Use normal saline, lactated Ringer's, or an antibiotic solution.
- • For wound dressings
  - ○ Woven gauze (sponges) – Absorbs exudate from the wound
  - ○ Nonadherent material – Does not stick to the wound bed
  - ○ Self-adhesive, transparent film – A temporary "second skin" ideal for small, superficial wounds
  - ○ Hydrocolloid – An occlusive dressing that swells in the presence of exudate; composed of gelatin and pectin, it forms a seal at the wound's surface to prevent evaporation of moisture from the skin
    - ▪ Maintains a granulating wound bed
    - ▪ May stay in place up to 7 days
  - ○ Hydrogel (Aquasorb) – Composition is mostly water; gels after contact with exudate, promoting autolytic debridement and cooling
    - ▪ For infected, deep wounds, or necrotic tissue
    - ▪ Not for moderately to heavily exudating wounds
    - ▪ Provides a moist wound bed
    - ▪ May stay in place for 3 days
- • Use the negative pressure of a vacuum-assisted closure.
- • Remove sutures and staples.
- • Administer analgesics and monitor for effective pain management.
- • Administer antimicrobials (topical, systemic) and monitor for effectiveness (reduced fever, increase in comfort, decreasing WBC count).
- • Document the location and type of wound and incision, the status of the wound and type of drainage, the type of dressing and materials, client teaching, and how the client tolerated the procedure.

Complications and Nursing Implications

- • Dehiscence is a partial or total rupture (separation) of a sutured wound, usually with separation of underlying skin layers. Evisceration is a dehiscence that involves the protrusion of visceral organs through a wound opening.
  - ○ Manifestations of dehiscence
    - ▪ A significant increase in the flow of serosanguineous fluid on the wound dressings
    - ▪ Immediate history of sudden straining (coughing, sneezing, vomiting)
    - ▪ The client reporting a change or "popping" or "giving way" in the wound area.
    - ▪ Visualization of viscera

  - ○ Risk factors
    - ▪ Chronic disease
    - ▪ Advanced age
    - ▪ Obesity

- Invasive abdominal cancer
- Vomiting
- Excessive straining, coughing, sneezing
- Dehydration, malnutrition
- Ineffective suturing
- Abdominal surgery

- ○ Evisceration and dehiscence require emergency treatment.
  - Call for help.
  - Stay with the client.
  - Cover the wound and any protruding organs with sterile towels or dressings soaked with sterile normal saline solution. Do not attempt to reinsert the organs.
  - Position the client supine with the hips and knees bent.
  - Observe for signs of shock.
  - Maintain a calm environment.
  - Keep the client NPO in preparation for returning to surgery.

- Infection
  - ○ Risk factors
    - Extremes in age (immature immune system, decrease in immune function)
    - Impaired circulation and oxygenation (COPD, peripheral vascular disease)
    - Wound condition and nature (gunshot wound vs. surgical incision)
    - Impaired or suppressed immune system
    - Malnutrition, such as with alcoholism
    - Chronic disease
    - Poor wound care, such as breaches in aseptic technique
  - ○ Manifestations (3 to 11 days after injury or surgery)
    - Purulent drainage
    - Pain
    - Redness, edema (in and around the wound)
    - Fever
    - Chills
    - Increased pulse, respiratory rate
    - Increase in WBC count
  - ○ Interventions
    - Prevent infection by using appropriate asepsis when performing dressing changes.
    - Provide optimal nutrition to promote the immune response.
    - Provide for adequate rest to promote healing.
    - Administer antibiotic therapy after collecting the appropriate specimens for culture and sensitivity testing.

PRESSURE ULCERS

- The National Pressure Ulcer Advisory Panel classifies pressure ulcers in six stages.

    ○ Suspected deep tissue injury – Discoloration but intact skin from damage to underlying tissue.

    ○ Stage I – Intact skin with an area of persistent, nonblanchable redness, typically over a bony prominence, that may feel warmer or cooler than the adjacent tissue. The tissue is swollen and has congestion, with possible discomfort at the site. With darker skin tones, the ulcer may appear blue or purple.

    ○ Stage II – Partial-thickness skin loss involving the epidermis and the dermis. The ulcer is visible and superficial and may appear as an abrasion, blister, or shallow crater. Edema persists, and the ulcer may become infected, possibly with pain and scant drainage.

    ○ Stage III – Full-thickness tissue loss with damage to or necrosis of subcutaneous tissue. The ulcer may extend down to, but not through, underlying fascia. The ulcer appears as a deep crater with or without undermining of adjacent tissue and without exposed muscle or bone. Drainage and infection are common.

    ○ Stage IV – Full-thickness tissue loss with destruction, tissue necrosis, or damage to muscle, bone, or supporting structures. There may be sinus tracts, deep pockets of infection, tunneling, undermining, eschar (black scab-like material), or slough (tan, yellow, or green scab-like material).

    ○ Unstageable – No determination of stage because eschar or slough obscures the wound.

 View Image: Stages of Pressure Ulcers

- The primary focus of prevention and treatment of pressure ulcers is to relieve the pressure and provide optimal nutrition and hydration.

- Assess all clients regularly for skin-integrity status and for risk factors that contribute to impaired skin integrity.

- Use a risk assessment tool (Braden, Norton scales) for periodic systemic monitoring for skin breakdown risk.

- Pressure ulcers are a significant source of morbidity and mortality among older adults and those who have limited mobility.

- Risk factors for developing pressure ulcers

    ○ Aging skin

    ○ Immobility

    ○ Incontinence, excessive moisture

    ○ Skin friction, shearing

    ○ Vascular disorders

    ○ Obesity

    ○ Inadequate nutrition, hydration

    ○ Anemia

    ○ Fever, dehydration

    ○ Impaired circulation

- ○ Edema
- ○ Sensory deficits
- ○ Impaired cognitive functioning, neurological disorders
- ○ Chronic diseases (diabetes mellitus, chronic renal failure, congestive heart disease, chronic lung disease)
- ○ Sedation that impairs spontaneous repositioning

Nursing Interventions

- Prevention
  - ○ Keep skin clean, dry, and intact. Provide a firm, wrinkle-free foundation with wrinkle-free linens.
  - ○ Use pressure-reducing surfaces and devices.
  - ○ Inspect the client's skin frequently and document the client's risk using a tool such as the Braden scale.
  - ○ Clean the skin with a mild cleansing agent and pat it dry immediately following urine or stool incontinence.
  - ○ Bathe with tepid water (not hot) and minimal scrubbing.
  - ○ Apply dimethicone-based moisture barrier creams or alcohol-free barrier films to the skin of clients who are incontinent.
  - ○ Do not use powder or cornstarch to prevent friction or repel moisture due to their abrasive grit and aspiration potential.
  - ○ Reposition the client in bed at least every 2 hr and every 1 hr in a chair. Document position changes.
  - ○ Keep the head of the bed at or below a 30° angle (or flat), unless contraindicated, to relieve pressure on the sacrum, buttocks, and heels.
  - ○ Use pressure-reducing devices (overlays; replacement mattresses; specialty beds; kinetic therapy; foam, gel, or air cushions).
  - ○ Keep clients from sliding down in bed, as this increases shearing forces that pull tissue layers apart and cause damage.
  - ○ Lift, rather than pull, clients up in bed or in a chair, because pulling creates friction that can damage the outer layer of skin (epidermis).
  - ○ Raise heels off of the bed to prevent pressure.
  - ○ Ambulate clients as soon as possible and as often as possible.
  - ○ Instruct clients who are mobile to shift their weight every 15 min when sitting.
  - ○ Implement active and passive exercises for clients who are immobile.
  - ○ Do not massage bony prominences.
  - ○ Provide adequate hydration (2,000 to 3,000 mL/day) and meet protein and calorie needs.
  - ○ Note if serum albumin levels are low (below 3.5 g/dL), because a lack of protein puts the client at greater risk for skin breakdown, slowed healing, and infection.
  - ○ Provide nutritional support as indicated, such as vitamin and mineral supplements (especially A, C, zinc, copper), nutritional supplements, and enteral and parenteral nutrition.

- Treatment

STAGE	INTERVENTIONS	
Suspected deep tissue injury and Stage I	› Relieve pressure. › Encourage frequent turning and repositioning. › Use pressure-relieving devices, such as an air-fluidized bed.	› Implement pressure-reduction surfaces (air mattress, foam mattress). › Keep the client dry, clean, well-nourished, and hydrated.
Stage II	› Maintain a moist healing environment (saline or occlusive dressing). › Promote natural healing while preventing the formation of scar tissue.	› Provide nutritional supplements. › Administer analgesics.
Stage III	› Clean and/or debride: » Prescribed dressing. » Surgical intervention. » Proteolytic enzymes.	› Provide nutritional supplements. › Administer analgesics. › Administer antimicrobials (topical and/or systemic).
Stage IV	› Clean and/or debride: » Prescribed dressing. » Surgical intervention. » Proteolytic enzymes. › Perform nonadherent dressing changes every 12 hr.	› Treatment may include skin grafts or specialized therapy such as hyperbaric oxygen. › Provide nutritional supplements. › Administer analgesics. › Administer antimicrobials (topical and/or systemic).
Unstageable	› Debride until staging is possible.	

Note: Do not use alcohol, Dakin's solution, acetic acid, povidone-iodine, hydrogen peroxide or any other cytotoxic cleansers on a pressure ulcer wound.

 View Image: Pressure-Relieving Device

Complications and Nursing Implications

- Deterioration to a Higher Stage Ulceration and/or Infection
  - Assess the ulcer frequently and report an increase in the size or depth of the lesion, changes in granulation tissue (color, texture), and changes in exudates (color, quantity, odor).
  - Follow the facility's protocol for ulcer treatment.
- Systemic Infection
  - Assess for sepsis (changes in level of consciousness, persistent recurrent fever, tachycardia, tachypnea, hypotension, oliguria, increase in WBC count).
  - Prevent infection by using asepsis when performing ulcer treatment and dressing changes.
  - Provide optimal nutrition to promote the immune response.
  - Provide for adequate rest to promote healing.
  - Administer antibiotic therapy after collecting the appropriate specimens for culture and sensitivity testing.

APPLICATION EXERCISES

1. An adolescent who has diabetes mellitus is 2 days postoperative following an appendectomy. The client is tolerating a regular diet. He has ambulated successfully around the unit with assistance. He requests pain medication every 6 to 8 hr while reporting pain at a 2 on a scale of 0 to 10 after receiving the medication. His incision is approximated and free of redness, with scant serous drainage on the dressing. Which of the following risk factors for poor wound healing does this client have? (Select all that apply.)

_____ A. Extremes in age

_____ B. Impaired circulation

_____ C. Impaired/suppressed immune system

_____ D. Malnutrition

_____ E. Poor wound care

2. A nurse is assessing a client who is 5 days postoperative following abdominal surgery. The surgeon suspects an incisional wound infection and has prescribed antibiotic therapy for the nurse to initiate after collecting wound and blood specimens for culture and sensitivity. Which of the following assessment findings should the nurse expect? (Select all that apply.)

_____ A. Increase in incisional pain

_____ B. Fever and chills

_____ C. Reddened wound edges

_____ D. Increase in serosanguineous drainage

_____ E. Decrease in thirst

3. A nursing instructor is reviewing the wound healing process with a group of nursing students. They should be able to identify which of the following alterations as a wound or injury that heals by secondary intention? (Select all that apply.)

_____ A. Stage III pressure ulcer

_____ B. Sutured surgical incision

_____ C. Casted bone fracture

_____ D. Laceration sealed with adhesive

_____ E. Open burn area

4. A client who had abdominal surgery 24 hr ago suddenly reports a pulling sensation and pain in his surgical incision. The nurse checks the client's surgical wound and finds the wound separated with viscera protruding. Which of the following interventions is appropriate? (Select all that apply.)

_____ A. Cover the area with saline-soaked sterile dressings.

_____ B. Apply an abdominal binder snugly around the abdomen.

_____ C. Use sterile gauze to apply gentle pressure to the exposed tissues.

_____ D. Position the client supine with his hips and knees bent.

_____ E. Offer the client a warm beverage, such as herbal tea.

5. A nurse is caring for an older adult client who is at risk for developing pressure ulcers. Which of the following interventions should the nurse use to help maintain the integrity of the client's skin? (Select all that apply.)

_____ A. Keep the head of the bed elevated 30 degrees.

_____ B. Massage the client's bony prominences frequently.

_____ C. Apply cornstarch liberally to the skin after bathing.

_____ D. Have the client sit on a gel cushion when in a chair.

_____ E. Reposition the client at least every 3 hr while in bed.

6. A nurse is teaching a group of nursing students about the National Pressure Ulcer Advisory Panel's classification system for pressure ulcers. Use the ATI Active Learning Template: Basic Concept to complete this item. Under Related Content, list the six pressure ulcer stages along with a brief description of the assessment findings typical for ulcers at each stage.

APPLICATION EXERCISES KEY

1. A. INCORRECT: The client is not at either extreme of the age spectrum.

    B. **CORRECT:** Diabetes mellitus places this client at risk for impaired circulation.

    C. **CORRECT:** Diabetes mellitus places this client at risk for impaired immune system function.

    D. INCORRECT: There is no indication that the client is malnourished.

    E. INCORRECT: There is no indication that there have been any breaches in aseptic technique during wound care.

    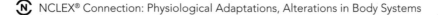 NCLEX® Connection: Health Promotion and Maintenance, High Risk Behaviors

2. A. **CORRECT:** Pain and tenderness at the wound site are expected findings with an incisional infection.

    B. **CORRECT:** Fever and chills are expected findings with an incisional infection.

    C. **CORRECT:** Reddened or inflamed wound edges are expected findings with an incisional infection.

    D. INCORRECT: Serosanguineous drainage is more common immediately after surgery. Purulent drainage is an expected finding with an incisional infection.

    E. INCORRECT: Changes in thirst have many causes. That finding alone does not indicate an incisional infection.

    NCLEX® Connection: Physiological Adaptations, Alterations in Body Systems

3. A. **CORRECT:** Open pressure ulcers heal by secondary intention, which is the process for wounds that have tissue loss and widely separated edges.

    B. INCORRECT: Sutured surgical incisions heal by primary intention, which is the process for wounds that have little or no tissue loss and well-approximated edges.

    C. INCORRECT: Unless the bone edges have pierced the skin, a casted bone fracture is an injury to underlying structures and does not require healing of the skin.

    D. INCORRECT: Lacerations sealed with tissue adhesive heal by primary intention, which is the process for wounds that have little or no tissue loss and well-approximated edges.

    E. **CORRECT:** Open burn areas heal by secondary intention, which is the process for wounds that have tissue loss and widely separated edges.

    NCLEX® Connection: Reduction of Risk Potential, System Specific Assessments

4.   A. **CORRECT:** The nurse should cover the wound with a sterile dressing soaked with sterile normal saline solution to keep the exposed organs and tissues moist until the surgeon can assess and intervene.

    B. INCORRECT: An abdominal binder can help prevent, not treat, a wound evisceration.

    C. INCORRECT: The nurse should not handle or apply pressure to any exposed organs or tissues because these actions increase the risks of trauma and perforation.

    D. **CORRECT:** This position minimizes pressure on the abdominal area.

    E. INCORRECT: The nurse must keep the client NPO in anticipation of the surgical team taking him back to the surgical suite for repair of the evisceration.

   NCLEX® Connection: Basic Care and Comfort, Mobility/Immobility

5.   A. **CORRECT:** Slight elevation reduces shearing forces that could tear sensitive skin on the sacrum, buttocks, and heels.

    B. INCORRECT: Massaging the skin over bony prominences can traumatize deep tissues.

    C. INCORRECT: Cornstarch can create gritty particles that can abrade sensitive skin.

    D. **CORRECT:** The client should sit on a gel, air, or foam cushion to redistribute weight away from ischial areas.

    E. INCORRECT: Frequent position changes are important for preventing skin breakdown, but every 3 hr is not frequent enough. The nurse should reposition the client at least every 2 hr.

   NCLEX® Connection: Basic Care and Comfort, Mobility/Immobility

6.   *Using the ATI Active Learning Template: Basic Concept*
- Related Content
  - Suspected deep tissue injury – Discolored but intact skin from damage to underlying tissue.
  - Stage I – Intact skin with an area of persistent, nonblanchable redness, typically over a bony prominence, that may feel warmer or cooler than adjacent tissue. The tissue is swollen and has congestion, with possible discomfort at the site. With darker skin tones, the ulcer may appear blue or purple.
  - Stage II – Partial-thickness skin loss involving the epidermis and the dermis. The ulcer is visible and superficial and may appear as an abrasion, blister, or shallow crater. Edema persists, and the ulcer may become infected, possibly with pain and scant drainage.
  - Stage III – Full-thickness tissue loss with damage to or necrosis of subcutaneous tissue. The ulcer may extend down to, but not through, underlying fascia. The ulcer appears as a deep crater with or without undermining of adjacent tissue and without exposed muscle or bone. Drainage and infection are common.
  - Stage IV – Full-thickness tissue loss with destruction, tissue necrosis, or damage to muscle, bone, or supporting structures. There may be sinus tracts, deep pockets of infection, tunneling, undermining, eschar (black scab-like material), or slough (tan, yellow, or green scab-like material).
  - Unstageable – No determination of stage because eschar or slough obscures the wound.

   NCLEX® Connection: Physiological Adaptations, Pathophysiology

UNIT 4   **PHYSIOLOGICAL INTEGRITY**
        SECTION: PHYSIOLOGICAL ADAPTATION

CHAPTER 56   **Bacterial, Viral, Fungal, and Parasitic Infections**

Overview

- Pathogens are the micro-organisms or microbes that cause infections.
    - Bacteria – most common type of pathogen (*Staphylococcus aureus, Escherichia coli, Mycobacterium tuberculosis*)
    - Viruses – organisms that use the host's genetic machinery to reproduce (rhinovirus, HIV, hepatitis, herpes zoster, herpes simplex)
    - Fungi – molds and yeasts (*Candida albicans,* Aspergillus)
    - Prions – protein particles that have the ability to cause infections (Creutzfeldt-Jakob disease)
    - Parasites – organisms that live on and often cause harm to a host organism
        - Protozoa (malaria, toxoplasmosis)
        - Helminths (worms [flatworms, roundworms])
        - Flukes (Schistosoma)
        - Arthropods (lice, mites, ticks)
- Virulence is the ability of a pathogen to invade the host and cause disease.
- Herpes zoster is a common viral infection that erupts years after exposure to chickenpox and invades a specific nerve tract.

Infection Process

- The infection process (chain of infection) includes:

    View Image: Chain of Infection

- Causative agent (bacteria, virus, fungus, prion, parasite)
- Reservoir (human, animal, water, soil, insects)
- Portal of exit from (means for leaving) the host
    - Respiratory tract (droplet, airborne)
        - *Mycobacterium tuberculosis* and Parainfluenza virus
    - Gastrointestinal tract
        - Shigella, *Salmonella enteritidis, Salmonella typhi,* hepatitis A, *Clostridium difficile*
    - Genitourinary tract
        - *Escherichia coli,* herpes simplex virus (type 1), HIV

- Skin/Mucous membranes
  - Herpes simplex virus and varicella
- Blood/Body fluids
  - HIV and hepatitis B and C
- Mode of transmission
  - Contact
    - Direct physical contact – person to person
    - Indirect contact with a vehicle of transmission – inanimate object, water, food, blood
    - Fecal-oral transmission – handling food after using a restroom and failing to wash hands
  - Droplet
    - Large droplets travel through the air up to 3 to 6 ft – sneezing, coughing, and talking
  - Airborne
    - Small droplets remain in the air and can travel extended distances depending on airflow – sneezing and coughing
  - Vector borne
    - Animals or insects as intermediaries (ticks transmit Lyme disease; mosquitoes transmit West Nile virus and malaria)
- Portal of entry to the host
  - Often the same as the portal of exit
- Susceptible host
  - Compromised defense mechanisms (immunosuppression, breaks in skin) leave the host more susceptible to infections.

Immune Defenses

- Nonspecific innate-native immunity allows the body to restrict entry or immediately respond to a foreign organism (antigen) through the activation of phagocytic cells, complement, and inflammation.
  - Nonspecific innate-native immunity provides temporary immunity but does not have memory of past exposures.
  - Intact skin is the body's first line of defense against microbial invasion.
  - The skin, mucous membranes, secretions, enzymes, phagocytic cells, and protective proteins work in concert to prevent infections.
  - Inflammatory response
    - Phagocytic cells (neutrophils, eosinophils, macrophages), the complement system, and interferons are involved.
    - An inflammatory response localizes the area of microbial invasion and prevents its spread.
- Specific adaptive immunity allows the body to make antibodies in response to a foreign organism (antigen).
  - Requires time to react to antigens
  - Provides permanent immunity due to memory of past exposures
  - Involves B and T lymphocytes
  - Produces specific antibodies against specific antigens (immunoglobulins [IgA, IgD, IgE, IgG, IgM]).

Assessment

- Risk Factors
  - Environmental factors
    - Excessive alcohol consumption
    - Nicotine use – smoking, smokeless tobacco
    - Malnutrition
  - Medication therapy (immunosuppressive agents)
    - Glucocorticosteroids
    - Antineoplastics
  - Chronic diseases
    - Diabetes mellitus
    - Cancer
    - HIV, AIDS
    - Peripheral vascular disease
    - Chronic pulmonary disease
  - Older adults are at increased risk for infections due to:
    - Slowed response to antibiotic therapy.
    - Slowed immune response – indicators of infection more difficult to identify, resulting in possible delays in diagnosis and treatment.
    - Loss of subcutaneous tissue and thinning of the skin.
    - Decreased vascularity and slowed wound healing.
    - Decreased cough and gag reflexes.
    - Chronic illnesses (diabetes mellitus, COPD, neurological or musculoskeletal impairments).
    - Decreased gastric acid production.
    - Decreased mobility.
    - Bowel/bladder incontinence.
    - Dementia.
    - Greater incidence of invasive devices (urinary catheters, feeding tubes, tracheostomies, intravenous lines).
    - Common indications of infection are not always present in the older adult client. Altered mental status, agitation, or incontinence may be present instead.
- Subjective Data
  - Chills
  - Sore throat
  - Fatigue and malaise
  - Change in level of consciousness, nuchal rigidity, photophobia, headache
  - Nausea, vomiting, anorexia, abdominal cramping, and diarrhea
  - Localized pain or discomfort

- Objective Data
  - Physical Assessment Findings
    - Fever
    - Increased pulse and respiratory rate, decreased blood pressure
    - Localized redness and edema
    - Enlarged lymph nodes
    - Dyspnea, cough, purulent sputum, and crackles in lung fields
    - Dysuria, urinary frequency, hematuria, and pyuria
    - Rash, skin lesions, purulent wound drainage, and erythema
    - Dysphagia, hyperemia, and enlarged tonsils
  - Laboratory Tests
    - White blood cell (WBC) count with differential
      - An elevated WBC count is an indicator of infection (expected reference range is 5,000 to 10,000/mm³)
      - The differential identifies specific types of WBCs that can assist in diagnosis of the severity of infection or the specific type of pathogen.
    - Culture and sensitivity
    - Erythrocyte sedimentation rate (ESR) – rate at which red blood cells settle out of plasma
      - An expected value for adults is 15 to 20 mm/hr.
      - An increase indicates an active inflammatory process or infection.
    - Immunoglobulin electrophoresis
      - Determines the presence and quantity of specific immunoglobulins (IgG, IgA, IgM).
      - Used to detect hypersensitivity disorders, autoimmune disorders, chronic viral infections, immunodeficiency, multiple myeloma, and intrauterine infections.
    - Antibody screening tests
      - Detect the presence of antibodies against specific causative agents (bacteria, fungi, viruses, parasites).
      - A positive antibody test indicates that the client has been exposed to and developed antibodies to a specific pathogen, but it does not provide information about whether or not the client is currently infected (HIV antibodies).
    - Auto-antibody screening tests
      - Detect the presence of antibodies against a person's own DNA (self-cells).
      - The presence of antibodies against self cells is associated with autoimmune conditions (systemic lupus erythematosus, rheumatoid arthritis).
    - Antigen tests
      - Detect the presence of a specific pathogen (HIV).
      - Used to identify certain infections or disorders.

- Stool for ova and parasites
  - Detects presence of ova and parasites, such as hookworm ova in stool.
  - Three separate stool specimens usually collected.
  - Each specimen must be transported to the laboratory while it is still warm.
- Diagnostic Procedures
  - Gallium scan
    - A nuclear scan that uses a radioactive substance to identify hot spots of WBCs within the client's body.
    - Radioactive gallium citrate is injected intravenously and accumulates in areas where inflammation is present.
  - X-rays, computed tomography (CT) scan, magnetic resonance imaging (MRI), and biopsies are used to determine the presence of infection, abscesses, and lesions.

Patient-Centered Care

- Nursing Care
  - Assess
    - Presence of risk factors for infection
    - Recent travel or exposure to an infectious disease
    - Behaviors that may put the client at increased risk
    - Increased temperature, heart and respiratory rate, thirst, anorexia
    - Presence of chills, which occur when temperature is rising, and diaphoresis, which occurs when temperature is decreasing
    - Presence of hyperpyrexia (greater than 105.8°), which can cause brain and organ damage
  - Implement infection control measures.
    - Perform frequent hand hygiene to prevent transmission of infection to other clients.
    - Maintain a clean environment.
    - Perform wound care measures such as sterile dressing changes.
    - Use personal protective equipment/barriers (gloves, masks, gowns, goggles).
    - Encourage recommended immunizations.
    - Implement protective precautions as needed.
      - Standard (implemented for all clients)
      - Contact (*Clostridium difficile*, herpes simplex virus, impetigo)
      - Droplet (Haemophilus influenzae type B, pertussis, plague, *streptococcal pneumoniae*)
      - Airborne (measles, varicella, tuberculosis)
  - Encourage adequate rest and nutrition.
  - Provide diversional activities if needed.
  - Encourage increased fluid intake or maintain intravenous fluid replacement to prevent dehydration.
  - Protect and maintain the client's protective barriers (skin, mucous membranes).

- Medications
  - Antipyretics
    - Antipyretics (acetaminophen and aspirin) are used for fever and discomfort as prescribed.
    - Nursing Considerations
      - Monitor fever to determine effectiveness of medication.
      - Graph the client's temperature fluctuations on the medical record for trending.
  - Antimicrobial therapy
    - Antimicrobial medications kill pathogens or prevent their growth. Anthelmintics are given for worm infestations. There are currently no treatments for prions.
    - Nursing Considerations
      - Administer antimicrobial therapy as prescribed.
      - Monitor for medication effectiveness (reduced fever, increased level of comfort, decreasing WBC count).
      - Maintain a medication schedule to assure consistent therapeutic blood levels of the antibiotic.
- Care After Discharge
  - Client Education
    - Teach the client regarding:
      - Any infection control measures needed at home.
      - Self-administration of medication therapy.
      - Complications that need to be reported immediately.

Complications

- Medication-resistant infections
  - Antimicrobials are becoming less effective for some strains of pathogens, due to the pathogen's ability to adapt and become resistant to previously sensitive antibiotics. This significantly limits the number of antibiotics that are effective against the pathogen. Use of antibiotics, especially broad-spectrum antibiotics, has significantly decreased to prevent new strains from evolving. Taking the measures below can ensure an antimicrobial is warranted and increase the effectiveness of treatment.
  - Methicillin-resistant *Staphylococcus aureus* (MRSA) is a strain of *S. aureus* that is resistant to all antibiotics, except vancomycin (Vancocin).
  - Vancomycin-resistant *Staphylococcus aureus* (VRSA) is a strain of *S. aureus* that is resistant to vancomycin but so far is sensitive to other antibiotics specific to the strain.
  - Nursing Actions
    - Obtain specimens for culture and sensitivity prior to initiation of antimicrobial therapy.
    - Monitor antimicrobial levels and ensure that therapeutic levels are maintained.
    - Implement precautions to prevent the spread of the infection.
  - Client Education
    - Complete the full course of antimicrobial therapy.
    - Avoid overuse of antimicrobials.

- Sepsis
  - A systemic inflammatory response syndrome resulting from the body's response to a serious infection, usually bacterial (peritonitis, meningitis, pneumonia, wound infections, urinary tract infections).
  - Risk factors for sepsis include very young age, very old age, weakened immune system, and severe injuries (trauma). Sepsis is a potentially life-threatening complication that can lead to widespread inflammation, blood clotting, organ failure, and shock.
  - Blood cultures definitively diagnose sepsis. Systemic antimicrobials are prescribed accordingly. Vasopressors and anticoagulants may be prescribed for shock and blood clotting manifestations. Mechanical ventilation, dialysis, and other interventions may be needed for treatment of specific organ failure.

Herpes Zoster (Shingles)

- Herpes zoster is a viral infection. It initially produces chickenpox, after which the virus lies dormant in the dorsal root ganglia of the sensory cranial and spinal nerves. It is then reactivated as shingles later in life.
  - Shingles is usually preceded by a prodromal period of several days, during which pain, itching, tingling, or burning may occur along the involved dermatome.
  - Shingles can be very painful and debilitating.
- Assessment
  - Risk Factors
    - Concurrent illness
    - Stress
    - Compromise to the immune system
    - Fatigue
    - Poor nutritional status
    - Possible immunocompromise makes older adult clients more susceptible to herpes zoster infection. Assess the client carefully for typical and atypical indications of infection.
  - Subjective Data
    - Paresthesia
    - Pain that is unilateral and extends horizontally along a dermatome
  - Objective Data
    - Physical Assessment Findings
      - Vesicular, unilateral rash (the rash and lesions occur on the skin area innervated by the infected nerve)
      - Changes in or loss of vision if the eye is affected
      - Rash that is erythematous, vesicular, pustular, or crusting (depending on the stage)
      - Rash that usually lasts several weeks
      - Low-grade fever

- Laboratory Tests
  - Cultures provide a definitive diagnosis (but the virus grows so slowly that cultures are often of minimal diagnostic use).
  - Occasionally, an immunofluorescence assay can be done.
- Patient-Centered Care
  - Nursing Care
    - Assess/Monitor
      - Pain
      - Condition of lesions
      - Presence of fever
      - Neurologic complications
      - Indications of infection
    - Use an air mattress or bed cradle for pain prevention/control of affected areas.
    - Isolate the client until the vesicles have crusted over.
    - Maintain strict wound care precautions.
    - The virus can be transmitted through direct contact, causing chickenpox. Avoid exposing the client to infants, pregnant women who have not had chickenpox, and clients who are immunocompromised.
    - Moisten dressings with cool tap water or 5% aluminum acetate (Burow's solution) and apply to the affected skin for 30 to 60 min, four to six times per day as prescribed.
    - Use lotions, such as calamine lotion, or recommend oatmeal baths to help relieve itching and discomfort.
    - Administer medications as prescribed.
  - Medications
    - Analgesics (NSAIDs, narcotics) enhance client comfort.
    - If started soon after the rash appears, antiviral agents, such as acyclovir (Zovirax), can decrease the severity of the infection and shorten the clinical course.
    - Recommend zoster vaccine live (Zostavax) for clients 50 and over to prevent shingles. This vaccine does not treat active shingles infections.
- Complications
  - Postherpetic neuralgia
    - Characterized by pain that persists for longer than 1 month following resolution of the vesicular rash.
    - Tricyclic antidepressants may be prescribed.
    - Postherpetic neuralgia is common in adults older than 60 years of age.

APPLICATION EXERCISES

1. A nurse is discussing the infection process at a staff education session. Which of the following examples are appropriate for the nurse to include when discussing the direct contact mode of transmission? (Select all that apply.)

    _____ A. A client vomits on a nurse's uniform.

    _____ B. A nurse has a needle stick injury.

    _____ C. A mosquito bites a hiker in the woods.

    _____ D. A nurse finds a hole in his glove while handling a soiled dressing.

    _____ E. A person fails to wash her hands after using the bathroom.

2. A nurse is preparing to admit a client who is suspected to have pulmonary tuberculosis. Which of the following actions should the nurse plan to perform first?

    A. Implement airborne precautions.

    B. Obtain a sputum culture.

    C. Administer prescribed antituberculosis medications.

    D. Recommend a screening test for family members.

3. A nurse in a primary care clinic is assessing a client who has a history of herpes zoster. Which of the following findings suggests the client is experiencing postherpetic neuralgia?

    A. Linear clusters of vesicles present on the client's right shoulder

    B. Purulent drainage from both of the client's eyes

    C. Decreased white blood cell count

    D. Report of continued pain following resolution of rash

4. A charge nurse is discussing the care of a client who has methicillin-resistant *Staphylococcus aureus* (MRSA) with a newly licensed nurse. Which of the following statements by the newly licensed nurse indicates an understanding of the teaching?

    A. "I should obtain a specimen for culture and sensitivity after the first dose of an antimicrobial."

    B. "MRSA is usually resistant to vancomycin, so another antimicrobial will be prescribed."

    C. "I will need to monitor the client's serum antimicrobial levels during the course of therapy."

    D. "To decrease resistance, antimicrobial therapy is discontinued when the client is no longer febrile."

5. A nurse in a residential care facility is assessing an older adult client. Which of the following findings should the nurse recognize as atypical indications of an infection? (Select all that apply.)

_____ A. Urinary incontinence

_____ B. Malaise

_____ C. Acute confusion

_____ D. Fever

_____ E. Agitation

6. A nurse is admitting a client who has a new diagnosis of bacterial meningitis. Use the ATI Active Learning Template: Systems Disorder and the Medical-Surgical Nursing Review Module to complete this item to include the following sections:

A. Description of Disorder/Disease Process: Identify the mode of transmission.

B. Assessment:
   - Risk Factors: Identify at least three risk factors for acquiring bacterial meningitis.
   - Objective and Subjective Data: Identify at least three indications of infection with bacterial meningitis.

C. Client Education: Identify information the nurse should provide the client and family about acquiring adaptive immunity for bacterial meningitis.

D. Patient-Centered Care: Identify three nursing interventions to prevent the transmission of bacterial meningitis.

APPLICATION EXERCISES KEY

1. A. **CORRECT:** Transmission from a client's emesis is identified as person-to-person or direct contact.

   B. INCORRECT: Transmission from a needle or other inanimate object is identified as indirect contact.

   C. INCORRECT: Transmission from an insect is identified as vector-borne.

   D. INCORRECT: Transmission from a soiled dressing or other inanimate object is identified as indirect contact.

   E. **CORRECT:** Transmission from a client's contaminated hands is identified as person-to-person or direct contact.

    NCLEX® Connection: Safety and Infection Control, Standard Precautions/Transmission-Based Precautions/Surgical Asepsis

2. A. **CORRECT:** The safety risk to the nurse and others is transmission of the infection. The first action is to place the client on airborne precautions.

   B. INCORRECT: Obtaining a sputum culture is an appropriate action, but it does not address the safety risk and therefore is not the first action the nurse should take.

   C. INCORRECT: Administering prescribed medications is an appropriate action, but it does not address the safety risk and therefore is not the first action the nurse should take.

   D. INCORRECT: Recommending screening tests for those in close contact with the client is an appropriate action, but it does not address the safety risk and therefore is not the first action the nurse should take.

    NCLEX® Connection: Safety and Infection Control, Standard Precautions/Transmission-Based Precautions/Surgical Asepsis

3. A. INCORRECT: Localized linear clusters of vesicles are an expected finding of herpes zoster rather than postherpetic neuralgia.

   B. INCORRECT: Eye infection is a potential complication of herpes zoster but does not suggest postherpetic neuralgia.

   C. INCORRECT: Immunosuppression increases the client's risk for herpes zoster but does not suggest postherpetic neuralgia.

   D. **CORRECT:** Pain that persists following resolution of the vesicular rash is an indication of postherpetic neuralgia.

    NCLEX® Connection: Physiological Adaptations, Illness Management

4. A. INCORRECT: The nurse should obtain a specimen for culture and sensitivity prior to the initiation of antimicrobial therapy.

    B. INCORRECT: MRSA is resistant to all antibiotics, except vancomycin.

    C. **CORRECT:** Monitoring antimicrobial levels ensures that therapeutic levels are maintained.

    D. INCORRECT: Discontinuing antimicrobial therapy prior to completing a full course of treatment increases the risk of producing resistant pathogens.

     NCLEX® Connection: Safety and Infection Control, Standard Precautions/Transmission-Based Precautions/Surgical Asepsis

5. A. **CORRECT:** Urinary incontinence is an atypical indication of infection in an older adult client.

    B. INCORRECT: Malaise is a typical indication of infection.

    C. **CORRECT:** Acute confusion is an atypical indication of infection in an older adult client.

    D. INCORRECT: Fever is a typical indication of infection.

    E. **CORRECT:** Agitation is an atypical indication of infection in an older adult client.

    NCLEX® Connection: Safety and Infection Control, Standard Precautions/Transmission-Based Precautions/Surgical Asepsis

6. *Using the ATI Active Learning Template: Systems Disorder*

    A. Description of Disorder/Disease Process
        - Droplet transmission

    B. Assessment
        - Risk Factors
            ○ Recent or current bacterial-based infections
            ○ Immunosuppression
            ○ Invasive procedures
            ○ Skull fracture or penetrating head wound
            ○ Overcrowded or communal living conditions
        - Objective and Subjective Data
            ○ Constant headache
            ○ Nuchal rigidity
            ○ Photophobia
            ○ Fever and chills
            ○ Altered level of consciousness
            ○ Red macular rash
            ○ Elevated WBC
            ○ CT or MRI identifies increased intracranial pressure

    C. Client Education
        - Infants should receive the *Haemophilus influenzae* type b (Hib) vaccine.
        - Adults and older adults at risk should receive the pneumococcal polysaccharide vaccine (PPSV).
        - Adolescents should receive the meningococcal vaccine on schedule and prior to living in a residential or communal setting.

    D. Patient-Centered Care
        - Implement droplet precautions.
        - Administer prescribed antibiotics.
        - Educate visitors about the need to wear a mask in the client's room.
        - Perform frequent hand hygiene.
        - Maintain a clean environment.

        Ⓝ NCLEX® Connection: Safety and Infection Control, Standard Precautions/Transmission-Based Precautions/Surgical Asepsis

chapter 57

Overview

- Fluids

  - Body fluids are distributed between intracellular (ICF) and extracellular (ECF) compartments.

  - Fluid can move between compartments (through selectively permeable membranes) by a variety of methods (diffusion, active transport, filtration, osmosis) in order to maintain homeostasis.

  - Fluid imbalances that the nurse should be familiar with are:

    - Fluid volume deficits

    - Fluid volume excess

- Electrolytes

  - Electrolytes are minerals (sometimes called salts) that are present in all body fluids. They regulate fluid balance and hormone production, strengthen skeletal structures, and act as catalysts in nerve response, muscle contraction, and the metabolism of nutrients.

  - When dissolved in water or another solvent, electrolytes separate into ions and then conduct either a positive (cations – magnesium, potassium, sodium, calcium) or negative (anions – phosphate, sulfate, chloride, bicarbonate) electrical current.

  - Electrolytes are distributed between ICF and ECF compartments. While laboratory tests can accurately reflect the electrolyte concentrations in plasma, it is not possible to directly measure electrolyte concentrations within cells.

FLUID VOLUME DEFICITS

- Fluid volume deficits (FVDs) include

  - Isotonic FVD is the loss of water and electrolytes from the ECF.

    - Isotonic FVD is often referred to as hypovolemia because intravascular fluid is also lost.

  - Dehydration is the loss of water from the body without the loss of electrolytes.

    - This hemoconcentration results in increases in Hct, serum electrolytes, and urine specific gravity.

- Compensatory mechanisms include sympathetic nervous system responses of increased thirst, antidiuretic hormone (ADH) release, and aldosterone release.

- Hypovolemia can lead to hypovolemic shock.

- Ⓖ Older adults have an increased risk for dehydration due to multiple physiological factors including a decrease in total body mass, which includes total body water content.

Assessment

- Risk Factors
  - Causes of isotonic FVD (hypovolemia)
    - Abnormal gastrointestinal (GI) losses – vomiting, nasogastric suctioning, diarrhea
    - Abnormal skin losses – diaphoresis
    - Abnormal renal losses – diuretic therapy, diabetes insipidus, kidney disease, adrenal insufficiency, osmotic diuresis
    - Third spacing – peritonitis, intestinal obstruction, ascites, burns
    - Hemorrhage
    - Altered intake – impaired swallowing, confusion, nothing by mouth (NPO)
  - Causes of dehydration
    - Hyperventilation
    - Prolonged fever
    - Diabetic ketoacidosis
    - Enteral feeding without sufficient water intake
- Subjective and Objective Data
  - Vital signs – hypothermia, tachycardia, thready pulse, hypotension, orthostatic hypotension, decreased central venous pressure, tachypnea (increased respirations), hypoxia
  - Neuromusculoskeletal – dizziness, syncope, confusion, weakness, fatigue
  - GI – thirst, dry mucous membranes, dry furrowed tongue, nausea/vomiting, anorexia, acute weight loss
  - Renal – oliguria (decreased production of urine)
  - Other clinical findings – diminished capillary refill, cool clammy skin, diaphoresis, sunken eyeballs, flattened neck veins, absence of tears, decreased skin turgor
    - Assessment of skin turgor in the older adult may not provide reliable findings due to a natural loss of skin elasticity.
- Laboratory Findings
  - Hct – Increased in both hypovolemia and dehydration unless the fluid volume deficit is due to hemorrhage.
  - Serum osmolarity
    - Dehydration – increased hemoconcentration osmolarity (greater than 300 mOsm/kg) – increased protein, BUN, electrolytes, glucose
  - Urine specific gravity and osmolarity
    - Dehydration – increased concentration (urine specific gravity greater than 1.030)
  - Serum sodium
    - Dehydration – increased hemoconcentration

Patient-Centered Care

- Nursing Care
  - Assess respiratory rate, symmetry, and effort.
  - Monitor for shortness of breath and dyspnea.
  - Check urinalysis, oxygen saturation (SaO_2), CBC, and electrolytes.
  - Administer supplemental oxygen as prescribed.
  - Measure the client's weight daily at same time of day using the same scale.
  - Observe for nausea and vomiting.
  - Assess and monitor the client's vital signs (check for hypotension and orthostatic hypotension).
  - Check neurological status to determine level of consciousness.
  - Assess heart rhythm (may be irregular or tachycardic).
  - Initiate and maintain IV access.
  - Place the client in shock position (on the back with the legs elevated).
  - Fluid replacement: Administer IV fluids as prescribed (isotonic solutions such as lactated Ringer's or 0.9% sodium chloride; blood transfusions).
  - Monitor I&O. Encourage fluids as tolerated. Alert the provider to a urine output less than 30 mL/hr.
  - Monitor level of consciousness and ensure client safety.
  - Assess level of gait stability.
  - Encourage the client to use the call light and ask for assistance.
  - Encourage the client to change positions slowly (rolling from side to side or standing up).
  - Check capillary refill (expected reference range less than 2 seconds).
  - Provide frequent oral care.
  - Prevent skin breakdown.

FLUID VOLUME EXCESSES

- Fluid volume excesses include
  - Fluid volume excess (FVE) is the isotonic retention of water and sodium in abnormally high proportions.
    - FVE is often referred to as hypervolemia because of the resulting increased blood volume.
  - Overhydration, or hypoosmolar fluid imbalance, is the gain of more water than electrolytes.
    - This hemodilution results in decreases in Hct, serum electrolytes, and protein.
- Severe hypervolemia can lead to pulmonary edema and heart failure.
- Compensatory mechanisms include an increased release of natriuretic peptides, resulting in increased excretion of sodium and water by the kidneys, and a decreased release of aldosterone.

Assessment

- Risk Factors
    - Causes of hypervolemia
        - Chronic stimulus to the kidney to conserve sodium and water (heart failure, cirrhosis, increased glucocorticosteroids)
        - Abnormal kidney function with reduced excretion of sodium and water (kidney failure)
        - Interstitial to plasma fluid shifts (hypertonic fluids, burns)
        - Age-related changes in cardiovascular and kidney function
        - Excessive sodium intake from IV fluids, diet, or medications (sodium bicarbonate antacids, hypertonic enema solutions)
    - Causes of overhydration
        - Water replacement without electrolyte replacement (strenuous exercise with profuse diaphoresis)
        - Syndrome of inappropriate antidiuretic hormone (SIADH), which is the excess secretion of ADH
        - Head injuries
        - Barbiturates
        - Anesthetics
- Subjective and Objective Data
    - Vital signs – tachycardia, bounding pulse, hypertension, tachypnea, increased central venous pressure
    - Neuromusculoskeletal – confusion, muscle weakness
    - GI – weight gain, ascites
    - Respiratory – dyspnea, orthopnea, crackles
    - Other clinical findings – edema, distended neck veins
- Laboratory Findings
    - Hct
        - Hypervolemia – decreased Hct
        - Overhydration – decreased Hct = hemodilution
    - Serum osmolarity
        - Overhydration – osmolarity less than 280 mOsm/kg
    - Serum sodium
        - Hypervolemia – sodium within expected reference range
    - Electrolytes, BUN, and creatinine
        - Overhydration/hypervolemia – decreased electrolytes, BUN, and creatinine
    - Arterial blood gases
        - Respiratory alkalosis – decreased $PaCO_2$ (less than 35 mm Hg), increased pH (greater than 7.45)
- Diagnostic Procedures
    - Chest x-rays may indicate pulmonary congestion.

Patient-Centered Care

- Nursing Care
  - Assess respiratory rate, symmetry, and effort.
  - Assess breath sounds in all lung fields. Lung sounds may be diminished with crackles.
  - Monitor for shortness of breath and dyspnea.
  - Check ABGs, SaO$_2$, CBC, and chest x-ray results.
  - Position the client in semi-Fowler's position.
  - Measure the client's weight daily.
  - Monitor and document edema (pretibial, sacral, periorbital).
  - Monitor I&O.
  - Implement prescribed restrictions for fluid and sodium intake.
    - Provide fluids in small glass to promote the perception of a full glass of fluid.
    - Set 1- to 2-hr short-term goals for the fluid restriction to promote client control and understanding.
  - Administer supplemental oxygen as needed.
  - Reduce IV flow rates.
  - Administer diuretics (osmotic, loop) as prescribed.
  - Monitor and document circulation to the extremities.
  - Reposition the client at least every 2 hr.
  - Support arms and legs to decrease dependent edema as appropriate.

ELECTROLYTES

- Major electrolytes in the body include sodium, potassium, chloride, magnesium, phosphorus, and calcium. Nurses monitor laboratory values to identify any electrolyte imbalances.
- It is important to recognize the clinical manifestations of electrolyte imbalance. Clients at greatest risk for electrolyte imbalance are infants and children, older adults, clients who have cognitive disorders, and clients who are chronically ill.

SODIUM IMBALANCES

- Sodium (Na+) is the major electrolyte found in ECF and is present in most body fluids or secretions.
- Sodium is essential for maintenance of acid-base and fluid balance, active and passive transport mechanisms, and irritability and conduction of nerve and muscle tissue.
- Expected serum sodium levels are between 136 and 145 mEq/L.

Hyponatremia

- Hyponatremia is a serum sodium level less than 136 mEq/L.

- Hyponatremia is a net gain of water or loss of sodium-rich fluids.

- Hyponatremia delays and slows the depolarization of membranes.

- Water moves from the ECF into the ICF, which causes cells to swell (cerebral edema).

- Serious complications can result from untreated acute hyponatremia (coma, seizures, respiratory arrest).

Assessment

- Risk Factors

  - Causes of hyponatremia (loss of sodium)

    - Deficient ECF volume

    - Abnormal GI losses – vomiting, nasogastric suctioning, diarrhea, tap water enemas

    - Renal losses – diuretics, kidney disease, adrenal insufficiency, excessive sweating

    - Skin losses – burns, wound drainage, gastrointestinal obstruction, peripheral edema, ascites.

    - Increased or normal ECF volume – excessive oral water intake, SIADH

    - Edematous states – heart failure, cirrhosis, nephrotic syndrome

    - Excessive hypotonic IV fluids

    - Inadequate sodium intake (NPO status)

    - Age-related risk factors – Older adult clients are at greater risk due to an increased incidence of chronic illnesses, use of diuretic medications, and risk for insufficient sodium intake.

- Subjective and Objective Data

  - Physical assessment findings – vary with a normal, decreased, or increased ECF volume

  - Vital signs – hypothermia, tachycardia, rapid thready pulse, hypotension, orthostatic hypotension

  - Neuromusculoskeletal – headache, confusion, lethargy, muscle weakness with possible respiratory compromise, fatigue, decreased deep tendon reflexes (DTRs), seizures, coma

  - GI – increased motility, hyperactive bowel sounds, abdominal cramping, anorexia, nausea, vomiting

- Laboratory Findings

  - Serum sodium

    - Decreased – less than 136 mEq/L

  - Serum osmolarity

    - Decreased – less than 280 mOsm/kg

Patient-Centered Care

- Nursing Care
  - Report abnormal laboratory findings to the provider.
  - Fluid overload – Restrict water intake as prescribed.
  - Acute hyponatremia:
    - Administer hypertonic oral and IV fluids as prescribed.
    - Encourage foods and fluids high in sodium (cheese, milk, condiments).
  - Restoration of normal ECF volume – Administer isotonic IV therapy (0.9% sodium chloride, lactated Ringer's).
  - Monitor I&O and weigh the client daily.
  - Monitor vital signs and level of consciousness, reporting abnormal findings.
  - Encourage the client to change positions slowly.
  - Follow any prescribed fluid restrictions.

Hypernatremia

- Hypernatremia is a serum sodium level greater than 145 mEq/L.
- Hypernatremia is a serious electrolyte imbalance. It can cause significant neurological, endocrine, and cardiac disturbances.
- Increased sodium causes hypertonicity of the serum. This causes a shift of water out of the cells, making the cells dehydrated.

Assessment

- Risk Factors
  - Water deprivation (NPO)
  - Heat stroke
  - Excessive sodium intake – dietary sodium intake, hypertonic IV fluids, hypertonic tube feedings, bicarbonate intake
  - Excessive sodium retention – kidney failure, Cushing's syndrome, aldosteronism, some medications (glucocorticosteroids)
  - Fluid losses – fever, diaphoresis, burns, respiratory infection, diabetes insipidus, hyperglycemia, watery diarrhea
  - Age-related changes, specifically decreased total body water content and inadequate fluid intake related to an altered thirst mechanism
  - Compensatory mechanisms – increased thirst and increased production of ADH

- Subjective and Objective Data
  - Vital signs – hyperthermia, tachycardia, orthostatic hypotension
  - Neuromusculoskeletal – restlessness, disorientation, irritability, muscle twitching, muscle weakness, seizures, decreased level of consciousness, reduced to absent DTRs
  - GI – thirst, dry mucous membranes, dry and swollen tongue that is red in color, increased motility, hyperactive bowel sounds, abdominal cramping, nausea
  - Other clinical findings – edema, warm flushed skin, oliguria
- Laboratory Findings
  - Serum sodium
    - Increased – greater than 145 mEq/L
  - Serum osmolarity
    - Increased – greater than 300 mOsm/kg

Patient-Centered Care

- Nursing Care
  - Report abnormal laboratory findings to the provider.
  - Fluid loss – based on serum osmolarity
    - Administer hypotonic IV fluids (0.225% sodium chloride).
  - Excess sodium
    - Encourage water intake and discourage sodium intake.
    - Administer diuretics (loop diuretics).

  - Monitor level of consciousness and ensure safety.
  - Provide oral hygiene and other comfort measures to decrease thirst.
  - Monitor I&O, and alert the provider if urinary output is inadequate.

POTASSIUM IMBALANCES

- Potassium (K+) is the major cation in ICF.
- Potassium plays a vital role in cell metabolism; transmission of nerve impulses; functioning of cardiac, lung, and muscle tissues; and acid-base balance.
- Potassium has reciprocal action with sodium.
- Expected serum potassium levels are 3.5 to 5 mEq/L.

Hypokalemia

- Hypokalemia is a serum potassium level below 3.5 mEq/L.
- Hypokalemia is the result of an increased loss of potassium from the body or movement of potassium into the cells.

Assessment

- Risk Factors
  - Abnormal GI losses – vomiting, nasogastric suctioning, diarrhea, inappropriate laxative use
  - Renal losses – excessive use of potassium-excreting diuretics such as furosemide (Lasix), corticosteroids
  - Skin losses – diaphoresis, wound losses
  - Hyperaldosteronism
  - Insufficient potassium
  - Inadequate dietary intake (rare)
  - Prolonged administration of non-electrolyte-containing IV solutions such as 5% dextrose in water
  - ICF – metabolic alkalosis, after correction of acidosis (treatment of diabetic ketoacidosis), during periods of tissue repair (burns, trauma, starvation), total parenteral nutrition
- Subjective and Objective Data
  - Vital signs – hyperthermia, weak irregular pulse, hypotension, respiratory distress
  - Neuromusculoskeletal – ascending bilateral muscle weakness with respiratory collapse and paralysis, muscle cramping, decreased muscle tone and hypoactive reflexes, paresthesias, mental confusion
  - ECG – premature ventricular contractions (PVCs), bradycardia, blocks, ventricular tachycardia, flattening T waves, and ST depression
  - GI – decreased motility, hypoactive bowel sounds, abdominal distention, constipation, ileus, nausea, vomiting, anorexia
  - Other clinical findings – polyuria (excretion of dilute urine)
- Laboratory Findings
  - Serum potassium
    - Decreased – Less than 3.5 mEq/L
  - Arterial blood gases
    - Metabolic alkalosis – pH greater than 7.45
- Diagnostic Procedures
  - Electrocardiogram (ECG) shows findings of dysrhythmias, such as PVCs, ventricular tachycardia, flattening T waves, and ST depression.

Patient-Centered Care

- Nursing Care
  - Report abnormal findings to the provider.
  - Treat the underlying cause.
  - Replace potassium.
    - Provide dietary education and encourage foods high in potassium (avocados, dried fruit, cantaloupe, bananas, potatoes, spinach).
    - Provide oral potassium supplementation.

○ IV potassium supplementation

■ Mixed by a pharmacist and double-checked by two nurses prior to administration.

■ The maximum recommended rate is 10 to 20 mEq/hr.

■ Never IV bolus (high risk of cardiac arrest)

○ Monitor for phlebitis (tissue irritant).

○ Monitor for and maintain an adequate urine output.

○ Monitor for shallow, ineffective respirations and diminished breath sounds.

○ Monitor the client's cardiac rhythm and intervene promptly as needed.

○ Monitor clients receiving digoxin. Hypokalemia increases the risk for digoxin toxicity.

○ Monitor level of consciousness and ensure safety.

○ Monitor bowel sounds and abdominal distention and intervene as needed.

Hyperkalemia

• Hyperkalemia is a serum potassium level greater than 5.0 mEq/L.

• Hyperkalemia is the result of an increased intake of potassium, movement of potassium out of the cells, or inadequate renal excretion.

• Hyperkalemia uncommon in clients who have adequate renal function.

• Hyperkalemia is potentially life-threatening due to the risk of cardiac arrhythmias and cardiac arrest.

Assessment

• Risk Factors

○ Increased total body potassium – IV potassium administration, salt substitutes, blood transfusion

○ ECF shift – decreased insulin, acidosis (diabetic ketoacidosis), tissue catabolism (sepsis, trauma, surgery, fever, myocardial infarction)

○ Hypertonic states – uncontrolled diabetes mellitus

○ Decreased excretion of potassium – kidney failure, severe dehydration, potassium-sparing diuretics, ACE inhibitors, adrenal insufficiency

○ Older adult clients – at greater risk due to decreased kidney function and medical conditions resulting in the use of salt substitutes, angiotensin-converting enzyme inhibitors, and potassium-sparing diuretics

• Subjective and Objective Data

○ Vital signs – slow, irregular pulse; hypotension

○ Neuromusculoskeletal – irritability, confusion, weakness with ascending flaccid paralysis, paresthesias, lack of reflexes

○ ECG – ventricular fibrillation, peaked T waves, widened QRS, cardiac arrest

○ GI – increased motility, diarrhea, abdominal cramps, hyperactive bowel sounds

○ Other clinical findings – oliguria

- Laboratory Findings
  - Serum potassium
    - Increased – Greater than 5 mEq/L
  - Arterial blood gases
    - Metabolic acidosis – pH less than 7.35
- Diagnostic Procedures
  - ECG will show dysrhythmias (ventricular fibrillation, peaked T waves, widened QRS).

Patient-Centered Care

- Nursing Care
  - Report abnormal findings to the provider.
  - Decrease potassium intake:
    - Stop infusion of IV potassium.
    - Withhold oral potassium.
    - Provide a potassium-restricted diet.
    - If potassium levels are extremely high, dialysis may be required.
  - Promote the movement of potassium from ECF to ICF:
    - Administer IV fluids with dextrose and regular insulin.
  - Monitor the client's cardiac rhythm and intervene promptly as needed.
  - Medications to increase potassium excretion:
    - Administer loop diuretics, such as furosemide (Lasix), if kidney function is adequate. Loop diuretics increase the excretion of potassium from the renal system.
    - Sodium polystyrene sulfonate (Kayexalate) is given orally or as an enema. Kayexalate increases the excretion of potassium from the gastrointestinal system.
  - Maintain IV access.
  - Prepare the client for dialysis if prescribed.

CALCIUM IMBALANCES

- Calcium is found in the body's cells, bones, and teeth. The expected total calcium level is 9 to 10.5 mg/dL.
- Calcium balance is essential for proper functioning of the cardiovascular, neuromuscular, and endocrine systems, as well as blood clotting and bone and teeth formation.

Hypocalcemia

- Hypocalcemia is a serum calcium level less than 9 mg/dL.

Assessment

- Risk Factors
  - ○ Increased calcium output
    - ▪ Chronic diarrhea
    - ▪ Steatorrhea as with pancreatitis (binding of calcium to undigested fat)
  - ○ Inadequate calcium intake or absorption:
    - ▪ Malabsorption syndromes, such as Crohn's disease
    - ▪ Vitamin D deficiency (alcohol use disorder, kidney failure)
  - ○ Calcium shift from extracellular fluid into bone or to an inactive form:
    - ▪ Repeated blood transfusion
    - ▪ Post-thyroidectomy
    - ▪ Hypoparathyroidism
- Subjective and Objective Data
  - ○ Muscle twitches/tetany
    - ▪ Numbness and tingling (extremities, circumoral)
    - ▪ Frequent, painful muscle spasms at rest that can progress to tetany
    - ▪ Hyperactive DTRs
    - ▪ Positive Chvostek's sign (tapping on the facial nerve triggering facial twitching)
    - ▪ Positive Trousseau's sign (hand/finger spasms with sustained blood pressure cuff inflation)
  - ○ Cardiovascular
    - ▪ Decreased myocardial contractility (decreased heart rate and hypotension)
  - ○ GI – hyperactive bowel sounds, diarrhea, abdominal cramping
  - ○ Central nervous system – seizures due to overstimulation of the CNS
- Laboratory Findings
  - ○ Calcium level less than 9 mg/dL
- Diagnostic Procedures
  - ○ ECG – Prolonged QT interval and ST segments

Patient-Centered Care

- Nursing Care
  - ○ Administer oral or IV calcium supplements. (Carefully monitor respiratory and cardiovascular status.)
  - ○ Initiate seizure precautions.
  - ○ Keep emergency equipment on standby.
  - ○ Encourage foods high in calcium, including dairy products and dark green vegetables.

Hypercalcemia

- Hypercalcemia is a serum calcium level greater than 10.5 mg/dL.

Assessment

- Risk Factors
  - Decreased calcium output
    - Thiazide diuretics
  - Increased calcium intake and absorption
  - Calcium shift from bone to extracellular fluid
    - Hyperparathyroidism
    - Bone cancer
    - Paget's disease
    - Chronic immobility
- Subjective and Objective Data
  - Neuromuscular
    - Decreased reflexes
    - Bone pain
    - Flank pain if renal calculi develop
  - Cardiovascular
    - Dysrhythmias
  - GI – anorexia, nausea, vomiting, constipation
  - Central nervous system
    - Weakness, lethargy
    - Confusion, decreased level of consciousness
- Laboratory Findings – Calcium level greater than 10.5 mg/dL
- Diagnostic Procedures
  - ECG – shortened QT interval and ST segment

Patient-Centered Care

- Nursing Care
  - Increase client activity level.
  - Limit dietary calcium.
  - Encourage fluids to promote urinary excretion.
  - Encourage fiber to promote bowel elimination.
  - Implement safety precautions if client is confused.
  - Monitor for pathologic fractures.

  - Encourage acid-ash fluids such as prune or cranberry juice to decrease the risk for renal calcium stone formation.

MAGNESIUM IMBALANCES

- Most of the body's magnesium is found in the bones. Magnesium in smaller amounts is found within the body cells. A very small amount is found in ECF. The expected magnesium level is 1.3 to 2.1 mEq/L

Hypomagnesemia

- Hypomagnesemia is a serum magnesium level less than 1.3 mEq/L.

Assessment

- Risk Factors
  - Increased magnesium output
    - GI losses (diarrhea, nasogastric suction)
    - Thiazide or loop diuretics
  - Inadequate magnesium intake or absorption:
    - Malnutrition
    - Alcohol use disorder
    - Laxative use
- Subjective and Objective Data
  - Neuromuscular – increased nerve impulse transmission (hyperactive DTRs, paresthesias, muscle tetany), positive Chvostek's and Trousseau's signs
  - GI – hypoactive bowel sounds, constipation, abdominal distention, paralytic ileus
  - Cardiovascular – dysrhythmias, tachycardia, hypertension
- Nursing Care
  - Discontinue magnesium-losing medications.
  - Administer oral or IV magnesium sulfate following safety protocols. IV route is used because IM can cause pain and tissue damage. Oral magnesium can cause diarrhea and increase magnesium depletion. Monitor closely.
  - Encourage foods high in magnesium, including whole grains and dark green vegetables.
  - Implement seizure precautions.

Hypermagnesemia

- Hypermagnesemia is a serum magnesium level greater than 2.1 mEq/L.

Assessment

- Risk Factors
  - Decreased magnesium output
    - Kidney failure
    - Adrenal insufficiency
  - Increased magnesium intake and absorption
    - Laxatives or antacids containing magnesium
- Subjective and Objective Data
  - Neuromuscular
    - Diminished DTRs
    - Muscle paralysis
    - Shallow respirations, decreased respiratory rate
  - Cardiovascular
    - Bradycardia, hypotension
    - Dysrhythmias, cardiac arrest
  - Central nervous system
    - Lethargy
- Laboratory Findings
  - Calcium level greater than 10.5 mg/dL
- Diagnostic Procedures
  - ECG – Shortened QT interval and ST segment

Patient-Centered Care

- Nursing Care – Perform frequent focused assessments (vital signs, level of consciousness, reflexes). Notify the provider of changes or absent reflexes.

APPLICATION EXERCISES

1. A nurse is performing an admission assessment on a client who has hypovolemia due to vomiting and diarrhea. Which of the following is an expected finding? (Select all that apply.)

_____ A. Hot, dry skin

_____ B. Hypertension

_____ C. Tachycardia

_____ D. Syncope

_____ E. Decreased skin turgor

2. A nurse is reviewing the laboratory test results for a client who is receiving treatment for septicemia with a prolonged fever. Which of the following indicates the client is developing dehydration? (Select all that apply.)

_____ A. Hct 55%

_____ B. Serum osmolarity 260 mOsm/kg

_____ C. Serum sodium 150 mEq/L

_____ D. Urine specific gravity 1.035

_____ E. Serum creatinine 0.6 mg/dL

3. A nurse on a medical-surgical unit is caring for a group of clients. Which of the following clients is at risk for hypervolemia?

A. A client who has a new diagnosis of adrenal insufficiency

B. A client who has heart failure

C. A client who is receiving treatment for diabetic ketoacidosis

D. A client who has abdominal ascites

4. A nurse is planning care for a client who has hypernatremia. Which of the following actions should the nurse anticipate including in the plan of care?

A. Infuse hypotonic IV fluids.

B. Implement a fluid restriction.

C. Increase sodium intake.

D. Administer sodium polystyrene sulfonate (Kayexalate).

5. A charge nurse is leading a staff education session about caring for a client who has hypocalcemia. Which of the following statements by a staff nurse indicates the need for further teaching?

    A. "I should monitor for hand spasms during blood pressure cuff inflation."

    B. "Clients who have a vitamin D deficiency are at risk for hypocalcemia."

    C. "Clients who have hypocalcemia are at risk for pathologic fractures."

    D. "I should implement seizure precautions for a client who has hypocalcemia."

6. A nurse is caring for a client who has hypokalemia as an adverse effect of furosemide (Lasix). Use the ATI Active Learning Template: System Disorder to complete this item to include the following sections:

    A. Description of Disorder/Disease Process

    B. Objective and Subjective Findings: Identify at least five expected findings.

    C. Patient-Centered Care: Identify two safety actions for the administration of IV potassium supplementation.

APPLICATION EXERCISES KEY

1. A. INCORRECT: Cool clammy skin is an expected finding of hypovolemia.

    B. INCORRECT: Hypotension is an expected finding of hypovolemia.

    C. **CORRECT:** Tachycardia is an expected finding of hypovolemia.

    D. **CORRECT:** Syncope is an expected finding of hypovolemia.

    E. **CORRECT:** Decreased skin turgor is an expected finding of hypovolemia.

    Ⓝ NCLEX® Connection: Physiological Adaptations, Fluid and Electrolyte Imbalances

2. A. **CORRECT:** An increased Hct is an indication of dehydration.

    B. INCORRECT: A serum osmolarity greater than 300 mOsm/kg is an indication of dehydration.

    C. **CORRECT:** An elevated serum sodium level is an indication of dehydration.

    D. **CORRECT:** An increased urine specific gravity is an indication of dehydration.

    E. INCORRECT: An elevated serum creatinine level is an indication of dehydration.

    Ⓝ NCLEX® Connection: Basic Care and Comfort, Nutrition and Oral Hydration

3. A. INCORRECT: A client who has adrenal insufficiency is at risk for isotonic fluid volume deficit (hypovolemia).

    B. **CORRECT:** A client who has heart failure is at risk for hypervolemia.

    C. INCORRECT: A client who has diabetic ketoacidosis is at risk for dehydration.

    D. INCORRECT: A client who has ascites is at risk for hypovolemia.

    Ⓝ NCLEX® Connection: Physiological Adaptations, Illness Management

4. A. **CORRECT:** Hypotonic IV fluids, such as 0.225% sodium chloride, are indicated for the treatment of hypernatremia related to fluid loss.

    B. INCORRECT: Increased fluid intake is indicated for the treatment of hypernatremia.

    C. INCORRECT: Decreased sodium intake is indicated for the treatment of hypernatremia.

    D. INCORRECT: Administration of Kayexalate is indicated for the treatment of hyperkalemia.

    Ⓝ NCLEX® Connection: Physiological Adaptations, Unexpected Response to Therapies

5.   A. INCORRECT: This statement does not require further teaching. Hand/finger spasms during sustained blood pressure cuff inflation (positive Trousseau's sign) are an indication of hypocalcemia.

   B. INCORRECT: This statement does not require further teaching. Vitamin D deficiency, such as with alcohol use disorder, increases the risk for hypocalcemia.

   C. **CORRECT:** This statement requires further teaching. Clients who have hypercalcemia are at risk for pathologic fractures.

   D. INCORRECT: This statement does not require further teaching. Clients who have hypocalcemia are at risk for seizures due to overstimulation of the central nervous system.

   Ⓝ NCLEX® Connection: Physiological Adaptations, Unexpected Response to Therapies

6.   *Using the ATI Active Learning Template: System Disorder*

   A. Description of Disorder/Disease Process

   • Hypokalemia is a serum potassium level below 3.5 mEq/L that can result from the increased loss of potassium from the body due to the use of potassium-excreting diuretics such as furosemide.

   B. Objective and Subjective Findings

   • Vital signs – hyperthermia, weak irregular pulse, hypotension, respiratory distress

   • Neuromusculoskeletal – ascending bilateral muscle weakness, muscle cramping, decreased muscle tone, hypoactive reflexes, paresthesias, mental confusion

   • GI – decreased motility, hypoactive bowel sounds, abdominal distention, constipation, nausea, vomiting, anorexia

   • Arrhythmias – PVCs, bradycardia, blocks, ventricular tachycardia, flattening T waves, ST depression

   • Polyuria

   C. Patient-Centered Care

   • Ensure all infusions containing potassium are mixed by the pharmacist.

   • Double check all infusions containing potassium with another nurse prior to administration.

   • Administer IV potassium infusions at a maximum rate of 10 to 20 mEq/hr.

   • Never administer potassium as an IV bolus.

   • Monitor the client's vital signs, cardiac and respiratory status closely during administration of IV potassium supplementation.

   Ⓝ NCLEX® Connection: Pharmacological and Parenteral Therapies, Expected Actions/Outcomes

Berman, A. J., & Snyder S. (2012). *Fundamentals of nursing: Concepts, process, and practice* (9th ed.). Upper Saddle River, NJ: Prentice-Hall.

Dudek, S. G. (2010). *Nutrition essentials for nursing practice* (6th ed.). Philadelphia: Lippincott Williams & Wilkins.

Eliopoulos, C. (2014). *Gerontological nursing* (8th ed.). Philadelphia: Lippincott Williams & Wilkins.

Grodner, M., Roth, S. L., & Walkingshaw, B. C. (2012). *Nutritional foundations and clinical applications of nutrition: A nursing approach* (5th ed.). St. Louis, MO: Mosby.

Ignatavicius, D. D., & Workman, M. L. (2013). *Medical-surgical nursing* (7th ed.). St. Louis, MO: Saunders.

Lehne, R. A. (2013). *Pharmacology for nursing care* (8th ed.). St. Louis: Saunders.

Potter, P. A., Perry, A. G., Stockert, P., & Hall, A. (2013). *Fundamentals of nursing* (8th ed.). St. Louis, MO: Mosby.

Touhy, T. A., & Jett, K. F. (2012) *Ebersole & Hess' toward healthy aging: Human needs and nursing response* (8th ed.). St. Lois, MO: Mosby.

Townsend, M. C. (2011). *Essentials of psychiatric mental health nursing: Concepts of care in evidence-based practice* (5th ed.). Philadelphia: F. A. Davis.

Varcarolis, E. M., Carson, V. B., & Shoemaker, N. C. (2010). *Foundations of psychiatric mental health nursing: A clinical approach* (6th ed.). St. Louis, MO: Saunders.

Wilson, B. A., Shannon, M. T., & Shields, K. M. (2013). *Pearson nurse's drug guide 2013*. Upper Saddle River, NJ: Prentice Hall.

CONTENT _____ REVIEW MODULE CHAPTER _____

TOPIC DESCRIPTOR_____

Related Content (e.g. delegation, levels of prevention, advance directives)	Underlying Principles	Nursing Interventions
		› Who?
		› When?
		› Why?
		› How?

Appendix

CONTENT _____ REVIEW MODULE CHAPTER _____

TOPIC DESCRIPTOR _____

DESCRIPTION OF PROCEDURE:

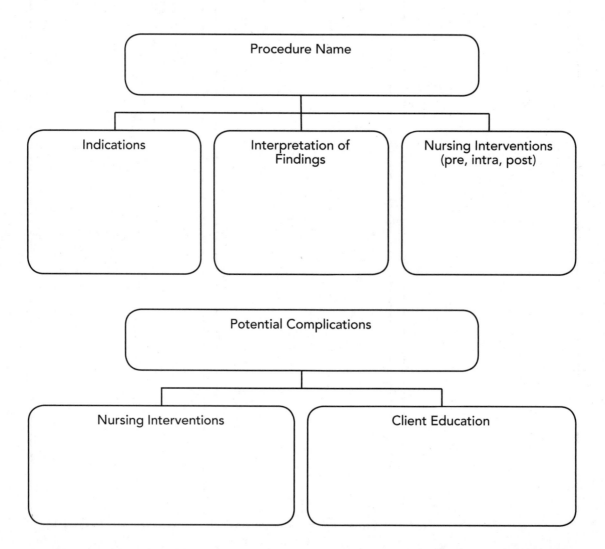

CONTENT _____ REVIEW MODULE CHAPTER _____

TOPIC DESCRIPTOR _____

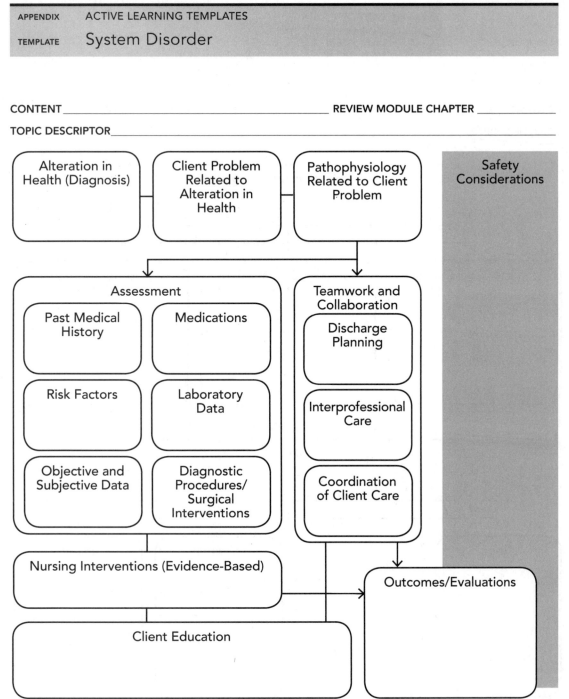

Appendix

CONTENT_____ REVIEW MODULE CHAPTER _____

TOPIC DESCRIPTOR_____

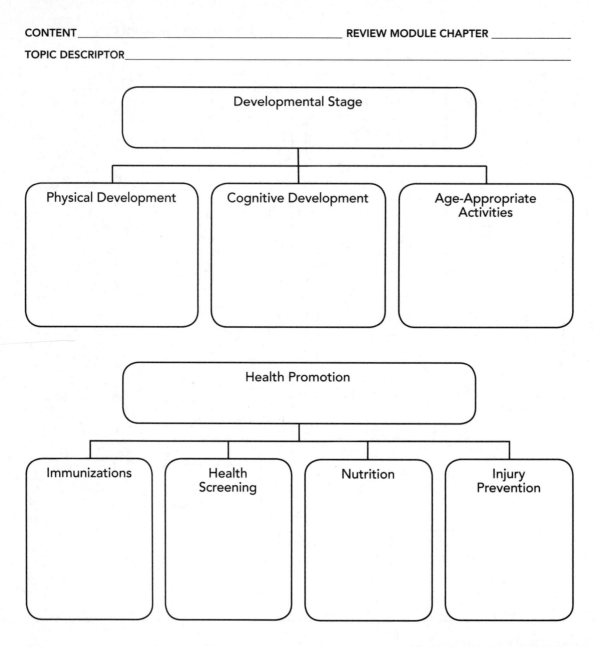

Developmental Stage

Physical Development

Cognitive Development

Age-Appropriate Activities

Health Promotion

Immunizations

Health Screening

Nutrition

Injury Prevention

CONTENT _____ REVIEW MODULE CHAPTER _____

TOPIC DESCRIPTOR_____

MEDICATION _____

EXPECTED PHARMACOLOGICAL ACTION:

Therapeutic Uses

Adverse Effects

Nursing Interventions

Contraindications

Client Education

Medication/Food Interactions

Medication Administration

Evaluation of Medication Effectiveness

Appendix

CONTENT _____ REVIEW MODULE CHAPTER _____

TOPIC DESCRIPTOR_____

DESCRIPTION OF SKILL:

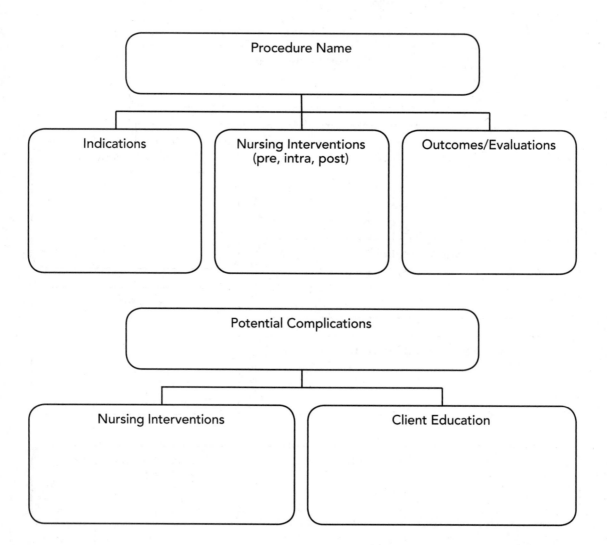

APPENDIX   ACTIVE LEARNING TEMPLATES

TEMPLATE   Therapeutic Procedure

CONTENT _____ REVIEW MODULE CHAPTER _____

TOPIC DESCRIPTOR_____

DESCRIPTION OF PROCEDURE:

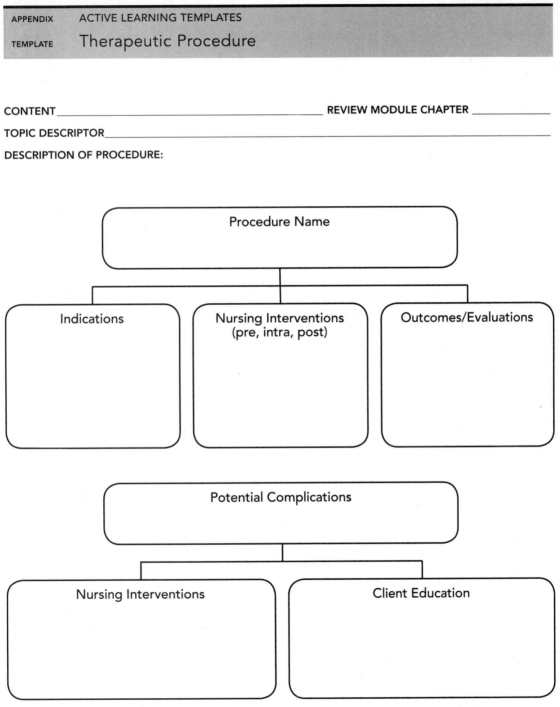

Procedure Name

Indications

Nursing Interventions
(pre, intra, post)

Outcomes/Evaluations

Potential Complications

Nursing Interventions

Client Education